# Adult Body MR

*Editor*

FRANK H. MILLER

# RADIOLOGIC CLINICS
# OF NORTH AMERICA

www.radiologic.theclinics.com

*Consulting Editor*
FRANK H. MILLER

July 2014 • Volume 52 • Number 4

**ELSEVIER**

1600 John F. Kennedy Boulevard • Suite 1800 • Philadelphia, Pennsylvania, 19103-2899

http://www.theclinics.com

**RADIOLOGIC CLINICS OF NORTH AMERICA Volume 52, Number 4**
**July 2014 ISSN 0033-8389, ISBN 13: 978-0-323-31171-7**

Editor: John Vassallo (j.vassallo@elsevier.com)
Developmental Editor: Donald Mumford

*Radiologic Clinics of North America* (ISSN 0033-8389) is published bimonthly by Elsevier Inc., 360 Park Avenue South, New York, NY 10010-1710. Months of issue are January, March, May, July, September, and November. Periodicals postage paid at New York, NY and additional mailing offices. Subscription prices are USD 460 per year for US individuals, USD 709 per year for US institutions, USD 220 per year for US students and residents, USD 535 per year for Canadian individuals, USD 905 per year for Canadian institutions, USD 660 per year for international individuals, USD 905 per year for international institutions, and USD 315 per year for Canadian and foreign students/residents. To receive student and resident rate, orders must be accompanied by name of affiliated institution, date of term and the signature of program/residency coordinatior on institution letterhead. Orders will be billed at individual rate until proof of status is received. Foreign air speed delivery is included in all *Clinics* subscription prices. All prices are subject to change without notice. **POSTMASTER:** Send address changes to *Radiologic Clinics of North America*, Elsevier Health Sciences Division, Subscription Customer Service, 3251 Riverport Lane, Maryland Heights, MO63043. **Customer Service: Telephone: 1-800-654-2452** (U.S. and Canada); **1-314-447-8871** (outside U.S. and Canada). **Fax: 1-314-447-8029. E-mail: journalscustomerservice-usa@elsevier.com** (for print support); **journalsonlinesupport-usa@elsevier.com** (for online support).

*Reprints.* For copies of 100 or more of articles in this publication, please contact the Commercial Reprints Department, Elsevier Inc., 360 Park Avenue South, New York, New York 10010-1710. Tel.: +1-212-633-3874; Fax: +1-212-633-3820; E-mail: reprints@elsevier.com.

*Radiologic Clinics of North America* also published in Greek Paschalidis Medical Publications, Athens, Greece.

*Radiologic Clinics of North America* is covered in *MEDLINE/PubMed (Index Medicus), EMBASE/Excerpta Medica, Current Contents/Life Sciences, Current Contents/Clinical Medicine, RSNA Index to Imaging Literature, BIOSIS, Science Citation Index,* and *ISI/BIOMED.*

Printed in the United States of America.

# Contributors

## CONSULTING EDITOR

**FRANK H. MILLER, MD**
Chief, Body Imaging Section and Fellowship
Program and GI Radiology; Medical Director
MRI; Professor, Department of Radiology,
Northwestern University, Feinberg School of
Medicine, Northwestern Memorial Hospital,
Chicago, Illinois

## EDITOR

**FRANK H. MILLER, MD**
Chief, Body Imaging Section and Fellowship
Program and GI Radiology; Medical Director
MRI; Professor, Department of Radiology,
Northwestern University, Feinberg School of
Medicine, Northwestern Memorial Hospital,
Chicago, Illinois

## AUTHORS

**BRIAN C. ALLEN, MD**
Assistant Professor of Radiology, Abdominal
Imaging, Department of Radiology, Wake
Forest Baptist Medical Center, Wake Forest
University School of Medicine, Winston-Salem,
North Carolina

**WIRANA ANGTHONG, MD**
Clinical Research Scholar of Magnetic
Resonance Imaging, Department of Radiology,
University of North Carolina Hospitals,
University of North Carolina at Chapel Hill,
Chapel Hill, North Carolina; Department of
Radiology, HRH Princess Maha Chakri
Sirindhorn Medical Center, Srinakharinwirot
University, Ongkharak, Nakhon Nayok,
Thailand

**JAD BOU AYACHE, MD**
Cardiovascular Imaging Fellow, Department of
Radiology, Northwestern University, Chicago,
Illinois

**JONATHAN R. COGLEY, MD**
Clinical Fellow, Section of Body Imaging,
Department of Radiology, Northwestern
University, Feinberg School of Medicine,
Northwestern Memorial Hospital, Chicago,
Illinois

**JEREMY D. COLLINS, MD**
Assistant Professor of Radiology,
Divisions of Cardiovascular Imaging and
Interventional Radiology, Department of
Radiology, Northwestern University, Feinberg
School of Medicine, Northwestern Memorial
Hospital, Chicago, Illinois

**AMIR H. DAVARPANAH, MD**
Department of Radiology, Yale-New Haven
Hospital, New Haven, Connecticut

**FLAVIUS F. GUGLIELMO, MD**
Assistant Professor, Department of Radiology,
Thomas Jefferson University Hospital, Thomas
Jefferson University, Philadelphia,
Pennsylvania

**SHIVA GUPTA, MD**
Assistant Professor, Department of Radiology,
The University of Texas MD Anderson Cancer
Center, Houston, Texas

**NANCY HAMMOND, MD**
Department of Radiology, Northwestern
University, Feinberg School of Medicine,
Northwestern Memorial Hospital, Chicago,
Illinois

**THOMAS A. HOPE, MD**
Assistant Professor, Department of Radiology
and Biomedical Imaging, University of
California San Francisco, San Francisco,
California

**GARY M. ISRAEL, MD**
Professor, Department of Radiology, Yale-New
Haven Hospital, New Haven, Connecticut

**YONG-HWAN JEON, MD**
Clinical Research Scholar of Magnetic
Resonance Imaging, Department of Radiology,
University of North Carolina Hospitals,
University of North Carolina at Chapel Hill,
Chapel Hill, North Carolina

**BONG SOO KIM, MD**
Professor, Department of Radiology, Jeju
National University Hospital, Jeju National
University School of Medicine, Jeju-si,
Jeju-do, Korea

**JOHN R. LEYENDECKER, MD**
Professor of Radiology, Abdominal Imaging,
Department of Radiology, Wake Forest Baptist
Medical Center, Wake Forest University School
of Medicine, Winston-Salem, North Carolina

**FRANK H. MILLER, MD**
Chief, Body Imaging Section and Fellowship
Program and GI Radiology; Medical Director
MRI; Professor, Department of Radiology,
Northwestern University, Feinberg School of
Medicine, Northwestern Memorial Hospital,
Chicago, Illinois

**DONALD G. MITCHELL, MD**
Director of MRI; Professor, Department of
Radiology, Thomas Jefferson University
Hospital, Thomas Jefferson University,
Philadelphia, Pennsylvania

**ERIN O'NEILL, MD**
Clinical Fellow, Department of Radiology,
Northwestern University, Feinberg School of
Medicine, Northwestern Memorial Hospital,
Chicago, Illinois

**MICHAEL A. OHLIGER, MD**
Assistant Professor, Department of Radiology
and Biomedical Imaging, University of
California San Francisco, San Francisco,
California

**AYTEKIN OTO, MD**
Professor, Department of Radiology, University
of Chicago, Chicago, Illinois

**ALIYA QAYYUM, MD**
Professor, Department of Diagnostic
Radiology, The University of Texas MD
Anderson Cancer Center, Houston, Texas

**CHRISTOPHER G. ROTH, MD**
Associate Professor and Vice Chairman,
Department of Radiology, Thomas Jefferson
University Hospital, Thomas Jefferson
University, Philadelphia, Pennsylvania

**KUMAR SANDRASEGARAN, MD**
Associate Professor, Department of Radiology,
Indiana University School of Medicine,
Indianapolis, Indiana

**RICHARD C. SEMELKA, MD**
Director of Magnetic Resonance
Imaging; Director of MFR Services;
Vice Chair of Quality and Safety; Professor,
Department of Radiology, University of
North Carolina Hospitals, University of
North Carolina at Chapel Hill, Chapel Hill,
North Carolina

**EVAN S. SIEGELMAN, MD**
Associate Professor, Department of
Radiology, Hospital of the University of
Pennsylvania, Perelman School of Medicine at
the University of Pennsylvania, Philadelphia,
Pennsylvania

**JOSEPH H. YACOUB, MD**
Assistant Professor, Department of Radiology,
Stritch School of Medicine, Loyola University
Chicago, Maywood, Illinois

**BENJAMIN L. YAM, MD**
Department of Radiology, Hospital of the
University of Pennsylvania, Perelman School of
Medicine at the University of Pennsylvania,
Philadelphia, Pennsylvania

# Contents

> Magnetic resonance (MR) imaging plays an important role in assessment of the full range of abdominal disease. The appropriate use of cooperative and motion-resistant protocols can allow accurate determination of the character of focal lesions in the abdomen under most circumstances. This article discusses current MR techniques and the proper use of MR imaging in the diagnostic evaluation of cooperative and noncooperative patients.

> Proper selection of a gadolinium-based contrast agent (GBCA) for body magnetic resonance imaging (MRI) cases requires understanding the indication for the MRI exam, the key features of the different GBCAs, and the effect that the GBCA has on the selected imaging protocol. The different categories of GBCAs require timing optimization on postcontrast sequences and adjusting imaging parameters to obtain the highest T1 contrast. Gadoxetate disodium has many advantages when evaluating liver lesions, although there are caveats and limitations that need to be understood. Gadobenate dimeglumine, a high-relaxivity GBCA, can be used for indications when stronger T1 relaxivity is needed.

> Focal liver lesions (FLLs) are commonly encountered on routine imaging studies. Most lesions detected are benign, but many are indeterminate at the time of initial imaging. This article reviews the important role of MR imaging for the detection and characterization of various benign FLLs while illustrating typical imaging appearances and potential pitfalls in interpretation. The utility of diffusion-weighted imaging and hepatocyte-specific contrast agents is also discussed.

> Magnetic resonance (MR) imaging surpasses all other imaging modalities in characterizing liver lesions by virtue of the exquisite tissue contrast, specificity for various tissue types, and extreme sensitivity to contrast enhancement. In addition to differentiating benign from malignant lesions, MR imaging generally discriminates between the various malignant liver lesions. Hepatocellular carcinoma constitutes most primary malignant liver lesions and usually arises in the setting of cirrhosis. Intrahepatic cholangiocarcinoma is a distant second and features distinctly different imaging features. Overall, metastases are the most common malignant liver lesions

and arise from several primary neoplasms; most commonly gastrointestinal, lung, breast, and genitourinary.

Over the past decade the role of MR imaging in the evaluation of diffuse liver disease has become common practice. Although detection of focal liver lesions remains the mainstay of liver imaging, a growing cohort of patients are referred for evaluation of hepatosteatosis, iron deposition diseases, and cirrhosis. In particular, multiecho sequences are becoming the gold standard for quantification of fat and iron. MR elastography allows for improved early detection of hepatic fibrosis. Unfortunately, a majority of the diffuse liver diseases lack specific features on MR imaging, yet a solid understanding of the different pathologic processes allows an informed interpretation.

Although ultrasound, computed tomography, and cholescintigraphy play essential roles in the evaluation of suspected biliary abnormalities, magnetic resonance (MR) imaging and MR cholangiopancreatography can be used to evaluate inconclusive findings and provide a comprehensive noninvasive assessment of the biliary tract and gallbladder. This article reviews standard MR and MR cholangiopancreatography techniques, clinical applications, and pitfalls. Normal biliary anatomy and variants are discussed, particularly as they pertain to preoperative planning. A spectrum of benign and malignant biliary processes is reviewed, emphasizing MR findings that aid in characterization.

Magnetic resonance (MR) imaging of the pancreas is useful as both a problem-solving tool and an initial imaging examination of choice. With newer imaging sequences such as diffusion-weighted imaging, MR offers improved ability to detect and characterize lesions and identify and stage tumors and inflammation. MR cholangiopancreatography can be used to visualize the pancreatic and biliary ductal system. In this article, the use of MR to evaluate the pancreas, including recent advances, is reviewed and the normal appearance of the pancreas on different imaging sequences, as well as inflammatory diseases, congenital abnormalities, and neoplasms of the pancreas, are discussed.

MR imaging has proven to be a versatile modality in evaluation of the kidneys, collecting system, and adrenal glands. By performing a comprehensive MR examination, it is not only possible to accurately characterize cystic and solid lesions of the kidneys, as well as urothelial masses, but also to provide important preoperative information to the surgeon. In addition, MR imaging can characterize many adrenal lesions and can frequently obviate biopsy. The continued development and growth of MR technology combined with the current trend toward minimally invasive surgery will expand the role of MR imaging in the future.

Magnetic resonance enterography (MRE) utilization has increased for the evaluation of small bowel diseases over the last several years. In addition to performing similarly to computed tomography enterography (CTE) in the evaluation of inflammatory bowel disease, MRE lacks ionizing radiation, can image the small bowel dynamically, and provides excellent soft tissue contrast resolution. This article reviews imaging protocols for MRE, normal MR imaging appearance of small bowel, and the imaging findings of small bowel Crohn disease. The importance of imaging findings for directing management in patients with small bowel Crohn disease is emphasized throughout.

Multiparametric magnetic resonance (MR) imaging of the prostate is gaining acceptance in the management of prostate cancer. Emerging indications of prostate MR imaging may expand its use in the work-up of localized prostate cancer. Improvements in the standardization of prostate MR imaging techniques and reporting are needed for further establishment of the emerging roles of prostate MR imaging. This article describes the prostate MR imaging techniques and provides an approach for interpretation of prostate MR imaging studies. Established and emerging indications for prostate MR imaging are also reviewed.

Magnetic resonance (MR) angiographic techniques optimize the visualization of the vasculature at MR imaging. MR angiography has several advantages over Doppler ultrsonography and computed tomographic angiography, with adaptable protocols to answer specific clinical questions. Novel noncontrast MR angiographic techniques now enable assessment of the abdominopelvic vasculature without administration of gadolinium-based contrast media. This article reviews MR angiographic techniques and discusses applications for arterial and venous evaluation in the abdomen and pelvis.

Magnetic resonance (MR) imaging is a robust imaging modality for evaluation of vascular diseases. Technological advances have made MR imaging widely available for accurate and time-efficient vascular assessment. In this article the clinical usefulness of MR imaging techniques and their application are reviewed, using examples of vascular abnormalities commonly encountered in clinical practice, including abdominal, pelvic, and thoracic vessels. Common pitfalls and problem solving in interpretation of vascular findings in body MR imaging are also discussed.

In this article, functional magnetic resonance (MR) imaging techniques in the abdomen are discussed. Diffusion-weighted imaging (DWI) increases the confidence in detecting and characterizing focal hepatic lesions. The potential uses of DWI in kidneys, adrenal glands, bowel, and pancreas are outlined. Studies have shown potential use of quantitative dynamic contrast-enhanced MR imaging parameters, such as $K^{trans}$, in predicting outcomes in cancer therapy. MR elastography is considered to be a useful tool in staging liver fibrosis. A major issue with all functional MR imaging techniques is the lack of standardization of the protocol.

## PROGRAM OBJECTIVE

The objective of the Radiologic Clinics of North America is to keep practicing radiologists and radiology residents up to date with current clinical practice in radiology by providing timely articles reviewing the state of the art in patient care.

## TARGET AUDIENCE

Practicing radiologists, radiology residents, and other health care professionals who provide patient care utilizing radiologic findings.

## LEARNING OBJECTIVES

Upon completion of this activity, participants will be able to:
1. Discuss magnetic resonance imaging of biliary system, prostate, kidneys, adrenal glands and abdomen.
2. Review techniques for body magnetic resonance imaging.
3. Describe methods for vascular conundrums with MRI.

## ACCREDITATION

The Elsevier Office of Continuing Medical Education (EOCME) is accredited by the Accreditation Council for Continuing Medical Education (ACCME) to provide continuing medical education for physicians.

The EOCME designates this enduring material for a maximum of 15 *AMA PRA Category 1 Credit*(s)™. Physicians should claim only the credit commensurate with the extent of their participation in the activity.

All other health care professionals requesting continuing education credit for this enduring material will be issued a certificate of participation.

## DISCLOSURE OF CONFLICTS OF INTEREST

The EOCME assesses conflict of interest with its instructors, faculty, planners, and other individuals who are in a position to control the content of CME activities. All relevant conflicts of interest that are identified are thoroughly vetted by EOCME for fair balance, scientific objectivity, and patient care recommendations. EOCME is committed to providing its learners with CME activities that promote improvements or quality in healthcare and not a specific proprietary business or a commercial interest.

**The planning committee, staff, authors and editors listed below have identified no financial relationships or relationships to products or devices they or their spouse/life partner have with commercial interest related to the content of this CME activity:**

Brian C. Allen, MD; Wirana Angthong, MD; Jad Bou Ayache, MD; Jonathan R. Cogley, MD; Jeremy D. Collins, MD; Amir H. Davarpanah, MD; Flavius F. Guglielmo, MD; Shiva Gupta, MD; Nancy Hammond, MD; Kristen Helm; Brynne Hunter; Gary M. Israel, MD; Yong-Hwan Jeon, MD; Bong Soo Kim, MD; Sandy Lavery; John R. Leyendecker, MD; Jill McNair; Frank H. Miller, MD; Donald G. Mitchell, MD; Michael A. Ohliger, MD; Erin O'Neill, MD; Aytekin Oto, MD; Kumar Sandrasegaran, MD; Richard C. Semelka, MD; Evan S. Siegelman, MD; Karthikeyan Subramaniam; John Vassallo; Joseph H. Yacoub, MD; Benjamin L. Yam, MD.

**The planning committee, staff, authors and editors listed below have identified financial relationships or relationships to products or devices they or their spouse/life partner have with commercial interest related to the content of this CME activity:**

Thomas A. Hope, MD is a consultant/advisor for Guerbet LLC and has a research grant from GE Healthcare.
Aliya Qayyum, MD has a research grant from Philips Healthcare.
Christopher G. Roth, MD is an author for Reed Elsevier.

## UNAPPROVED/OFF-LABEL USE DISCLOSURE

The EOCME requires CME faculty to disclose to the participants:
1. When products or procedures being discussed are off-label, unlabelled, experimental, and/or investigational (not US Food and Drug Administration (FDA) approved); and
2. Any limitations on the information presented, such as data that are preliminary or that represent ongoing research, interim analyses, and/or unsupported opinions. Faculty may discuss information about pharmaceutical agents that is outside of FDA-approved labelling. This information is intended solely for CME and is not intended to promote off-label use of these medications. If you have any questions, contact the medical affairs department of the manufacturer for the most recent prescribing information.

## TO ENROLL

To enroll in the *Radiologic Clinics of North America* Continuing Medical Education program, call customer service at 1-800-654-2452 or sign up online at http://www.theclinics.com/home/cme. The CME program is available to subscribers for an additional annual fee of USD $315.

## METHOD OF PARTICIPATION

In order to claim credit, participants must complete the following:
1. Complete enrolment as indicated above.
2. Read the activity.
3. Complete the CME Test and Evaluation. Participants must achieve a score of 70% on the test. All CME Tests and Evaluations must be completed online.

## CME INQUIRIES/SPECIAL NEEDS

For all CME inquiries or special needs, please contact elsevierCME@elsevier.com.

# RADIOLOGIC CLINICS OF NORTH AMERICA

# Preface

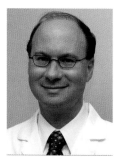

Frank H. Miller, MD
*Editor*

Body Magnetic Resonance (MR) imaging is a topic that needs frequent updating given the rapid advances in the field. There are numerous potential applications and growth areas for body MR. In addition, the lack of radiation has motivated physicians and patients to consider using MR instead of CT scans for follow-up exams, especially in younger patients. The scanner time for body MR has been reduced significantly with the use of breath-hold and parallel imaging and dynamic contrast-enhanced imaging so that the routine exam times are reasonable, less than 30 minutes. My hope is that body MR will be more widely adapted and that this issue will educate and motivate radiologists to perform these exams.

Body MR imaging is one of the largest growth areas in Northwestern's Department of Radiology. We currently use abdominal and pelvic MR as primary imaging modalities and not just for "problem" solving. It has been widely accepted by referring physicians, allowing us to perform over 10,000 exams per year. The exceptional contrast resolution and ability to make definitive diagnoses, avoiding biopsies and other tests, are unsurpassed in many of the abdominal and pelvic organs. The lack of radiation of MR has increased its utility in patients who previously required multiple follow-up CT scans. In addition, newer techniques, including diffusion and perfusion-weighted imaging and MR elastography, allow not only assessment of anatomic imaging features but also functional information. As the field continues to grow, updates such as this issue of the *Radiologic Clinics of North America* become extremely important.

I would like to thank the world-class talented contributors to the issue for their outstanding and timely contributions. As anticipated, they made my work a pleasure. Topics covered in this issue include practical technical articles, including articles entitled "fast, efficient, and comprehensive protocols" and "gadolinium contrast agent selection and optimal uses." In addition, important abdominal and pelvic MR organs are discussed, including the following: liver, pancreas, gallbladder and biliary (MRCP), kidney and adrenal glands, bowel (MR enterography), prostate, and vascular imaging. Several topics, including female pelvic imaging, were recently covered by the *Radiologic Clinics of North America* and as result were not included in this issue. Newer functional MR imaging techniques, which are becoming mainstream and routinely used, such as diffusion-weighted imaging, are included.

I would like to thank my chairman, Dr Eric Russell, and my section at Northwestern University, for their invaluable friendship and for making Northwestern a great place for academic pursuits. I would like to thank John Vassallo, Adrianne Brigido, Donald Mumford, Nicole Congleton, and the team at Elsevier, for their invaluable support, not only for this issue but also for the outstanding *Radiologic Clinics of North America* series. I would like to acknowledge the hard work by David Botos and Holly Harper at Northwestern in preparation of the articles. I would also like to thank my family for their love and continuous encouragement and support.

Frank H. Miller, MD
Department of Radiology
Northwestern University Feinberg School of
Medicine
Northwestern Memorial Hospital
676 North Saint Clair Street, Suite 800
Chicago, IL 60611, USA

E-mail address:
fmiller@northwestern.edu

radiologic.theclinics.com

# Body MR Imaging
## Fast, Efficient, and Comprehensive

 CrossMark

Bong Soo Kim, MD[a], Wirana Angthong, MD[b],
Yong-Hwan Jeon, MD[b], Richard C. Semelka, MD[b],*

KEYWORDS

- Abdominal MR imaging • Uncooperative patient • Motion-resistant MR imaging
- New MR imaging techniques • Artifacts

KEY POINTS

- Magnetic resonance (MR) imaging of the abdomen should be performed in a fast, efficient, and comprehensive fashion and provide consistent image quality and display of disease processes.
- Separation of protocols for cooperative and cooperation-challenged patients is necessary because inability of noncooperative patients to hold their breath impairs the image quality on abdominal MR imaging.
- Motion-resistant protocols including fast imaging and radial acquisition techniques radically improve imaging quality in noncooperative patients.

## INTRODUCTION

A major strength of magnetic resonance (MR) imaging is the variety of types of information that it is able to generate. As a result, abdominal MR imaging can provide comprehensive information on organ systems and disease entities. The use of fast scanning techniques provides consistently high image quality and good conspicuity of disease with a decrease of imaging times.[1–3] Examination time is critical because the longer MR studies could result in worsening of imaging quality because of motion, which tends to progress through the course of the study from patient exhaustion. The sequence acquisition time in routine MR protocols could generally be too long for high-diagnostic-quality abdominal MR imaging in noncooperative patients such as those who are agitated, sedated, or unconscious. Therefore,

it is necessary to develop separate protocols for noncooperative patients,[4–6] distinct from a standard cooperative protocol. To provide appropriate abdominal MR work-up in cooperative and noncooperative patients, this article provides basic information about different sequences and core information about image interpretation.

## COOPERATIVE PROTOCOL

In practice, it is important to recognize which technique is the most consistent in showing various diseases in order to target lesions in an imaging protocol. Attention to length of examination is critical because longer examinations result in fewer patients who can be examined and a decreased in patient cooperation. The different sequences used should ideally be of short duration and breath held or breathing independent. Another

---

Disclosure: None of the authors has a conflict of interest.
[a] Department of Radiology, Jeju National University Hospital, Jeju National University School of Medicine, 1753-3, Ara-1-dong, Jeju-si, Jeju-do 690-716, Korea; [b] Department of Radiology, University of North Carolina Hospitals, University of North Carolina at Chapel Hill, CB 7510, 2001 Old Clinic Building, Chapel Hill, NC 27599-7510, USA
* Corresponding author.
*E-mail address:* richsem@med.unc.edu

Radiol Clin N Am 52 (2014) 623–636
http://dx.doi.org/10.1016/j.rcl.2014.02.007
0033-8389/14/$ – see front matter © 2014 Elsevier Inc. All rights reserved.

radiologic.theclinics.com

consideration is reproducibility of examination protocols, because efficient operation of an MR imaging system requires the use of set protocols, which serves to speed up examinations, render examinations reproducible, and increases use by familiarity with a standard approach. **Table 1** lists the parameters of the MR sequences used in cooperative patients on 1.5-T and 3.0-T scanners. For most patients, it is possible to complete the core sequences within 15 minutes.

## T1-Weighted Sequences

### In-phase two-dimensional spoiled gradient echo sequence

In-phase imaging has become a routine part of liver MR imaging for investigating disease of the abdomen. This sequence is primarily used to provide the following information: presence of subacute blood or concentrated protein, which both have high signal intensity (**Fig. 1**); presence of fat as high-signal-intensity tissue (**Fig. 2**); and abnormally increased fluid content or

fibrous tissue content, which appear as low signal intensity.

### Out-of-phase two-dimensional spoiled gradient echo sequence

Out-of-phase images show a sharply defined black rim around organs with a fat-water interface, and the kidneys are a good organ to look for this. Out-of-phase sequences are helpful for the recognition of diseased tissue in which fat and water protons are present within the same voxel. Signal loss is maximal when fat content approaches 50%. This sequence plays an important role in detecting the presence of fat (steatosis) within the liver and lipid within adrenal masses to characterize them as adenomas, which are shown as loss of signal intensity relative to the in-phase sequence (**Fig. 3**). In addition, it is important to use in-phase/out-of-phase sequences to show magnetic susceptibility effects from the presence of iron (exogenous or endogenous) or air. Examples include iron storage diseases, such as hemochromatosis or

**Table 1**
**Parameters for cooperative patients used at 1.5 T and 3.0 T on MR imaging scanners**

| Parameter (T) | Precontrast Sequences | | | | Postcontrast Sequences | |
|---|---|---|---|---|---|---|
| | T1-weighted 2D-SGE In Phase/Out of Phase | | T2-weighted SS-ETSE | | Dynamic T1-weighted 3D-GRE[a] | |
| | 3.0 | 1.5 | 3.0 | 1.5 | 3.0 | 1.5 |
| Plane of acquisition | Axial | Axial | Axial, coronal | Axial, coronal | Axial, coronal | Axial, coronal |
| TR (ms) | 169 | 142 | 2000 | 1500 | 3.07 | 4.3 |
| TE (ms) | 2.5/1.58 | 4.4/2.2 | 95 | 90 | 1.32 | 1.6 |
| Flip angle (°) | 57 | 70 | 150 | 180 | 13 | 10 |
| Echo-train length | — | — | 179 | 156 | — | — |
| BW/pixel (Hz) | 400 | 490 | 781 | 651 | 500 | 350 |
| Matrix (phase × frequency) | 204 × 256 | 192 × 256 | 204 × 256 | 192 × 256 | 192 × 256 | 160 × 320 |
| FOV (mm) | 400 × 400 | 350 × 350 | 350 × 350 | 400 × 400 | 400 × 400 | 360 × 360 |
| No. of section | 28 | 19 | 30 | 20 | 72 | 72 |
| Section thickness (mm) | 8 | 8 | 8 | 8 | 3 | 3.5 |
| Intersectional gap (mm) | 1.6 | 1.6 | 1.6 | 1.6 | 0 | 0 |
| No. of signal acquisition | 1 | 1 | 1 | 1 | 1 | 1 |
| Fat suppression | None | None | Fat saturation for axial, none for coronal | | Fat saturation | Fat saturation |
| Respiratory control | BH | BH | BI | BI | BH | BH |

*Abbreviations:* BH, breath-holding; BI, breathing-independent; BW, bandwidth; FOV, field of view; GRE, gradient echo; Hz, hertz; sat, saturation; SGE, spoiled gradient echo; SS-ETSE, single-shot echo-train spin-echo; TE, echo time; TR, repetition time; 2D, two dimensional; 3D, three dimensional.

[a] Dynamic 3D-GRE sequences were used to acquire all 3 postcontrast phases in 3.0-T and 1.5-T scanners.

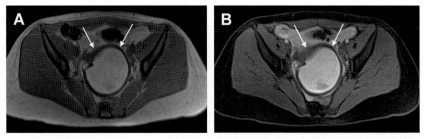

**Fig. 1.** MR images in a 27-year-old woman with a hemorrhagic corpus luteal cyst. Axial T1-weighted two-dimensional (2D) SGE in-phase (*A*) and T1-weighted fat-suppressed three-dimensional (3D) GRE (*B*) images show high signal intensity within an ovarian cystic mass (*arrows*) in the pelvic cavity, suggesting a hemorrhagic cyst. Hemoperitoneum is also visualized in the pelvic cavity.

hemosiderosis. Susceptibility effects increase with increase in echo time (TE) because of pronounced decay of transverse magnetization, which appears as lower-signal tissue on longer TE sequences (**Fig. 4**).[7,8]

### Coronal two-dimensional spoiled gradient echo sequence

Coronal T1-weighted images are obtained for an overview of the abdomen. Coronal MR images allow an additional perspective that may not clearly be shown on transverse images, and increase the confidence of diagnosis. Coronal images are useful for viewing the aorta, para-aortic lymph nodes, and mesenteric vessels, which display the vascular structures along their longitudinal axes. The coronal views should also be used to inspect the lung bases and the inferior and superior surfaces of the liver for the presence of metastases and other disease processes.

### Fat-suppressed T1-weighted three-dimensional gradient recalled echo sequence

Three-dimensional (3D) gradient recalled echo (GRE) sequences in combination with fat-suppression techniques provide high-quality imaging and very thin sections with adequate volume coverage in a single breath-hold imaging time. 3D GRE is suitable for dynamic contrast-enhanced MR studies because of its excellent inherent fat suppression and sensitivity to enhancement in tissues after gadolinium-based contrast agents (GBCAs) are given. Fat-suppression techniques are useful for the diagnosis of diseased tissues composed predominantly of fat, such as ovarian dermoid cyst, angiomyolipoma, lipoma, and myelolipoma (see **Fig. 2**), which are confidently diagnosed by showing the lesion to show high signal on in-phase images and dark on noncontrast fat-suppressed GRE images.[9] Fat-suppression technique improves the delineation of pancreatic borders and the pancreas, which appears homogeneously bright compared with surrounding low-signal-intensity fat and other abdominal organs (see **Fig. 2**). It is excellent for identifying chronic pancreatitis (less intense than normal high-intensity pancreas) and pancreatic masses such as small ductal adenocarcinoma (**Fig. 5**) and pancreatic neuroendocrine tumors.[10,11] The fat-suppression technique also allows the best visualization of renal corticomedullary differentiation, which is reduced in renal transplant rejection and chronic renal insufficiency.[12]

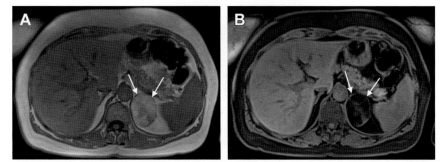

**Fig. 2.** MR images in a 56-year-old woman with an adrenal myelolipoma. Axial T1-weighted 2D SGE in-phase image (*A*) shows a lesion with high signal intensity (*arrows*) in left adrenal gland with suppression (*arrows*) on the T1-weighted fat-suppressed 3D GRE image (*B*). The normal pancreas is well shown as high signal intensity on axial T1-weighted fat-suppressed 3D GRE image.

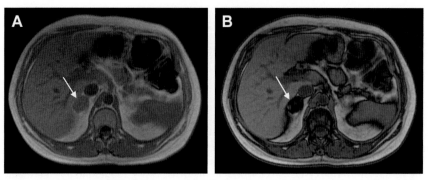

**Fig. 3.** MR images in a 51-year-old man with an adrenal adenoma. A right adrenal mass (*arrow*) has substantial signal reduction from the axial T1-weighted 2D SGE in-phase image (*A*) to the axial T1-weighted 2D SGE out-of-phase image (*B*).

## T2-weighted Sequences

### Single-shot echo-train spin-echo sequence

The important information that T2-weighted images provide includes (1) the presence of abnormal increased fluid content in diseased tissue and fluid-containing tumors (cysts, hamartomas, and hemangiomas), which results in high signal intensity; (2) the presence of chronic fibrotic tissue, which results in low-signal-intensity lesions, and the presence of low-fluid-content lesions, which results in a range of signal intensity from mildly low to mildly high; (3) the presence of iron deposition, which appears as markedly low signal intensity (see **Fig. 4**); and (4) the presence of lymph nodes in the porta hepatis, which have high signal intensity compared with liver parenchyma (**Fig. 6**). Fat suppression should generally be applied for at least one set of T2-weighted images of the liver, and it may also be helpful to perform this in a different plane, to obtain an additional benefit from a second data acquisition. One common circumstance in which fat suppression is useful on T2-weighted sequences is when the patient may have liver metastases and the background liver has steatosis. Without fat suppression, fatty liver has high signal intensity on a

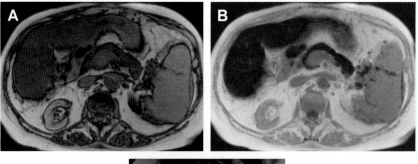

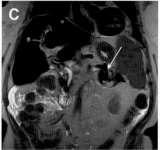

**Fig. 4.** MR images in a 62-year-old woman with idiopathic hemochromatosis. Axial T1-weighted 2D SGE out-of-phase image (echo time of 2.2 ms) (*A*) and axial T1-weighted 2D SGE in-phase image (echo time of 4.4 ms) (*B*) show a marked reduction in signal intensity in the liver, pancreas, and focal areas of the spleen in the image with the longer echo time. There is decreased signal intensity of liver and pancreas (*arrow*) on coronal T2-weighted fat-suppressed SS-ETSE (*C*).

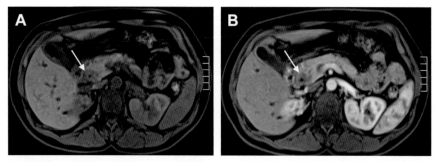

**Fig. 5.** MR images in a 49-year-old man with a small pancreatic cancer. Axial T1-weighted fat-suppressed 3D GRE image (*A*) shows a small mass arising in the pancreatic head, which invades the common bile duct and is shown as a low-signal-intensity lesion (*arrow*) with normal pancreas appearing bright. On the axial T1-weighted fat-suppressed 3D GRE arterial dominant phase image (*B*), a low-signal-intensity tumor (*arrow*) is identified in the head, clearly demarcated from uniformly well-enhancing normal pancreatic tissue.

standard single-shot echo-train spin-echo (SS-ETSE) sequence, because fat signal is high with this technique, thereby diminishing contrast with most liver lesions, whereas with fat suppression the liver becomes darker, ensuring optimal contrast with lesions that show mildly intrinsic high T2 signal. Coronal T2-weighted images are also obtained for an overall review of the abdomen. They are particularly useful for viewing the structures of the bowel and biliary system.

An additional advantage is that this sequence is resistance to susceptibility artifact. As a result, the bowel wall can clearly be seen and susceptibility artifact from metallic devices is minimal. In these settings it may be important to not use fat suppression to minimize susceptibility effects. Often a more complex fat-suppression sequence is important to minimize persistent fat signal on this sequence, such as combining fat suppression with inversion recovery.

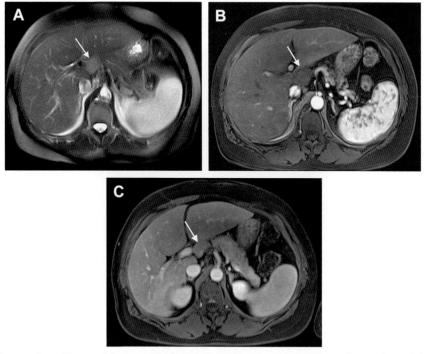

**Fig. 6.** MR images in a 45-year-old man with chronic liver disease and an enlarged porta hepatis lymph node. Axial T2-weighted fat-suppressed SS-ETSE image (*A*) shows the best delineation of a lymph node (*arrow*) in porta hepatis, compared with axial T1-weighted fat-suppressed 3D GRE arterial dominant phase (*B*) and early hepatic venous phase images (*C*). On the axial T2-weighted fat-suppressed SS-ETSE image, lymph nodes have moderately high signal intensity and both liver and background fat are low signal, rendering excellent conspicuity.

## Contrast-enhanced Fat-suppressed T1-weighted 3D GRE Sequence

### Hepatic arterial dominant phase

The hepatic arterial dominant (capillary) phase (HADP) is the single most important data set when using a nonspecific extracellular GBCA.[13] Capillary phase image acquisition is achieved by using a short-duration sequence initiated immediately after gadolinium injection. These images are identified by the presence of contrast in hepatic arteries and portal veins and its absence in the hepatic veins. Greater enhancement of normal pancreas than the liver can be reliably judged on HADP. Hypervascular liver tumors, especially hepatocellular carcinomas, focal nodular hyperplasia (Fig. 7), and hypervascular metastases are well recognized as intensely enhancing lesions on HADP, compared with background liver. HADP images are essential to observe hepatic perfusion abnormalities, such as are present in the full range of inflammatory conditions (Fig. 8). The pancreas shows uniform capillary blush on HADP, which renders it markedly high in signal intensity. In general, pancreatic adenocarcinoma usually appears as a focal hypovascular mass that is readily detected and characterized on HADP (see Fig. 5). In these instances, the tumor is well demarcated from adjacent uninvolved pancreas, which shows greater enhancement.

### Early hepatic venous phase

Images for this phase are acquired 45 to 60 seconds after initiation of the GBCA and are recognized by the presence of contrast in hepatic and portal veins. In this phase, the hepatic parenchyma is maximally enhanced so that hypovascular lesions such as cysts, hypovascular metastases, and scar tissue are most clearly identified as regions of absent or diminished enhancement. This phase is also useful in lesion characterization of hypervascular tumors, such as hepatocellular carcinoma, which show washout (that is, they become darker than liver) on early hepatic venous phase, and focal nodular hyperplasia, which shows fading (that is, it becomes isointense with liver) (see Fig. 7). This phase also clearly shows patency or thrombosis of portal and hepatic veins. The perfusion abnormalities on HADP such as compromised portal venous flow, acute-on-chronic hepatitis, inflammatory reactions to adjacent infection (eg, acute cholecystitis, liver abscess), and Budd-Chiari syndrome usually disappear on early hepatic venous or interstitial phases (see Fig. 8) and this often forms an important part of the diagnostic criteria for a phenomenon being vascular or inflammatory-vascular in nature.

### Interstitial phase

This phase is acquired 90 seconds to 5 minutes after initiation of the contrast material injection. The interstitial phase shows computed tomography (CT)–like images when performed with fat suppression. Late enhancement features of focal liver lesions are shown, which aid in lesion characterization. These findings assist in establishing a diagnosis of hepatocellular carcinoma by showing washout and delayed capsular enhancement; mass-forming intrahepatic cholangiocarcinoma, which shows progressive enhancement; and hemangioma, which shows coalescence and centripetal progression of enhancing nodules. Enhancement of peritoneal metastasis, inflammatory disease, and pulmonary nodules are well shown at this phase. The coronal interstitial images are acquired after 3 sets of transverse images. These images provide a general survey view of the abdomen from a surgeon's vantage point. These images are useful for detecting metastases of the musculoskeletal system (especially

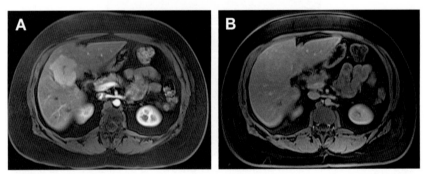

**Fig. 7.** MR images in a 41-year-old woman with a focal nodular hyperplasia. Axial T1-weighted fat-suppressed 3D GRE arterial dominant phase image (*A*) shows an intensely enhancing mass in the liver with central scar shown by low signal intensity. On early hepatic venous phase image (*B*), the tumor fades to near isointensity with background parenchyma and a central scar showing delayed enhancement.

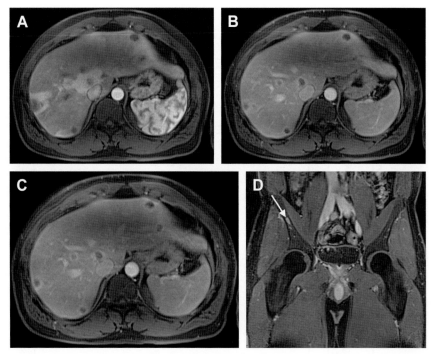

**Fig. 8.** MR images in a 40-year-old man with multiple liver and bone metastases from pancreatic head cancer. This patient has multiple ringlike enhancing metastases in the liver. On axial T1-weighted fat-suppressed 3D GRE arterial dominant phase imaging (*A*), sharply demarcated wedge-shaped perilesional enhancements are shown with disappearance on early hepatic venous (*B*) and interstitial phases (*C*), suggesting perfusion abnormalities. Coronal T1-weighted fat-suppressed 3D GRE interstitial phase image (*D*) shows a small enhancing metastasis (*arrow*) in the right ilium.

thoracolumbar spines, pelvis, and femoral heads) (see **Fig. 8**),[14] peritoneal disease, retroperitoneal disease, and metastases of lung bases. The coronal interstitial images also provide valuable information about bowel and mesenteric abnormalities and may be used to define abnormal enhancement in tumoral and inflamed regions of bowel. Direct coronal imaging (rather than reformatting transverse images) is strongly advised at this phase to substantiate the patency or thrombosis of the portal vein and superior mesenteric veins, which is important for the assessment of liver cirrhosis and pancreatic cancer. Artifacts, including flow artifacts, are a more serious problem with MR than with CT, and an important means for compensating for this is to acquire images in orthogonal planes. If a defect in a vessel represents thrombosis rather than flow, it should be apparent, with the same anticipated location, from one plane to the next. Flow artifacts show different morphologies from one plane to the next.

## MOTION-RESISTANT PROTOCOLS

Motion-resistant protocols achieve improved image quality in settings of noncooperation by either acquiring the critical data for image creation during only a small fraction of the time for free breathing, rendering this technique insensitive to the patient's motion (single-shot approaches) or by modifying the data acquisition to minimize effects of motion (eg, radial acquisition, multiple data averages). To facilitate patient throughput at our center, the primary individual determining whether a motion-resistant protocol should be performed is the scanning technologist, who decides whether the patient is following commands or whether they have difficulty breathing holding, and, if they are having difficulty, then the scanning technologist implements the motion-resistant protocol. To perform an adequate MR examination in noncooperative patients, it is useful to obtain the following sequences: T1-weighted dual-echo magnetization-prepared rapid-acquisition gradient echo (MP-RAGE), T1-weighted MP-RAGE before and after gadolinium, T1-weighted water excitation MP-RAGE (WE-MP-RAGE) after gadolinium, T1-weighted radial GRE sequence before and after gadolinium, and T1-weighted SS-ETSE. **Table 2** provides the MR imaging parameters for motion-resistant protocols on 1.5-T and 3.0-T scanners.

**Table 2**
Parameters for motion-resistant protocol used on 1.5-T and 3.0-T MR imaging scanners

| Parameter (T) | Precontrast Sequences | | | | Postcontrast Sequences | | | | | |
|---|---|---|---|---|---|---|---|---|---|---|
| | T1-weighted 2D MP-RAGE In Phase/Out of Phase | | T2-weighted SS-ETSE | | T1-weighted MP-RAGE | | T1-weighted WE-MP-RAGE | | T1-weighted Radial 3D-GRE | |
| | 3.0 | 1.5 | 3.0 | 1.5 | 3.0 | 1.5 | 3.0 | 1.5 | 3.0 | 1.5 |
| Plane of acquisition | Axial | Axial | Axial, coronal | Axial, coronal | Axial | Axial | Axial, coronal | Axial, coronal | Axial, coronal | Axial, coronal |
| TR (ms) | 1800 | 1540 | 2000 | 1500 | 2000 | 2000 | 2000 | 2000 | 600 | 350 |
| TE (ms) | 2.3/3.6 | 4.1/2.3 | 95 | 90 | 2.5 | 1.7 | 2.8 | 6.2 | 3.8 | 1.6 |
| TI (ms) | 1200 | 900 | — | — | 1200 | 700 | 1200 | 700 | — | — |
| Flip angle (°) | 20 | 15 | 150 | 180 | 20 | 15 | 20 | 15 | 10 | 10 |
| Echo-train length | — | — | 179 | 156 | — | — | — | — | — | — |
| BW/pixel (Hz) | 190/180 | 180/150 | 781 | 651 | 600 | 180 | 600 | 180 | 600 | 350 |
| Matrix (phase × frequency) | 256 × 189 | 256 × 156 | 204 × 256 | 192 × 256 | 180 × 256 | 180 × 256 | 180 × 256 | 128 × 192 | 380 × 380 | 380 × 380 |
| FOV (mm) | 380 × 380 | 380 × 380 | 350 × 350 | 400 × 400 | 400 × 400 | 350 × 350 | 400 × 400 | 350 × 350 | 380 × 380 | 380 × 380 |
| No. of sections | 40 | 38 | 30 | 20 | 28 | 20 | 28 | 20 | 72 | 80 |
| Section thickness (mm) | 5 | 6 | 8 | 8 | 8 | 8 | 8 | 8 | 3.0 | 3.0 |
| Intersectional gap (mm) | 1.0 | 1.2 | 1.6 | 1.6 | 1.6 | 1.6 | 1.6 | 1.6 | 0 | 0 |
| No. of signal acquisition | 1 | 2 | 1 | 1 | — | — | — | — | 1 | 1 |
| Fat suppression | None | None | Fat sat for axial, none for coronal | | None | None | Fat sat | Fat sat | Fat sat | Fat sat |
| Respiratory control | BI | BI | BI | BI | BI | BI | BI | BI | FB | FB |

*Abbreviations:* FB, free breathing; MP-RAGE, magnetization-prepared rapid-acquisition gradient echo; sat, saturation; TI, inversion time; WE-MP-RAGE, water excitation magnetization-prepared rapid-acquisition gradient echo.

## T1-weighted Sequences

### Two-dimensional MP-RAGE sequence

MP-RAGE, for example turbo fast low-angle shot (FLASH), is a single shot–type sequence that operates as a slice-by-slice single-shot technique and can generate T1-weighted images that are resistant to deterioration from respiratory motion (**Figs. 9** and **10**). This sequence can be used to obtain motion-free and moderate-quality images with acquisition times as short as 1 second. It has the intrinsic issue that signal/noise ratio (SNR) and contrast/noise ratio (CNR) are lower than in regular gradient echo images.[15] An inversion pulse leads to the longitudinal magnetization that creates the T1 contrast. The sequence acquires data using a very short repetition time (TR) and low flip-angle excitation pulses to reduce acquisition time and maintain the prepared magnetization.

Standard in-phase/out-of-phase GRE imaging are performed as multislice GRE acquisitions that require patients to suspend respiration, because sequences are generally 10 to 20 seconds in duration. New implementations of MP-RAGE in-phase/out-of-phase images are able to show the presence of fat, which is necessary to evaluate the liver and also adrenal masses in patients who cannot cooperate with standard in-phase/out-of-phase GRE imaging, such as in the elderly, the severely debilitated, and young children (see **Fig. 10; Fig. 11**).[16–18] Image quality and lesion conspicuity of MP-RAGE in-phase/out-of-phase imaging are also comparable with standard in-phase/out-of-phase GRE imaging.[18]

### Two-dimensional WE-MP-RAGE

Spatial-spectral selective water excitation is a newer fat-attenuation technique that selectively

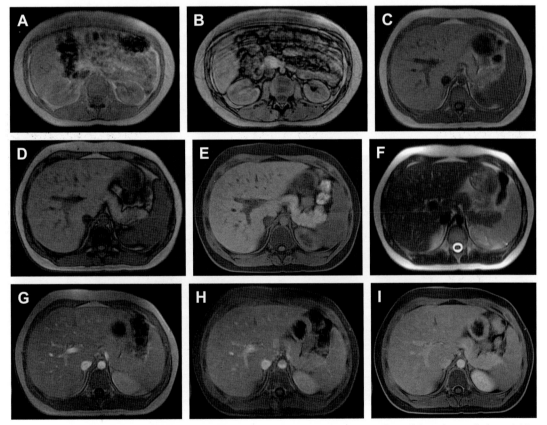

**Fig. 9.** MR images in a 10-year-old boy. Standard axial T1-weighted 2D SGE in-phase (*A*) and out-of-phase (*B*) images shows motion artifacts caused by respiration. In this patient, who could not suspend respiration, the study was switched to a motion-resistant protocol because unacceptable image quality was expected. The motion-resistant protocol included axial T1-weighted 2D MP-RAGE in-phase (*C*), axial T1-weighted 2D MP-RAGE out-of-phase (*D*), axial T1-weighted radial 3D GRE (*E*), axial T2-weighted fat-suppressed SS-ETSE (*F*), contrast-enhanced axial T1-weighted 2D MP-RAGE (*G*), contrast-enhanced axial T1-weighted 2D-WE-MP-RAGE (*H*), and contrast-enhanced axial T1-weighted radial 3D GRE images (*I*). This protocol shows substantially reduced artifacts and motion-free high-quality images in this difficult-to-scan child.

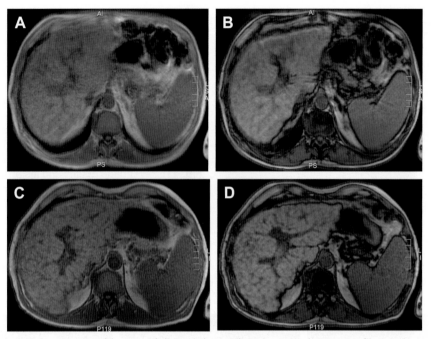

Fig. 10. MR images in a 64-year-old man with liver cirrhosis. There is a reticular pattern fibrosis through the liver, which has low signal intensity on T1-weighted images. Axial 2D SGE in-phase (*A*) and axial out-of-phase (*B*) images show motion artifacts caused by breathing and parallel imaging artifacts. No motion artifacts are present on axial 2D MP-RAGE in-phase (*C*) and out-of-phase (*D*) images. The fine pattern of fibrosis is particularly well shown on the axial 2D MP-RAGE out-of-phase image.

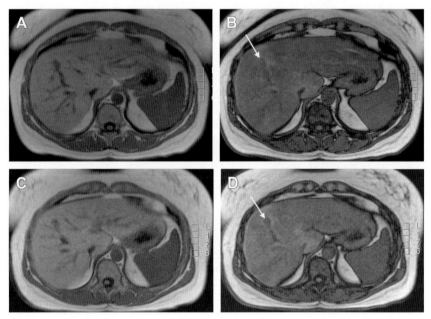

Fig. 11. MR images in a 48-year-old woman with liver steatosis and liver metastasis. The liver shows a reduction of signal intensity on the axial 2D SGE out-of-phase image (*B*) compared with the axial 2D SGE in-phase image (*A*). This reduction of signal intensity is also visualized on axial 2D MP-RAGE out-of-phase imaging (*D*), comparing with axial 2D MP-RAGE in-phase imaging (*C*). A small liver metastasis (*arrow*) is appreciated in S8 of the liver, better depicted in axial 2D MP-RAGE out-of-phase (*D*) than in axial 2D SGE out-of-phase (*B*) imaging.

excites water protons leaving protons in fat unperturbed, rather than exciting all protons and then spoiling the signal from fat protons. This is a faster fat-attenuating scheme than conventional exciting-spoiling fat suppression, and this speed is necessary for use on a rapid gradient technique such as MP-RAGE. WE-MP-RAGE can provide fat-attenuated contrast-enhanced T1-weighted images (**Fig. 12**). WE-MP-RAGE at 3 T can achieve better image quality and fat attenuation than at 1.5 T because of the intrinsic properties of the higher field strength, such as higher SNR and CNR, and increased chemical frequency shift between fat and water that reduces the duration of WE-radiofrequency pulses and data acquisition time.[4] This sequence, similar to fat-suppressed

spoiled gradient echo (SGE), could be used to detect abnormally increased fluid content or fibrous tissue content that appears as low signal intensity, and presence of subacute blood or concentrated protein, which are both high signal intensity.

### 3D radial GRE sequence

Standard T1-weighted GRE sequences acquire k-space data on a horizontal-filling line-by-line basis, which is a scheme that is sensitive to motion artifacts. Radial acquisition technique (projection reconstruction) has higher sampling density for central k-space (which contributes the bulk of the signal in images), because it acquires data in a radial spoke-wheel fashion, and undersamples

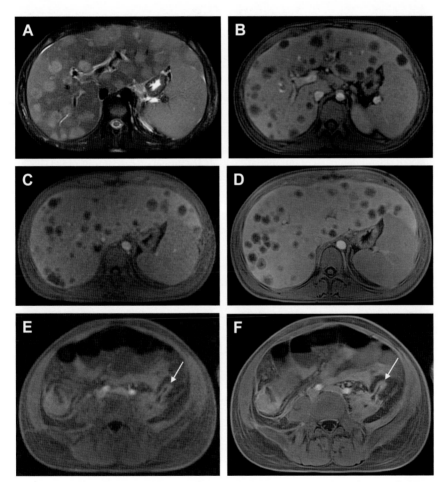

Fig. 12. MR images in a 25-year-old man with Crohn disease and abscess involving liver and psoas muscle. Multiple abscesses in liver are clearly shown in a noncooperative patient on axial T2-weighted fat-suppressed SS-ETSE (*A*), contrast-enhanced axial 2D MP-RAGE (*B*), contrast-enhanced axial 2D WE-MP-RAGE (*C*), and contrast-enhanced axial 3D radial GE (*D*) images. The abscess in psoas muscle (*arrow*) is well visualized on contrast-enhanced axial 2D WE-MP-RAGE (*E*), and contrast-enhanced axial 3D radial GE (*F*) images. Mild pixel graininess is present on contrast-enhanced axial 2D MP-RAGE (*B*) and contrast-enhanced axial 2D WE-MP-RAGE (*C, E*) images. Axial 3D radial GRE images (*D, F*) show clear definition of abdominal structure and lesion conspicuity by using a higher matrix and the thinner section slice in this sequence.

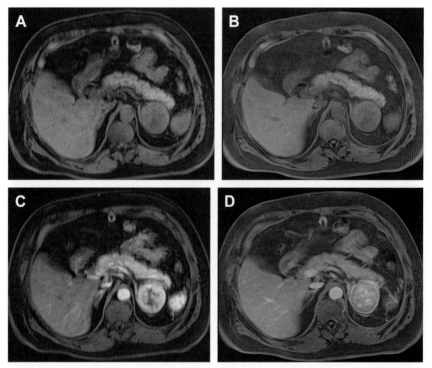

**Fig. 13.** MR images in a 68-year-old man with an oncocytoma in the left kidney. MR images on precontrast T1-weighted fat-suppressed 3D GRE (*A*) and T1-weighted fat-suppressed 3D GRE at arterial dominant phase (*C*) show blurred resolution of the tumor and pancreatic margin caused by motion. Better sharpness of tumor and pancreatic edge and clearer depiction of intrahepatic vessels are shown on precontrast radial GRE and interstitial phase radial GRE images (*B, D*).

the margins of k-space, with the net effect that images are less sensitive to motion artifacts from phase errors.[19–24] In clinical practice, free-breathing fat-suppressed 3D radial GRE sequence can provide excellent motion-controlled images with high spatial resolution in noncooperative patients, especially sedated children (see **Fig. 12**; **Fig. 13**).[5] 3D radial GRE sequence can generate streak artifacts, which are not seen with conventional rectilinear 3D GRE sequence, but these artifacts are usually of a mild degree and the images are of good diagnostic quality despite their presence.[5] They are most apparent in large patients, and are virtually absent in children (**Fig. 14**). The lesser presence of streak artifacts in pediatric patients relates to their smaller abdominal transverse

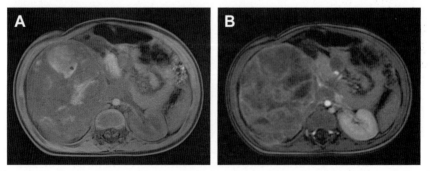

**Fig. 14.** MR images in a 2-year-old boy with a neuroblastoma in the right adrenal gland. Precontrast T1-weighted fat-suppressed axial 3D radial GRE image (*A*) shows a bulky, heterogenous, solid mass with hemorrhagic component. The mass extends across the midline adjacent to the aorta at the level of the renal arteries and displaces the inferior vena cava and pancreatic head on contrast-enhanced T1-weighted fat-suppressed axial 3D radial GRE imaging (*B*). Radial 3D GRE imaging shows high image quality with minimal motion artifacts in this difficult-to-scan child.

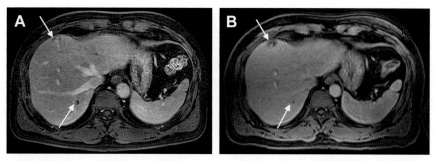

**Fig. 15.** MR images in a 51-year-old man with 2 small hemangiomas in the liver. Gadolinium-enhanced 3D GRE at 3 T (*A*) shows more increased conspicuity of hemangiomas (*arrows*) than at 1.5 T (*B*) because of higher SNR and CNR at 3.0 T compared with 1.5 T. MR images show more characteristics of hemangiomas (peripheral globular enhancement) at 3.0 T than at 1.5 T. Higher SNR at 3.0 T improves visualization of portal veins and hepatic veins beyond those at 1.5 T.

dimensions compared with adults. In the near future, the development of compressed sensing, parallel technique and radial sampling in radial 3D GRE may make it possible to achieve image acquisition at high temporal resolution using a smaller number of radial spokes, which will allow dynamic gadolinium-enhanced imaging, including in the hepatic arterial phase, in clinical practice.[25]

### T2-weighted Sequences

#### SS-ETSE sequence

The SS-ETSE sequence is a breathing-independent technique that is useful both in standard and motion-resistant protocols. This technique acquires the full image after a single excitation pulse. A variety of strategies compensate for the entire k-space not being acquired over this short time period, and what is described as half-acquisition is a common approach that samples approximately 60% of k-space in the horizontal filling approach, and uses the added 10% to correct for the undersampling by filling in the remaining 40% of k-space. Images are obtained in less than a second with virtually no motion artifact even during free breathing (see **Fig. 12**).[15] This sequence is discussed in more detail earlier.

### HIGH-RESOLUTION IMAGES
#### Parallel MR Imaging

Parallel MR imaging with suitable phased-array coils can be used in combination with most MR sequences to reduce scan time. Parallel imaging is often used to increase spatial resolution, decrease data acquisition time, and most often a combination of both. This technique makes high temporal resolution possible in noncooperative patients, as well as higher spatial resolution (useful in the pelvis), reduced effective interecho spacing (eg, less image blurring and image distortion in

SS-ETSE), and reduced specific absorption rate caused by shorter echo trains at 3 T.

### 3.0-T MR Imaging

3-T MR imaging can provide higher SNR and CNR than 1.5-T MR imaging, which leads to improved image resolution.[26,27] The higher SNR combined with higher in-plane and through-plane spatial resolution at 3 T improves lesion conspicuity on gadolinium-enhanced 3D GRE sequences (**Fig. 15**). 3-T MR images have many advantages compared with 1.5-T images, including use in small children because of the higher SNR on MP-RAGE, small-volume disease in general, and concurrent vascular imaging with tissue imaging (visualization of arteries especially but also venous structures) using the tissue-imaging sequence of 3D-GRE alone.

### SUMMARY

To achieve routine use in clinical practice, abdominal MR imaging must consistently provide both superior and important information on organ systems and disease entities. The suppression of, or compensation for, motion artifacts is the most important determinant of diagnostic efficacy in upper abdominal MR imaging. This suppression or compensation can largely be achieved by the use of separate protocols for cooperative and noncooperative patients. The clinical MR study should be performed in a fast, efficient, and comprehensive fashion, should focus on the benefit to the patient, and should emphasize clinically essential strategies.

### REFERENCES

1. Gaa J, Hatabu H, Jenkins RL, et al. Liver masses: replacement of conventional T2-weighted spin-echo

MR imaging with breath-hold MR imaging. Radiology 1996;200(2):459–64.

2. Semelka RC, Balci NC, Op de Beeck B, et al. Evaluation of a 10-minute comprehensive MR imaging examination of the upper abdomen. Radiology 1999;211(1):189–95.

3. Semelka RC, Kelekis NL, Thomasson D, et al. HASTE MR imaging: description of technique and preliminary results in the abdomen. J Magn Reson Imaging 1996;6(4):698–9.

4. Altun E, Semelka RC, Dale BM, et al. Water excitation MPRAGE: an alternative sequence for postcontrast imaging of the abdomen in noncooperative patients at 1.5 Tesla and 3.0 Tesla MRI. J Magn Reson Imaging 2008;27(5):1146–54.

5. Azevedo RM, de Campos RO, Ramalho M, et al. Free-breathing 3D T1-weighted gradient-echo sequence with radial data sampling in abdominal MRI: preliminary observations. AJR Am J Roentgenol 2011;197(3):650–7.

6. Sharma P, Martin DR, Dale BM, et al. Diagnostic approach to protocoling and interpreting MR studies of the abdomen and pelvis. In: Semelka RC, editor. Abdominal-pelvic MRI. Hoboken (NJ): Wiley-Blackwell; 2010. p. 1–43 Chapter 1.

7. Merkle EM, Nelson RC. Dual gradient-echo in-phase and opposed-phase hepatic MR imaging: a useful tool for evaluating more than fatty infiltration or fatty sparing. Radiographics 2006;26(5):1409–18.

8. Kierans AS, Leonardou P, Shaikh F, et al. Body MR imaging: sequences we use and why. Appl Radiol 2009;38(5):7–12.

9. Delfaut EM, Beltran J, Johnson G, et al. Fat suppression in MR imaging: techniques and pitfalls. Radiographics 1999;19(2):373–82.

10. Gallix BP, Bret PM, Atri M, et al. Comparison of qualitative and quantitative measurements on unenhanced T1-weighted fat saturation MR images in predicting pancreatic pathology. J Magn Reson Imaging 2005;21(5):583–9.

11. Pamuklar E, Semelka RC. MR imaging of the pancreas. Magn Reson Imaging Clin N Am 2005; 13(2):313–30.

12. Kettritz U, Semelka RC, Brown ED, et al. MR findings in diffuse renal parenchymal disease. J Magn Reson Imaging 1996;6(1):136–44.

13. Semelka RC, Helmberger TK. Contrast agents for MR imaging of the liver. Radiology 2001;218(1):27–38.

14. Northam M, de Campos RO, Ramalho M, et al. Bone metastases: evaluation of acuity of lesions using dynamic gadolinium-chelate enhancement, preliminary results. J Magn Reson Imaging 2011;34(1):120–7.

15. Semelka RC, Martin DR, Balci NC. Magnetic resonance imaging of the liver: how I do it. J Gastroenterol Hepatol 2006;21(4):632–7.

16. Ramalho M, Heredia V, de Campos RO, et al. In-phase and out-of-phase gradient-echo imaging in abdominal studies: intra-individual comparison of three different techniques. Acta Radiol 2012;53(4): 441–9.

17. Ferreira A, Ramalho M, de Campos RO, et al. Comparison of T1-weighted in- and out-of-phase single shot magnetization-prepared gradient-recalled-echo with three-dimensional gradient-recalled-echo at 3.0 Tesla: preliminary observations in abdominal studies. J Magn Reson Imaging 2012;35(5):1187–95.

18. Heredia V, Ramalho M, de Campos RO, et al. Comparison of a single shot T1-weighted in- and out-of-phase magnetization prepared gradient recalled echo with a standard two-dimensional gradient recalled echo: preliminary findings. J Magn Reson Imaging 2011;33(6):1482–90.

19. Chandarana H, Block TK, Rosenkrantz AB, et al. Free-breathing radial 3D fat-suppressed T1-weighted gradient echo sequence: a viable alternative for contrast-enhanced liver imaging in patients unable to suspend respiration. Invest Radiol 2011;46(10): 648–53.

20. Rasche V, de Boer RW, Holz D, et al. Continuous radial data acquisition for dynamic MRI. Magn Reson Med 1995;34(5):754–61.

21. Song HK, Dougherty L. Dynamic MRI with projection reconstruction and KWIC processing for simultaneous high spatial and temporal resolution. Magn Reson Med 2004;52(4):815–24.

22. Spuentrup E, Katoh M, Buecker A, et al. Free-breathing 3D steady-state free precession coronary MR angiography with radial k-space sampling: comparison with Cartesian k-space sampling and Cartesian gradient-echo coronary MR angiography–pilot study. Radiology 2004;231(2):581–6.

23. Kim KW, Lee JM, Jeon YS, et al. Free-breathing dynamic contrast-enhanced MRI of the abdomen and chest using a radial gradient echo sequence with K-space weighted image contrast (KWIC). Eur Radiol 2012;23(5):1352–60.

24. Bamrungchart S, Tantaway EM, Midia EC, et al. Free breathing three-dimensional gradient echo-sequence with radial data sampling (radial 3D-GRE) examination of the pancreas: comparison with standard 3D-GRE volumetric interpolated breathhold examination (VIBE). J Magn Reson Imaging 2013;38(6):1572–7.

25. Chandarana H, Feng L, Block TK, et al. Free-breathing contrast-enhanced multiphase MRI of the liver using a combination of compressed sensing, parallel imaging, and golden-angle radial sampling. Invest Radiol 2013;48(1):10–6.

26. Chang KJ, Kamel IR, Macura KJ, et al. 3.0-T MR imaging of the abdomen: comparison with 1.5 T. Radiographics 2008;28(7):1983–98.

27. Erturk SM, Alberich-Bayarri A, Herrmann KA, et al. Use of 3.0-T MR imaging for evaluation of the abdomen. Radiographics 2009;29(6):1547–63.

# Gadolinium Contrast Agent Selection and Optimal Use for Body MR Imaging

Flavius F. Guglielmo, MD[a,*], Donald G. Mitchell, MD[a], Shiva Gupta, MD[b]

## KEYWORDS

- Gadolinium-based contrast agents • Extracellular space agents
- Hepatocyte-specific contrast agents • Blood pool agents • Postgadolinium pulse sequences
- Gadolinium chelate structure and stability

## KEY POINTS

- Proper selection of a gadolinium-based contrast agent requires understanding the indication for the magnetic resonance (MR) imaging examination, the key features of the different types of commercially available contrast agents, and the effect that the contrast agent has on the selected imaging protocol.
- The timing is different for each category of gadolinium contrast, and therefore, protocols must be created that optimize the timing based on the type of gadolinium contrast agent administered.
- Gadoxetate disodium has many advantages when evaluating liver lesions. However, there are important caveats and limitations that need to be understood before selecting this agent.
- A high-relaxivity contrast agent such as gadobenate dimeglumine can be used when stronger T1 relaxivity is needed, such as for MR angiography, MR enterography, MR venography, pelvis fistula MR imaging, and combined abdomen and pelvis MR imaging. Gadobenate dimeglumine, at reduced dose, is also ideal for MR urography, because of the high relaxivity in plasma versus urine.

## INTRODUCTION

Choosing the optimal gadolinium contrast agent for body magnetic resonance (MR) imaging cases requires the following:

1. Knowing the patient's clinical information to determine the appropriate examination indication and whether intravenous gadolinium administration is needed
2. Knowing the relevant properties of the chosen gadolinium contrast agent
3. Understanding the effect that intravenous gadolinium has on body MR imaging pulse sequences

This article describes how to combine these factors when choosing an intravenous gadolinium contrast agent to perform efficient and high-quality body MR imaging examinations.

## GADOLINIUM GENERAL INFORMATION
### Gadolinium Mechanism of Action

Gadolinium is highly paramagnetic because of its 7 unpaired electrons.[1] Although the iodine molecule directly increases computed tomography (CT) attenuation, the effect of the gadolinium molecule is indirect. This leads to an

Funding Sources: None (F.F. Guglielmo, S. Gupta); CMC Contrast AB (Consultant) (D.G. Mitchell).
Conflict of Interest: None (F.F. Guglielmo, S. Gupta); CMC Contrast AB (Consultant) (D.G. Mitchell).
a Department of Radiology, Thomas Jefferson University Hospital, 132 South 10th Street, Philadelphia, PA 19107, USA; b Department of Radiology, The University of Texas MD Anderson Cancer Center, 1400 Pressler Street, Unit 1473, FCT15.5013, Houston, TX 77030, USA
* Corresponding author.
E-mail address: flavius.guglielmo@jefferson.edu

Radiol Clin N Am 52 (2014) 637–656
http://dx.doi.org/10.1016/j.rcl.2014.02.004
0033-8389/14/$ – see front matter © 2014 Elsevier Inc. All rights reserved.

amplification effect, because one gadolinium atom can facilitate relaxation of many adjacent water molecules. Gadolinium acts by shortening T1, T2, and T2* relaxation times of adjacent water protons.[1–4] This relaxation primarily causes increased signal intensity (enhancement) on T1-weighted images (**Fig. 1**). However, T2 shortening can predominate and cause decreased signal intensity on T2-weighted images (**Fig. 2**) and, in high gadolinium concentrations, can cause decreased signal intensity on T1-weighted images, as a result of dominant T2 shortening if the echo time (TE) is high enough (**Fig. 3**). Examples in which particularly high gadolinium concentration can be found include urine or first-pass venous injection into the superior vena cava. In short tau inversion recovery (STIR) sequences, the T1 shortening from gadolinium results in a loss of signal intensity (**Fig. 4**).[1,4]

## GADOLINIUM-BASED CONTRAST AGENTS

There are currently 9 different commercially available gadolinium-based contrast agents (GBCAs) that can be used for body MR imaging cases. The decision about which agent to use can be simplified by first considering which category of GBCA is needed for the examination indication. The 3 categories include extracellular space agents, hepatocyte-specific contrast agents, and blood pool agents.[1,2,5] After selecting the proper category for the indicated body MR imaging examination, it is important to understand some of the characteristics of each of the agents. Although each agent has many differentiating characteristics the key features for selecting the optimal GBCA are highlighted in **Table 1**.[4,6–12]

### *Extracellular Space Agents (ECSAs)*

#### *Available agents*
There are 6 approved ECSAs, including gadoterate meglumine (Dotarem, Guerbet, Villepinte, France), gadobutrol (Gadovist/Gadavist, Bayer HealthCare, Leverkusen, Germany), gadopentetate dimeglumine (Magnevist, Bayer HealthCare, Leverkusen, Germany), gadodiamide (Omniscan, GE Healthcare, Chalfont St Giles, England), gadoversetamide (OptiMARK, Mallinckrodt, St Louis, MO), and gadoteridol (ProHance, Bracco Diagnostics, Princeton, NJ) (see **Table 1**). Although an hepatocyte-specific contrast agent, because of its relatively low (5%) hepatocellular uptake, gadobenate dimeglumine is used primarily as an ECSA, and its high relaxivity makes it a good choice for several ECSA indications (see later discussion).

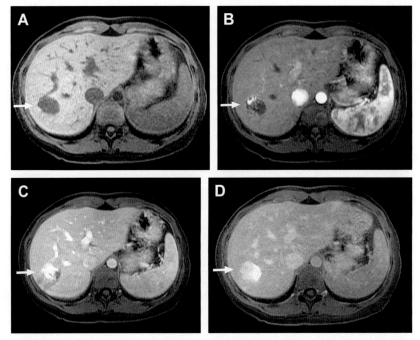

**Fig. 1.** Axial pregadolinium (*A*), arterial phase (*B*), portal venous phase (*C*), and delayed phase (*D*) fat-suppressed 3D gradient-echo (GRE) images showing an enhancing right-lobe liver lesion with discontinuous nodular peripheral and progressive centripetal enhancement consistent with a hemangioma (*arrows*) (*A–C*: repetition time [TR] = 4, echo time [TE] = 1.8, flip angle [FA] 12) (*D*: TR = 3.5, TE = 1.7, FA 15).

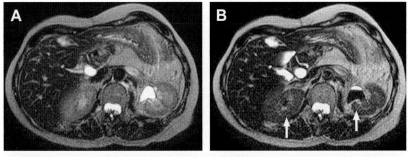

**Fig. 2.** Axial pregadolinium (*A*) and postgadolinium (*B*) heavily T2-weighted images. Shortened T2 relaxivity primarily causes decreased signal intensity in the renal collecting systems (*arrows*). There is little or no change in other tissues (repetition time 760, echo time 178).

## Mechanism of action

ECSAs are rapidly distributed to the extracellular space, which includes the vascular space plus the interstitial space. ECSAs require evaluation of the different phases of contrast enhancement, including the arterial, blood pool (venous), and extracellular (delayed) phase. ECSAs remain in the extracellular space and are rapidly eliminated with 100% renal excretion (which differs from the hepatocyte-specific contrast agent, gadobenate dimeglumine, which has 95% renal excretion and 5% hepatobiliary excretion).[13] Choosing the best ECSA among the numerous available agents takes into account the differentiating characteristics, including relaxivity, safety considerations, and cost.

## ECSA indications

- Abdominal and/or pelvic pain
- Abdominal and/or pelvic mass
- Cardiac MR imaging
- Cirrhotic liver-hepatocellular carcinoma [HCC] screening/evaluation
- Mediastinum

- MR cholangiopancreatography
- Tumor staging or follow-up

### ECSA indications for which gadobenate dimeglumine (ie, a high-relaxivity agent) is preferred

- Combined abdomen/pelvis MR imaging
- MR angiography
- MR enterography
- MR urography
- MR venography
- Pelvis fistula MR imaging

## Hepatocyte-Specific Contrast Agents (HSCAs)

### Available agents

Hepatocyte-specific contrast agents (HSCAs) are also known as combined hepatobiliary/extracellular space agents. Two HSCAs are commercially available, including gadoxetate disodium (Eovist/Primovist; Bayer HealthCare, Leverkusen, Germany), marketed as Eovist in the United States and Primovist elsewhere worldwide; and gadobenate dimeglumine (MultiHance; Bracco

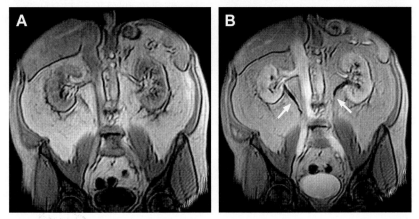

**Fig. 3.** Coronal (*A*) pregadolinium and (*B*) postgadolinium T1-weighted images on 0.7-T MR imaging (repetition time 248, echo time 8, flip angle 70). The high gadolinium concentration in the proximal ureters leads to decreased signal intensity on T1-weighted images (*arrows*).

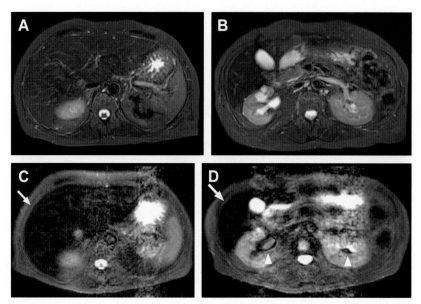

**Fig. 4.** Axial pregadolinium (*A, B*) and postgadolinium (*C, D*) STIR images obtained after the intravenous administration of gadoxetate disodium. In STIR sequences, the T1 shortening property of gadolinium results in a loss of signal intensity. Note the darkening of the liver (*arrow* in *C, D*) and renal collecting systems (*arrowheads* in *D*) on postcontrast images (repetition time 880, echo time 67, inversion time 80).

Diagnostics Inc., Princeton, NJ). HSCAs are excreted through a combination of biliary and renal routes.[14–16] Because of the 50% biliary excretion of gadoxetate disodium compared with 5% biliary excretion for gadobenate dimeglumine, the hepatobiliary phase imaging delay time is shorter for gadoxetate disodium and thus shortens total acquisition time for the study. For this reason, combined with a similar safety profile,[11] gadoxetate disodium has replaced gadobenate dimeglumine in North America for most applications that call for hepatobiliary effects. However, the high relaxivity of gadobenate dimeglumine makes this agent useful for many extracellular space indications, as indicated earlier.

*Mechanism of action*
HSCAs also include properties of extracellular space contrast agents, allowing hepatic arterial and portal venous phase imaging, with delayed hepatocyte uptake and excretion into the biliary system. Gadoxetate disodium and gadobenate dimeglumine are taken up by hepatocytes (at approximate rates of 50% and 5%, respectively) by the organic anion transporting protein (OATP-1), and are then excreted into bile canaliculi by the canalicular multispecific organic anion transporter. This combination of hepatocyte uptake and biliary excretion results in an additional hepatocellular phase of imaging, which occurs approximately 20 minutes after intravenous injection for

gadoxetate disodium (and between 45 minutes and 3 hours after injection of gadobenate dimeglumine).[1,2,14,17] Bilirubin competes with gadoxetate disodium for uptake via OATP-1, and therefore, patients with hyperbilirubinemia may have reduced gadoxetate disodium uptake and excretion.[17,18]

*Approved HSCA indications*

- Characterize focal nodular hyperplasia (FNH) or differentiate FNH from adenoma (**Fig. 5**)[14,19]
- Cirrhotic liver-HCC screening/evaluation (as an alternative to an ECSA)
- Rule out liver metastases or reevaluate known metastatic disease

*Off-label HSCA indications*

- Bile duct imaging, including presurgical or postsurgical evaluation (**Fig. 6**)[5,17]
- Gallbladder cystic duct obstruction

*Gadoxetate disodium caveats and limitations*

- The arterial and venous phases with gadoxetate disodium have weaker enhancement than with extracellular contrast agents, because of the lower dose of gadoxetate disodium. Also, the lower injection volume compared with ECSAs can lead to errors timing the dynamic postcontrast series and

**Table 1**
Characteristics of gadolinium-based contrast agents needed for protocoling body MR imaging cases

| Category | Generic Name | Product or Trade Name | Structure | Charge | T1 Relaxivity at 1.5 T | Hepatic Excretion (%) | Concentration (mmol/mL) | Recommended Dosage (mmol/kg) |
|---|---|---|---|---|---|---|---|---|
| ECSA | Gadoterate meglumine | Dotarem | Cyclic | Ionic | 3.4–3.8 | 0 | 0.5 | 0.1 |
| | Gadobutrol | Gadavist/Gadovist | Cyclic | Nonionic | 4.9–5.5 | 0 | 1 | 0.1 |
| | Gadopentetate dimeglumine | Magnevist | Linear | Ionic | 3.9–4.3 | 0 | 0.5 | 0.1 |
| | Gadodiamide | Omniscan | Linear | Nonionic | 4–4.6 | 0 | 0.5 | 0.1 |
| | Gadoversetamide | Optimark | Linear | Nonionic | 4.4–5 | 0 | 0.5 | 0.1 |
| | Gadoteridol | ProHance | Cyclic | Nonionic | 3.9–4.3 | 0 | 0.5 | 0.1 |
| HSCA | Gadoxetate disodium | Eovist/Primovist | Linear | Ionic | 6.5–7.3 | 50 | 0.25 | 0.025 |
| | Gadobenate dimeglumine | MultiHance | Linear | Ionic | 6–6.6 | 4–5 | 0.5 | 0.1 |
| BPA | Gadofosveset trisodium | Ablavar/Vasovist | Linear | Ionic | 18–20 | 5 | 0.25 | 0.03 |

*Abbreviation:* BPA, blood pool agents; ECSA, extracellular space agents; HSCA, hepatocyte-specific contrast agents; mmol/kg, millimoles per kilogram; mmol/mL, millimoles per milliliter; T, tesla.

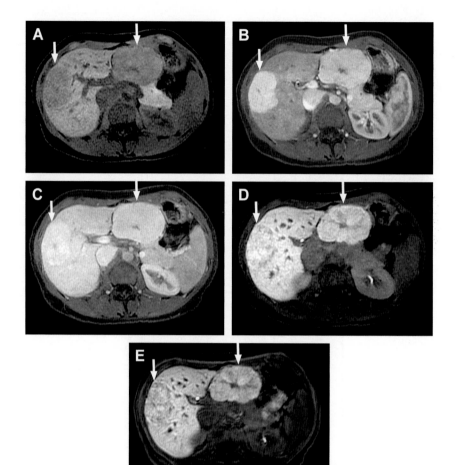

**Fig. 5.** Axial pregadolinium (*A*), arterial (*B*), portal venous (*C*), and late dynamic (*D*) and hepatobiliary phase (*E*) 3D gradient-echo images obtained after the intravenous administration of gadoxetate disodium show enhancing lesions in the right and left hepatic lobes consistent with FNH (*arrows*) (*A–C*: repetition time [TR] = 4, echo time [TE] = 1.8, flip angle [FA] 12) (*D*: TR = 3.5, TE = 1.7, FA 15) (*E*: TR = 4.5, TE = 1.7, FA 30).

truncation artifacts.[17] There are several theoretic ways to address this problem:

1. Use a double dose of gadoxetate disodium (ie, 0.05 mmol/kg), which is an off-label dose.
2. Obtain double or triple arterial phases to optimally time the bolus, to improve the arterial phase. However, this does not affect the venous or later phases.
3. Lowering the injection rate from the standard 2 mL/s to 1 mL/s.[20]
4. Diluting with saline to a total volume of 20 mL to obtain a more optimal 2 mL/s injection rate.[21]

- Motion artifact can occur during the early arterial phase in many patients, because of a self-limiting acute transient dyspnea, significantly limiting evaluation for arterial enhancing lesions (**Fig. 7**).[22] This situation can be avoided by using a different contrast agent for repeat or subsequent studies or can be potentially decreased by obtaining more arterial phase sequences (by undersampling k-space).[22]

- Arterial phase hyperenhancement, the most defining feature for LI-RADS 5 lesions (definitely HCC), is not as well seen with gadoxetate disodium as with ECSAs, because of the lower dose administered and the more frequent transient respiratory motion artifact. Also, washout appearance on delayed phase images, a major LI-RADS feature, is useful only with ECSAs, not gadoxetate disodium. With gadoxetate disodium, washout appearance is valid only on venous phase images; hypointensity on hepatobiliary phase images is an ancillary feature, not sufficiently specific to be a major feature. For these reasons,

A

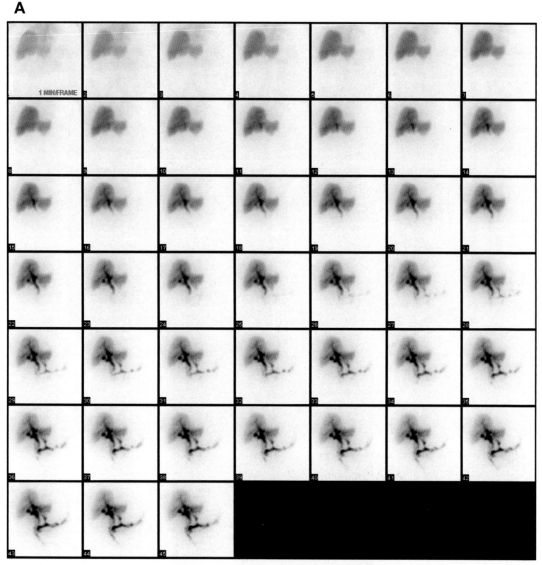

**Fig. 6.** Bile leak after cholecystectomy. Hepatobiliary iminodiacetic acid (HIDA) scan (*A*) and axial pregadolinium (*B*), arterial (*C*), late dynamic (*D*), and hepatobiliary phase (*E*) and coronal hepatobiliary phase (*F*) 3D gradient-echo images obtained after the intravenous administration of gadoxetate disodium. HIDA scan shows a bile leak in the gallbladder fossa. On MR imaging, the bile leak is noted on hepatobiliary delayed images (*arrow* in *E* and *F*). Note that the leak is not visible until the biliary system contains contrast (*arrowhead* in *E*) (*B, C*: repetition time [TR] = 4.1, echo time [TE] = 2.0, flip angle [FA] 10) (*D–F*: TR = 4.1, TE = 2.0, FA 20).

using gadoxetate disodium likely reduces sensitivity for detecting and characterizing LI-RADS 5 lesions; many of these lesions are likely characterized as LI-RADS 3 (intermediate probability for HCC) or LI-RADS 4 (probably HCC).[23]

- Preliminary results for HCC show that using gadoxetate disodium increases sensitivity and specificity for diagnosing HCC,[19,24] but a small percentage of lower-grade lesions may be characterized as benign,

because of delayed hepatobiliary uptake by well or moderately differentiated HCC (**Fig. 8**).[5,19,25–27]

- Some patients with reduced hepatobiliary function have suboptimal gadoxetate disodium enhancement.[16] This situation is particularly likely if the direct bilirubin is greater than 2.18 mg/dL (**Fig. 9**).[18]
- With previous ablative treatment such as radiofrequency ablation or chemoembolization designed to infarct tumor, ECSAs provide

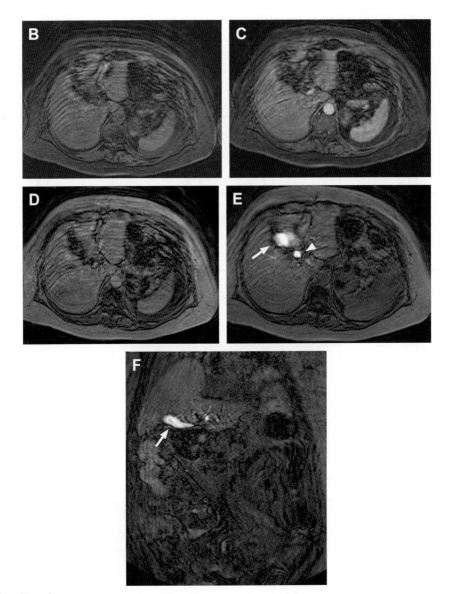

**Fig. 6.** *(continued)*

better contrast for distinguishing between infarcted and viable tumor in treated areas, because of the stronger and more sustained enhancement of tumor using these agents (**Fig. 10**). However, gadoxetate disodium provides greater sensitivity for detecting new foci of tumor. Therefore, the decision about which agent to use should be guided by whether evaluation of the treated lesion, or detection of new lesions, is prioritized. This topic is discussed further later.

- Interstitial enhancement on later phases (eg, fibrosis, edema) is minimal, because the agent is cleared early from the vascular space and only a small amount accumulates in the interstitial space. Therefore, gadoxetate disodium is suboptimal for suspected abscess, inflammation, or fibrosis. Also, evaluation of abdominal organs other than the liver is less than optimal.
- For certain hepatic lesions, such as confirming a hemangioma, an ECSA is preferred, predominantly because of the contributions of the delayed phase for showing persistent hyperenhancement (see **Fig. 1**).
- Gadoxetate disodium generally should not be used for abdomen and pelvis combination studies, unless the clinical indication is such that optimal postcontrast images are not critical for the pelvic portion. Gadobenate

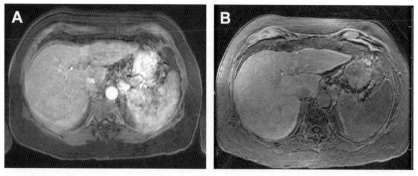

**Fig. 7.** Axial arterial phase (repetition time [TR] = 4, echo time [TE] = 1.8, flip angle [FA] 12) (*A*) and hepatobiliary phase (TR = 4.5, TE = 1.7, FA 30) (*B*) fat-suppressed 3D gradient-echo images. There is significant motion artifact on the arterial phase with minimal artifact on the hepatobiliary phase and other series (*not shown*), likely caused by the transient dyspnea related to gadoxetate disodium dynamic injection.

dimeglumine 0.1 mmol/kg can be used for these cases, because of its higher relaxivity and greater extracellular properties.

## Blood Pool Agents (BPAs)

### Available agents
Gadofosveset trisodium is currently the only commercially available BPA.[8,28–30]

### Mechanism of action
Gadofosveset trisodium (Vasovist/Ablavar; Lantheus Medical Imaging, North Billerica, MA) works by reversibly binding to albumin, which increases T1 relaxivity and results in a prolonged vascular phase. During the steady state (equilibrium phase), which lasts up to 1 hour, the increased T1 relaxivity and prolonged vascular phase allow high-resolution three-dimensional

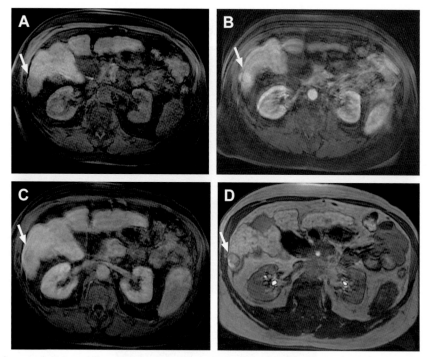

**Fig. 8.** Axial pregadolinium (*A*), arterial phase (*B*), portal venous phase (*C*), and hepatobiliary phase (*D*) fat-suppressed 3D gradient-echo images showing an early arterial enhancing right-lobe liver lesion with portal venous phase washout and heterogeneous hyperenhancement on the hepatobiliary phase (*arrows*). Pathology confirmed well-differentiated hepatocellular carcinoma (*A–C*: repetition time [TR] = 4, echo time [TE] = 1.8, flip angle [FA] 12) (*D*: TR = 4.3, TE = 1.5, FA 30).

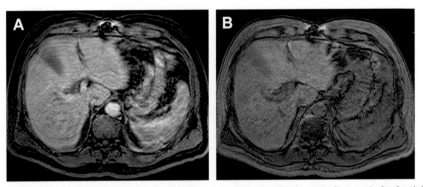

**Fig. 9.** Axial portal venous phase (repetition time [TR] = 4.1, echo time [TE] = 2.0, flip angle [FA] 10) (*A*) and hepatobiliary delayed phase (TR = 4.2, TE = 2, FA 20) (*B*) fat-suppressed 3D gradient-echo images in a patient with acute cholecystitis. On the day of the study, the patient's direct and total bilirubin levels were 2.4 mg/dL and 5.6 mg/dL, respectively. On the hepatobiliary phase, there is no biliary excretion of contrast.

(3D) MR angiography and MR venography to be performed.[28,30–33] Gadofosveset trisodium has approximately 5 times the relaxivity of extracellular space contrast agents, which allows first-pass MR angiography to be performed with similar image quality as ECSAs while administering a lower dose.[28,30] The standard dose for MR angiography is 0.03 mmol/kg, which results in a lower injection volume, despite its lower concentration (0.25 mmol/mL) compared with ECSAs. To obtain the same bolus profile as ECSAs, gadofosveset trisodium should be injected at a slower rate (ie, one-half to one-third the rate) than ECSAs.[34]

*BPA indications approved by the US Food and Drug Administration*

- Aortoiliac occlusive disease with known or suspected peripheral vascular disease

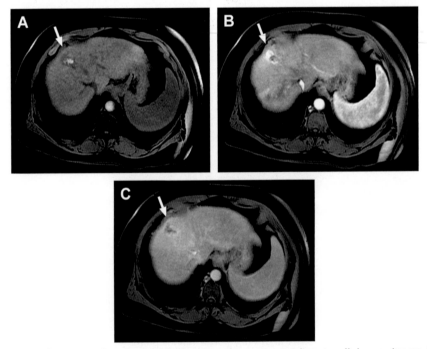

**Fig. 10.** Ablation cavity status after chemoembolization of a segment 8 hepatocellular carcinoma (HCC). Axial pregadolinium (*A*), arterial (*B*), and delayed postgadolinium (*C*) 3D gradient-echo images using 20 mL of gadobenate dimeglumine showing nodular early arterial enhancement in the ablation cavity with delayed washout (*arrows*) consistent with recurrent HCC (repetition time 6.6, echo time 3.1, flip angle 12).

*Off-label BPA indications*

- Abdominal aortic aneurysm or dissection
- Renal artery stenosis and fibromuscular dysplasia
- Potential renal donors
- Pulmonary embolism
- MR venography for lower extremity deep venous thrombosis
- Arteriovenous malformation evaluation
- Lower extremity arterial occlusive disease

## TIMING OF POSTGADOLINIUM CONTRAST 3D GRADIENT-ECHO SEQUENCES

Precontrast and postcontrast T1-weighted fat-suppressed 3D gradient-echo (3D GRE) sequences are often the most important series for making a diagnosis in body MR imaging cases.[35] Optimizing contrast enhancement for each different category of gadolinium and understanding the differences in timing for each category are critical.

### Baseline Precontrast Images

Baseline precontrast images are essential to determine if technical quality and anatomic coverage are adequate. Also, these images provide a basis of comparison to determine the presence or absence of enhancement, which in turn allows confident differentiation between solid tissue and fluid or other inert material.

### Optimal Timing for 3D GRE Sequences Performed with ECSAs

#### Arterial phase

Early arterial phase images show arterial structures, whereas late arterial phase images show hypervascular tissues. In the abdomen, during the late arterial phase, there is intense enhancement of the pancreas, spleen, and renal cortex, and minimal liver enhancement (see **Fig. 1**).[23,35,36] For agents that are injected at lower volume, such as gadobutrol, the contrast bolus can be prolonged either by injecting at a slower rate or by diluting with saline, or the scan acquisition time can be decreased. This strategy can avoid artifacts that can result when the duration of injection is shorter than the image acquisition time.[2,20,21]

#### Blood pool phase

The blood pool phase is also known as the portal venous phase or venous phase in abdominal imaging. Maximal hepatic enhancement occurs during this phase (see **Fig. 1**).[23,35,36]

#### Extracellular phase

The extracellular phase is also known as the delayed or equilibrium phase. This phase occurs 3 to 5 minutes after contrast injection. During this phase, contrast diffuses into the tissue interstitium (see **Fig. 1**).[23,35,36]

### Optimal Timing for 3D GRE Sequences Performed with Gadoxetate Disodium

#### Arterial and blood pool phase

Arterial and portal venous phase series are similar to the series obtained with extracellular space contrast agents. However, these phases are less than optimal, because of the lower dose of contrast used, and because of early hepatocyte uptake during the venous phase (see **Fig. 5**).

#### Late dynamic phase

When using gadoxetate disodium, a set of images is generally obtained 3 to 5 minutes after injection. Although the timing of this phase is similar to the extracellular (equilibrium) phase described earlier for ECSAs, these images do not represent equilibrium of contrast agent distribution, and the term delayed is ambiguous because later images (usually at 20 minutes after injection) are acquired. One common term for this phase is "late dynamic", although alternative acceptable terms include "transitional" and "early postdynamic" phases (see **Fig. 5**).[23]

#### Hepatobiliary phase

A delayed hepatobiliary phase approximately 20 minutes after injection is usually obtained with gadoxetate disodium (see **Fig. 5**). In some patients with normal hepatocyte function, a 10-minute postcontrast image may be adequate for detecting and characterizing liver lesions, although depiction of bile ducts (an off-label application of gadoxetate disodium) is more reliable at 20 minutes or longer, if needed.[4] When the clinical indication is to exclude a bile duct leak, delayed images need to be obtained until biliary contrast reaches the duodenum (see **Fig. 6**). With gadobenate dimeglumine, hepatobiliary phase series can be obtained between 45 minutes and 3 hours after contrast injection, but this is rarely practiced in North America because of difficulties with examination room scheduling.

### 3D GRE Sequences Specific for BPAs

#### Equilibrium (steady state) phase

With BPAs, a first-pass MR angiographic phase is obtained in similar manner as with extracellular space contrast agents. However, a high-resolution equilibrium (also known as a steady state) sequence can be obtained for up to 1 hour after injection, which is a major advantage with BPAs (**Fig. 11**).

## GADOLINIUM CHELATE STRUCTURE AND STABILITY

Free gadolinium is highly toxic. Thus, strong binding of a chelate helps prevent the toxic effects of gadolinium.[4,6] The stability of gadolinium is determined by the molecular structure and the ionicity.[4,6] There are 2 different molecular structures of GBCAs. Macrocyclic molecules bind strongly to gadolinium in an organized rigid ring. Linear molecules are open chains with weaker binding to gadolinium (**Table 2**). In vivo stability is higher for macrocyclic agents than for linear agents.[3,4,6,13,37–40] GBCAs can be ionic or nonionic. Among linear GBCAs, ionic agents have higher stability than nonionic GBCAs. Ionic-macrocyclic agents are the most stable GBCAs. GBCAs with the lowest thermodynamic stability are the linear, nonionic agents. These agents

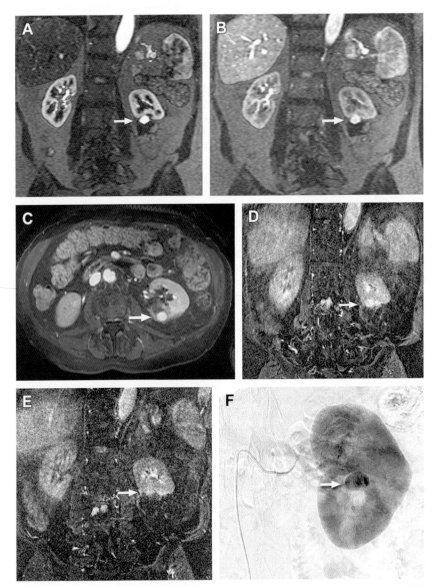

**Fig. 11.** Coronal and axial 3D GRE images obtained during the early arterial phase (*A*), late arterial phase at 22 seconds (*B*), venous phase at 2 minutes (*C*), equilibrium phase at 6 minutes (*D*), and equilibrium phase at 12 minutes (*E*) after the intravenous administration of gadofosveset trisodium. An enhancing mass in the left kidney lower pole is consistent with a renal artery pseudoaneurysm status after renal cell carcinoma cryoablation (*arrows*). Corresponding angiogram showing the enhancing pseudoaneurysm (*arrow*) (*F*) (*A, B*: repetition time [TR] = 3.1, echo time [TE] = 1.0, flip angle [FA] 30) (*C*: TR = 3, TE = 1.5, FA 15) (*D, E*: TR = 5.6, TE = 2.2, FA 20).

**Table 2**
**Molecular structure and ionicity of the 9 available gadolinium-based contrast agents**

|  | Nonionic | Ionic |
|---|---|---|
| Linear | Gadodiamide | Gadopentetate |
|  | Gadoversetamide | dimeglumine |
|  |  | Gadoxetate disodium |
|  |  | Gadobenate dimeglumine |
|  |  | Gadofosveset trisodium |
| Macrocyclic | Gadobutrol | Gadoterate |
|  | Gadoteridol | meglumine |

Ionic agents are more stable than nonionic agents. Macrocyclic agents are more stable than linear agents. Linear nonionic GBCAs have the lowest stability.

have been associated with most reported nephrogenic systemic fibrosis (NSF) cases. To decrease the toxic free gadolinium in the pharmaceutical solutions during their shelf-lives, the nonionic linear GBCAs include excess chelate. The stability of GBCAs is probably an important factor in NSF pathogenesis. Low-stability GBCAs are more likely to undergo transmetallation, releasing free gadolinium that deposits in tissues, thus attracting fibrocytes and initiating the process of fibrosis.[3,4,6,37,38,40,41] Few, if any, NSF cases have been reported after the exclusive use of the more stable macrocyclic GBCAs.[4,6,37,42]

## GADOLINIUM DOSAGE

- The recommended dose of ECSAs for most clinical indications is 0.1 mmol/kg of body weight, and the most commonly recommended injection rate is 2 mL/s. Higher doses (0.2–0.3 mmol/kg), have been used for MR angiography or for detection of cerebral metastases, although this practice has become less common in recent years.[3,7] For specific applications, gadodiamide and gadoteridol are approved for a dose up to 0.3 mmol/kg, although gadodiamide is linear and nonionic and therefore has lower in vivo stability than most other agents.[37]
- The standard dose for gadobenate dimeglumine is 0.1 mmol/kg when performing combined abdomen/pelvis MR imaging, MR enterography, and pelvis fistula MR imaging. For MR angiography and MR venography, a higher off-label dose of 0.15 mmol/kg may be more effective. For MR urography, a lower off-label dose of 0.07 mmol/kg allows

adequate renal enhancement and decreases hyperconcentration in the urine compared with the standard dose.
- Gadoxetate disodium is approved for a dose of 0.025 mmol/kg, although a common off-label modification is to round up to the nearest increment of 10 mL vials (ie, 10 or 20 mL).[2]
- Gadofosveset is approved for MR angiography of the abdominal and extremity vasculature at a dose up to 0.03 mmol/kg.[37] An even lower volume is administered because of its lower dose than ECSAs. To obtain a similar bolus profile as ECSAs, gadofosveset trisodium should be injected at one-half to one-third the rate of ECSAs.
- The Food and Drug Administration–approved indications restrict the marketing and sale of contrast agents, whereas physician usage depends on the medical literature and the standard of practice.

## GADOLINIUM DOSE, CONCENTRATION, AND INJECTION VOLUME

- The volume of gadolinium to inject depends on the gadolinium concentration, the gadolinium dose, and the patient's weight (see **Table 1**). The following formula can be used to calculate the GBCA volume to inject...

$$V = \frac{D \times W}{C}$$

V = volume (mL); D = dose by weight (mmol/kg); W = weight (kg); C = concentration (mmol/mL)

- Gadobutrol, which has the highest concentration of all ECSAs (1.0 vs 0.5 mmol/mL), has a lower volume to inject.
- Gadoxetate disodium is injected at a lower dose than all HSCAs and ECSAs (0.25 vs 0.1 mmol/kg) and has a lower injection volume, despite its lower concentration (0.25 mmol/mL).
- Gadofosveset trisodium is given at a lower dose than gadobenate dimeglumine (0.03 vs 0.1 mmol/kg) and has a lower injection volume, despite its lower concentration (0.25 mmol/mL).

## PULSE SEQUENCES RELATIVE TO THE TIMING OF INTRAVENOUS GADOLINIUM ADMINISTRATION

Unlike CT, in which the advantage of multiple postcontrast phases must be weighed against the added radiation dose from each phase, with MR imaging, standard practice is to obtain multiple postcontrast phases. To improve the efficiency of body MR imaging cases and to allow injection of contrast as early as possible, some pulse sequences can be performed during the interval between the early postcontrast (eg, arterial and venous phases) and the delayed postcontrast 3D GRE sequences.[36] The choice of postcontrast sequences that can be performed after the initial early postbolus phases depends on which gadolinium agent has been used, taking care that these images are not degraded by the contrast agent injection. As indicated later, some sequences may have improved diagnostic quality after giving intravenous gadolinium, some have a neutral effect, and some can have a negative effect.

### Pulse Sequences that May Have Improved Diagnostic Quality After Intravenous Gadolinium

- Two-dimensional (2D) radial slab MR cholangiopancreatography and high-resolution 3D MR cholangiopancreatography (**Fig. 12**)
- Moderately T2-weighted fat-suppressed series (**Fig. 13**)
- 2D gradient echo (2D GRE) series (**Fig. 14**)
- STIR after gadoxetate disodium (see **Fig. 4**)

A benefit of obtaining 2D radial slab MR cholangiopancreatography sequences after contrast is that gadolinium reduces the signal intensity of the kidneys and renal collecting systems, which improves visualization of the biliary and pancreatic ducts (see **Fig. 12**). Because gadoxetate disodium and gadobenate dimeglumine have 50% and 5% biliary excretion, respectively, the 2D radial slab MR cholangiopancreatography must be performed either before or within 5 minutes of contrast injection. Otherwise, the biliary excretion may darken the bile ducts and degrade biliary duct visualization, potentially rendering these images nondiagnostic. High-resolution 3D MR cholangiopancreatography generally cannot be completed within 5 minutes of contrast injection, and therefore should be performed before giving gadoxetate disodium or not at all.[17]

With moderately T2-weighted fat-suppressed sequences, a TE of 80 to 100 milliseconds is considered moderately T2 weighted. The advantages of performing this sequence after gadolinium administration include reduced signal of the kidneys and urinary collecting system and slightly reduced signal intensity of abdominal organs (see **Fig. 13**). The combination of fat suppression and intravenous gadolinium may increase the conspicuity of solid lesions and lymph nodes.[43]

The advantage of performing 2D GRE sequences after gadolinium administration is that the combined time-of-flight effect and gadolinium may increase the signal intensity of blood vessels (see **Fig. 14**).

STIR images feature inverse T1 weighting, reducing signal of fat and depicting tissues with long T1 as high signal intensity. For body MR imaging, we recommend that STIR images be moderately T2 weighted, with TE of about 60 milliseconds, so that T1 and T2 contrast are additive for depicting most focal liver lesions. Tissues that enhance postcontrast conversely have shorter T1, and therefore lower signal intensity. With gadoxetate disodium, postcontrast STIR images can be obtained so that the shortened T1 of hepatic parenchyma causes suppression of liver

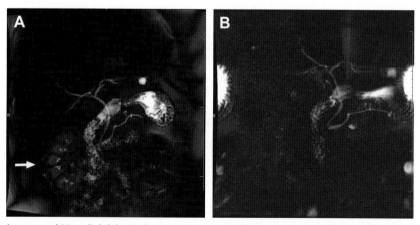

**Fig. 12.** Rotating coronal 2D radial slab MR cholangiopancreatography sequences obtained (*A*) without intravenous gadolinium at 3 T (repetition time [TR] 4000, echo time [TE] 735, thickness 30 mm), and (*B*) after administering 0.1 mmol/kg gadobutrol at 1.5 T (TR 2502, TE 1096, thickness 40 mm). Without gadolinium, the right kidney and calyces are visible (*arrow* in *A*) and can obscure the biliary and pancreatic ducts. After gadolinium (*B*), the kidney and collecting systems are darkened.

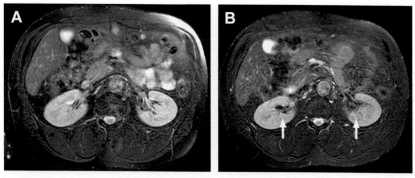

**Fig. 13.** Axial pregadolinium (*A*) and postgadolinium (*B*) moderately T2-weighted fat-suppressed images with intravenous administration of 20 mL of gadoxetate disodium. The main effect is darkening of the renal collecting systems (*arrows*). There is minimal effect on the remainder of the image (*A*, repetition time [TR] 2417, echo time [TE] 84) (*B*, TR 9230, TE 88).

signal, accentuating contrast between normal liver parenchyma and liver lesions (see **Fig. 4**). When using extracellular space agents, STIR images should be obtained only before administering gadolinium, because signal from enhancing tissues is suppressed after contrast.

### *Pulse Sequences that Can Be Performed Either Before or After Administering Gadolinium*

- Balanced steady-state free-precession (eg, True-FISP, FIESTA, BFFE) (**Fig. 15**)
- Diffusion-weighted images (**Fig. 16**)[2]

For sequences listed earlier, gadolinium has minimal effect on the images. We therefore recommend that these images be obtained after the dynamic series for efficiency. With diffusion-weighted images, the only caveat for performing this series after gadolinium is that susceptibility artifact from gadolinium in the urinary system may interfere with evaluation of adjacent structures.

### *Pulse Sequences that Should Not Be Performed After Administering Gadolinium*

- Dual gradient echo (Dual GRE) in-phase and out-of-phase series (**Fig. 17**)
- High-resolution 3D MR cholangiopancreatography after gadoxetate disodium administration
- STIR images after ECSA administration
- Single shot fast spin echo heavily T2 weighted sequences

Similar to contrast-enhanced CT scan, obtaining images after administering gadolinium may compromise evaluation of a fatty liver or fat-containing lesion with dual GRE in-phase and out-of-phase sequences. Also, as noted earlier, high-resolution 3D MR cholangiopancreatography should be performed before giving gadoxetate disodium or not at all, whereas STIR images should not be acquired after ECSA administration. Single shot fast spin echo heavily T2 weighted sequences should ideally be performed before contrast, which will more reliably

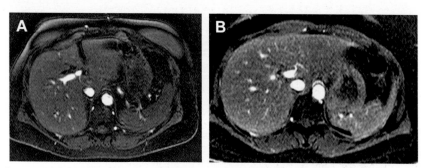

**Fig. 14.** Axial pregadolinium (*A*) and postgadolinium (*B*) 2D gradient echo images (PROSET) (repetition time 12, echo time 7) obtained before and after the intravenous administration of an extracellular contrast agent. The advantage of performing this sequence after gadolinium administration is that the combined time-of-flight effect and gadolinium may increase the signal intensity of blood vessels.

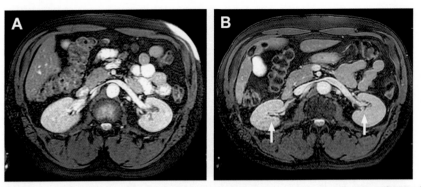

**Fig. 15.** Axial fat-saturated balanced steady-state free-precession images without gadolinium (FIESTA) (repetition time [TR] 3.6, echo time [TE] 1.5) (*A*) and after administering 20 mL of gadoxetate disodium (FIESTA) (TR 3.8, TE 1.7) (*B*). The main effect is minimal susceptibility artifact in the renal collecting systems from hyperconcentrated gadolinium (*arrows*).

show the high signal intensity of liver hemangiomas and allow evaluation of the renal collecting systems without the T2 shortening effects of excreted gadolinium (see **Fig. 2**).

## HIGH-RELAXIVITY CONTRAST AGENTS

Gadobenate dimeglumine (which is an hepatocyte-specific contrast agent) has a higher T1 relaxivity than the agents currently used for extracellular space enhancement, increasing enhancement for a given gadolinium dose on all postcontrast phases.[44] Therefore, this agent can be used for extracellular space indications in which stronger than routine enhancement is needed, such as MR angiography (**Fig. 18**), MR enterography, MR urography, MR venography, pelvis fistula MR imaging, and combined abdomen/pelvis MR imaging. For MR urography, there are also theoretic advantages to using gadobenate dimeglumine, but at a lower dose. It has double relaxivity in plasma, but not in urine. Thus, in the urinary system, there is

decreased enhancement of half-dose gadobenate dimeglumine compared with a full-dose of ECSAs, which is an advantage, to reduce signal loss from hyperconcentration.

## WHEN TO USE GADOXETATE DISODIUM AFTER HEPATOCELLULAR CARCINOMA (OR OTHER NEOPLASM) IS TREATED WITH CHEMOEMBOLIZATION OR RADIOEMBOLIZATION

For initial posttreatment studies (ie, within the first 2–3 months of treatment), an ECSA or gadobenate dimeglumine is best for showing nodular or masslike enhancement to indicate residual viable tumor (see **Fig. 10**). This statement remains true, if the most recent MR imaging study shows residual or possible residual viable tumor in the ablation cavity. When the most recent MR imaging shows no residual viable tumor in the ablation cavity, or if the predominate concern is to evaluate for tumor in untreated areas, gadoxetate disodium may be preferred.

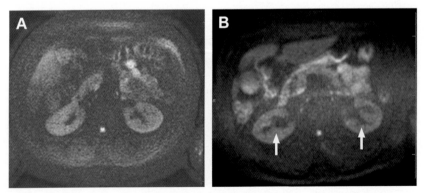

**Fig. 16.** Axial diffusion (repetition time [TR] 5200, echo time [TE] 77, b value 800) from a noncontrast MR imaging (*A*) and axial diffusion (TR 2440, TE 71, b value 800) 9 minutes after administering 20 mL of gadoxetate disodium (*B*). The main effect is minimal susceptibility artifact in the renal collecting systems from hyperconcentrated gadolinium (*arrows*).

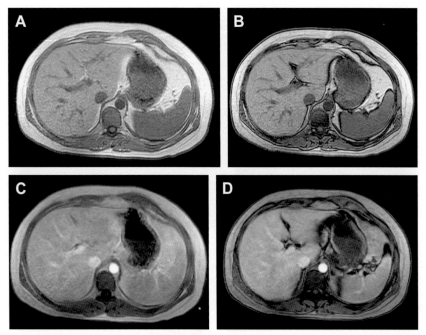

**Fig. 17.** Axial 2D dual GRE in-phase (*A*) and out-of-phase (*B*) images (repetition time [TR] 290, echo time [TE] 4.3/2.0) obtained precontrast and axial 3D dual GRE in-phase (*C*) and-out-of-phase (*D*) images (TR 6.2, TE 4.2/2.1) after administering intravenous gadolinium. The administration of gadolinium may compromise evaluation of signal intensity differences between the in-phase and out-of-phase sequences.

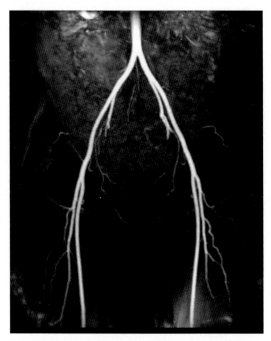

**Fig. 18.** Coronal MIP image from a normal lower extremity MR angiogram performed with 13 mL of ga-dobenate dimeglumine (repetition time 3, echo time 1.1, flip angle 25). The higher relaxivity of gadobenate dimeglumine allows optimal vascular enhancement compared with extracellular space contrast agents.

## WHAT IS THE OPTIMAL FLIP ANGLE FOR EACH GBCA?

The optimal flip angle chosen depends on the indication and the type of contrast that is chosen.

### Soft Tissue Evaluation Flip Angle

When the repetition time is 5 milliseconds or less, for pregadolinium, arterial, and portal venous phase sequences, the flip angle should be 10° to 15°. For delayed phase (with ECSAs) or late dynamic phase (with HSCAs) sequences, a flip angle of ~20° can be used, because postgadolinium T1s are shorter.[45]

### MR Angiography Flip Angle

A flip angle of 30° to 40° accentuates the contrast between arteries and background. This flip angle is appropriate for extracellular space contrast agents, gadobenate dimeglumine, and BPAs (**Fig. 19**).

### Gadoxetate Disodium (Hepatobiliary Phase) Flip Angle

Because of the marked T1 shortening of hepatic parenchyma on hepatobiliary phase images, increasing the flip angle to 25° or 30° is recommen-ded to optimize T1 contrast (see **Figs. 5–9**).[2,45]

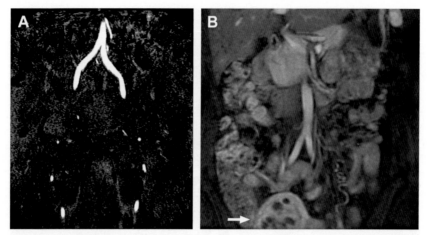

**Fig. 19.** (*A*) MR angiogram performed with a 30° flip angle (repetition time [TR] 2.8, echo time [TE] 1, flip angle 30) using 40 mL gadobenate dimeglumine. (*B*) MR angiogram from a different patient performed with a 15° flip angle (TR 3.6, TE 1.6, flip angle 15) using 10 mL gadobenate dimeglumine. There is an enhancing fibroid in the pelvis (*arrow*). In (*A*) the arteries are accentuated, whereas in (*B*), the soft tissues are highlighted.

## *Gadofosveset Trisodium (Steady State/Equilibrium Phase) Flip Angle*

The optimal flip angle for steady-state imaging is less than that for first-pass MR angiography, approximately 20° (see **Fig. 11**).[34]

## ALLERGIC REACTIONS TO GBCAS
### *General*

Although much time and effort are directed to reducing the risk of NSF in high-risk patients, allergic-type reactions, although rare, are more common.[46,47] According to the American College of Radiology *Manual of Contrast Media*, Version 9, 2013, "the frequency of all acute adverse events after an injection of 0.1 or 0.2 mmol/kg of gadolinium chelate ranges from 0.07% to 2.4%. The vast majority of these reactions are mild, including coldness at the injection site, nausea with or without vomiting, headache, warmth or pain at the injection site, paresthesias, dizziness, and itching. Reactions resembling an 'allergic' response are very unusual and vary in frequency from 0.004% to 0.7%."[42]

In a study by Jung and colleagues[46] in *Radiology* in August, 2012, there were a total of 112 immediate hypersensitivity reactions (0.079% of 141,623 total doses) in 102 patients (0.121% of 84,367 total patients). Patients with a previous history of hypersensitivity reactions to GBCAs had a higher rate of recurrence on subsequent gadolinium injection (30%).

There have been suggestions that the rate of allergic-type reactions is different between the different contrast agents.[46,48] However, this theory is difficult to substantiate, because of the low incidence of these reactions and limited attempts to control all other variables.

## *Precautionary Measures that Can Be Taken in a Patient with Risk Factors for Allergic-Type Reactions*

Determine if a GBCA is absolutely necessary. Otherwise, noncontrast MR imaging (with diffusion-weighted imaging) or another modality can be performed. A different brand of gadolinium might be considered, although there is lack of evidence validating an increase of safety.[47] A steroid preparation and possibly an antihistamine preparation could be initiated.[42,46]

## STRATEGIES FOR ADJUSTING BODY MR IMAGING PROTOCOLS FOR PATIENTS WITH REDUCED ESTIMATED GLOMERULAR FILTRATION RATES
### *Liver MR Imaging*

- Perform noncontrast MR imaging, but include diffusion-weighted images.
- Consider ultrasonography or CT scan.
- If contrast is still needed, use no more than a standard dose of 0.1 mmol/kg, preferably with a high-stability agent such as gadobutrol, gadoteridol or gadoterate meglumine, or try using a higher-relaxivity agent such as gadoxetate disodium at a dose of 0.025 mmol/kg.

### *Renal MR Angiography*

- Try using noncontrast techniques such as 2D or 3D steady-state free-precession, 3D phase contrast, or a more advanced version of time-of-flight that allows a longer time for inflow after an inversion pulse.
- If contrast is still needed, use no more than a standard dose of 0.1 mmol/kg or try

using a higher-relaxivity agent such as gadofosveset trisodium at a dose of 0.03 mmol/kg.

## SUMMARY

Choosing the optimal gadolinium contrast agent for body MR imaging cases requires knowing the patient history to determine if gadolinium administration is necessary to answer the clinical question, knowing the relevant properties of the chosen gadolinium contrast agent, and understanding the effect that gadolinium has on body MR imaging pulse sequences. The different categories of GBCAs require timing optimization on postcontrast sequences and adjusting imaging parameters to obtain the highest T1 contrast. Although a good choice for many liver-specific indications, there are several caveats and limitations that need to be considered when choosing gadoxetate disodium. High-relaxivity GBCAs are useful for examinations requiring stronger T1 relaxivity, such as MR angiography, MR enterography, MR venography, MR urography, combined abdomen/pelvis MR imaging, and pelvis fistula MR imaging. Macrocyclic GBCAs are the most stable and can decrease the risk of developing NSF caused by intravenous gadolinium administration.

## REFERENCES

1. Gandhi SN, Brown MA, Wong JG, et al. MR contrast agents for liver imaging: what, when, how. Radiographics 2006;26(6):1621–36.
2. Ringe KI, Husarik DB, Sirlin CB, et al. Gadoxetate disodium–enhanced MRI of the liver: part 1, protocol optimization and lesion appearance in the noncirrhotic liver. Am J Roentgenol 2010;195(1):13–28.
3. Prince MR, Zhang HL, Prowda JC, et al. Nephrogenic systemic fibrosis and its impact on abdominal imaging. Radiographics 2009;29(6):1565–74.
4. Hao D, Ai T, Goerner F, et al. MRI contrast agents: basic chemistry and safety. J Magn Reson Imaging 2012;36(5):1060–71.
5. Seale MK, Catalano OA, Saini S, et al. Hepatobiliary-specific MR contrast agents: role in imaging the liver and biliary tree. Radiographics 2009;29(6):1725–48.
6. Morcos S. Extracellular gadolinium contrast agents: differences in stability. Eur J Radiol 2008;66(2):175–9.
7. van der Molen AJ, Bellin MF. Extracellular gadolinium-based contrast media: differences in diagnostic efficacy. Eur J Radiol 2008;66(2):168–74.
8. Caravan P, Comuzzi C, Crooks W, et al. Thermodynamic stability and kinetic inertness of MS-325, a new blood pool agent for magnetic resonance imaging. Inorg Chem 2001;40(9):2170–6.
9. Uggeri F, Aime S, Anelli PL, et al. Novel contrast agents for magnetic resonance imaging. Synthesis and characterization of the ligand BOPTA and its Ln(III) complexes (Ln = Gd, La, Lu). X-ray structure of disodium (TPS-9-145337286-CS)-[4-carboxy-5, 8, 11-tris (carboxymethyl)-1-phenyl-2-oxa-5, 8, 11-triazatridecan-13-oato (5-)] gadolinate (2-) in a mixture with its enantiomer. Inorg Chem 1995;34(3):633–43.
10. Schmitt-Willich H, Brehm M, Ewers CL, et al. Synthesis and physicochemical characterization of a new gadolinium chelate: the liver-specific magnetic resonance imaging contrast agent Gd-EOB-DTPA. Inorg Chem 1999;38(6):1134–44.
11. Shellock FG, Parker JR, Pirovano G, et al. Safety characteristics of gadobenate dimeglumine: clinical experience from intra-and interindividual comparison studies with gadopentetate dimeglumine. J Magn Reson Imaging 2006;24(6):1378–85.
12. White D, DeLearie L, Moore D, et al. The thermodynamics of complexation of lanthanide (III) DTPA-bisamide complexes and their implication for stability and solution structure. Invest Radiol 1991; 26:S226–8.
13. Reiter T, Ritter O, Prince MR, et al. Minimizing risk of nephrogenic systemic fibrosis in cardiovascular magnetic resonance. J Cardiovasc Magn Reson 2012;14(1):31.
14. Bieze M, van den Esschert JW, Nio CY, et al. Diagnostic accuracy of MRI in differentiating hepatocellular adenoma from focal nodular hyperplasia: prospective study of the additional value of gadoxetate disodium. Am J Roentgenol 2012;199(1):26–34.
15. Schuhmann-Giampieri G, Mahler M, Roll G, et al. Pharmacokinetics of the liver-specific contrast agent Gd-EOB-DTPA in relation to contrast-enhanced liver imaging in humans. J Clin Pharmacol 1997;37(7):587–96.
16. Tamada T, Ito K, Higaki A, et al. Gd-EOB-DTPA-enhanced MR imaging: evaluation of hepatic enhancement effects in normal and cirrhotic livers. Eur J Radiol 2011;80(3):e311–6.
17. Van Beers BE, Pastor CM, Hussain HK. Primovist, Eovist: what to expect? J Hepatol 2012;57(2):421–9.
18. Lee NK, Kim S, Kim GH, et al. Significance of the "delayed hyperintense portal vein sign" in the hepatobiliary phase MRI obtained with Gd-EOB-DTPA. J Magn Reson Imaging 2012;36(3):678–85.
19. Goodwin MD, Dobson JE, Sirlin CB, et al. Diagnostic challenges and pitfalls in MR imaging with hepatocyte-specific contrast agents. Radiographics 2011;31(6):1547–68.
20. Zech CJ, Vos B, Nordell A, et al. Vascular enhancement in early dynamic liver MR imaging in an animal model: comparison of two injection regimen and two different doses Gd-EOB-DTPA

(gadoxetic acid) with standard Gd-DTPA. Invest Radiol 2009;44(6):305–10.

21. Motosugi U, Ichikawa T, Sou H, et al. Dilution method of gadolinium ethoxybenzyl diethylenetriaminepentaacetic acid (Gd-EOB-DTPA)-enhanced magnetic resonance imaging (MRI). J Magn Reson Imaging 2009;30(4):849–54.

22. Davenport MS, Viglianti BL, Al-Hawary MM, et al. Comparison of acute transient dyspnea after intravenous administration of gadoxetate disodium and gadobenate dimeglumine: effect on arterial phase image quality. Radiology 2013; 266(2):452–61.

23. American College of Radiology. Liver Imaging Reporting and Data System version 2013.1. Available at: http://www.acr.org/Quality-Safety/Resources/LIRADS/. Accessed November 21, 2013.

24. Haradome H, Grazioli L, Tinti R, et al. Additional value of gadoxetic acid-DTPA-enhanced hepatobiliary phase MR imaging in the diagnosis of early-stage hepatocellular carcinoma: comparison with dynamic triple-phase multidetector CT imaging. J Magn Reson Imaging 2011;34(1): 69–78.

25. Lee SA, Lee CH, Jung WY, et al. Paradoxical high signal intensity of hepatocellular carcinoma in the hepatobiliary phase of Gd-EOB-DTPA enhanced MRI: initial experience. Magn Reson Imaging 2011; 29(1):83–90.

26. Narita M, Hatano E, Arizono S, et al. Expression of OATP1B3 determines uptake of Gd-EOB-DTPA in hepatocellular carcinoma. J Gastroenterol 2009; 44(7):793–8.

27. Kitao A, Zen Y, Matsui O, et al. Hepatocellular carcinoma: signal intensity at gadoxetic acid–enhanced MR imaging–correlation with molecular transporters and histopathologic features. Radiology 2010; 256(3):817–26.

28. Lewis M, Yanny S, Malcolm PN. Advantages of blood pool contrast agents in MR angiography: a pictorial review. J Med Imaging Radiat Oncol 2012; 56(2):187–91.

29. Goyen M. Gadofosveset-enhanced magnetic resonance angiography. Vasc Health Risk Manag 2008; 4(1):1.

30. Hadizadeh DR, Gieseke J, Lohmaier SH, et al. Peripheral MR angiography with blood pool contrast agent: prospective intraindividual comparative study of high-spatial-resolution steady-state MR angiography versus standard-resolution first-pass MR angiography and DSA. Radiology 2008;249(2): 701–11.

31. Albrecht T, Willinek WA. Peripheral vascular imaging with a blood pool contrast agent: imaging strategies and influence on patient management. Eur Radiol Suppl 2008;18:27–34.

32. Meaney J, Goyen M. Recent advances in contrast-enhanced magnetic resonance angiography. Eur Radiol 2007;17:B2.

33. Prince MR, Meaney JF. Expanding role of MR angiography in clinical practice. Eur Radiol Suppl 2006;16:3–8.

34. Hartmann M, Wiethoff A, Hentrich HR, et al. Initial imaging recommendations for Vasovist angiography. Eur Radiol Suppl 2006;16:15–23.

35. Mitchell D, Cohen M. MRI principles. Philadelphia: Elsevier; 2004.

36. Semelka RC, Helmberger TK. Contrast agents for MR imaging of the liver. Radiology 2001;218(1):27–38.

37. Bellin MF, Van Der Molen AJ. Extracellular gadolinium-based contrast media: an overview. Eur J Radiol 2008; 66(2):160–7.

38. Idée JM, Port M, Raynal I, et al. Clinical and biological consequences of transmetallation induced by contrast agents for magnetic resonance imaging: a review. Fundam Clin Pharmacol 2006;20(6):563–76.

39. Laurent S, Elst LV, Muller RN. Comparative study of the physicochemical properties of six clinical low molecular weight gadolinium contrast agents. Contrast Media Mol Imaging 2006;1(3):128–37.

40. Morcos S. Nephrogenic systemic fibrosis following the administration of extracellular gadolinium based contrast agents: is the stability of the contrast agent molecule an important factor in the pathogenesis of this condition? Br J Radiol 2007;80(950):73–6.

41. Cacheris WP, Quay SC, Rocklage SM. The relationship between thermodynamics and the toxicity of gadolinium complexes. Magn Reson Imaging 1990;8(4):467–81.

42. Cohan R, Davenport M, Dillman J, et al. ACR Manual on Contrast Media Version 9, 2013.

43. Jeong YY, Mitchell DG, Holland GA. Liver lesion conspicuity: T2-weighted breath-hold fast spin-echo MR imaging before and after gadolinium enhancement–initial experience. Radiology 2001;219(2):455–60.

44. Shellock FG, Parker JR, Venetianer C, et al. Safety of gadobenate dimeglumine (MultiHance): summary of findings from clinical studies and postmarketing surveillance. Invest Radiol 2006;41(6):500.

45. Kim S, Mussi TC, Lee LJ, et al. Effect of flip angle for optimization of image quality of gadoxetate disodium–enhanced biliary imaging at 1.5 T. Am J Roentgenol 2013;200(1):90–6.

46. Jung JW, Kang HR, Kim MH, et al. Immediate hypersensitivity reaction to gadolinium-based MR contrast media. Radiology 2012;264(2):414–22.

47. Murphy KJ, Brunberg JA, Cohan R. Adverse reactions to gadolinium contrast media: a review of 36 cases. Am J Roentgenol 1996;167(4):847–9.

48. Prince MR, Zhang H, Zou Z, et al. Incidence of immediate gadolinium contrast media reactions. Am J Roentgenol 2011;196(2):W138–43.

# MR Imaging of Benign Focal Liver Lesions

Jonathan R. Cogley, MD[a], Frank H. Miller, MD[b],*

## KEYWORDS

- Liver • Hepatic MR imaging • Diffusion-weighted imaging • Hemangioma
- Focal nodular hyperplasia (FNH) • Hepatic adenoma • Liver abscess • Biliary cystadenoma

## KEY POINTS

- Magnetic resonance (MR) imaging is helpful for definitive characterization of various solid and cystic hepatic lesions.
- MR imaging also provides important information about the background liver parenchyma, biliary tree, and hepatic vasculature.
- Diffusion-weighted imaging in the liver can be particularly helpful for detection of otherwise subtle lesions and for the diagnosis of pyogenic abscesses.
- Diffusion-weighted imaging alone cannot differentiate between solid benign hepatocellular lesions and malignant lesions, as both can exhibit restricted diffusion with overlap between their respective apparent diffusion coefficient values.
- Hepatocyte-specific contrast agents are helpful for the differentiation of focal nodular hyperplasia and hepatocellular adenoma, two lesions with overlapping imaging features and patient populations, but with potential management implications depending on the diagnosis.

## INTRODUCTION

Focal liver lesions are increasingly encountered during routine imaging studies because of advances in technology and more widespread use of imaging. The great majority of lesions are benign in patients with noncirrhotic livers; however, many are indeterminate at the time of initial discovery. Definitive characterization by magnetic resonance (MR) imaging may alleviate patient anxiety, drastically alter management in someone undergoing staging for malignancy, and help avoid unnecessary biopsy or costly follow-up imaging.

MR imaging offers important advantages over computed tomography (CT), such as the lack of ionizing radiation and improved soft tissue contrast. The American College of Radiology Appropriateness Criteria[1] assigns the highest rating to MR imaging without and with contrast for characterization of indeterminate liver lesions, regardless of whether the patient is otherwise healthy, has liver disease, or has a known extrahepatic malignancy. This review presents a standardized approach to liver MR imaging while detailing common and less common benign focal liver lesions and their imaging characteristics.

## MR IMAGING TECHNIQUE
### Protocol

The goal of a dedicated liver MR imaging is to fully assess any focal lesions and provide valuable information about the background liver parenchyma, biliary system, and vasculature. This is

Funding Source: None.
Conflict of Interest: None.

[a] Section of Body Imaging, Department of Radiology, Northwestern Memorial Hospital, Northwestern University Feinberg School of Medicine, 676 North Saint Clair Street, Suite 800, Chicago, IL 60611, USA; [b] Department of Radiology, Northwestern University Feinberg School of Medicine, Northwestern Memorial Hospital, 676 North Saint Clair Street, Suite 800, Chicago, IL 60611, USA
* Corresponding author.
*E-mail address:* fmiller@northwestern.edu

Radiol Clin N Am 52 (2014) 657–682
http://dx.doi.org/10.1016/j.rcl.2014.02.005
0033-8389/14/$ – see front matter © 2014 Elsevier Inc. All rights reserved.

radiologic.theclinics.com

accomplished by using a wide range of fluid-sensitive and anatomic pulse sequences, including dynamic contrast-enhanced images that allow for improved lesion detection and characterization (**Table 1**). Enhancement depends on both the nature of the lesion and timing of imaging with respect to the contrast bolus.[2] Images are routinely obtained during hepatic arterial, portal venous, and equilibrium (equal distribution of contrast among the intravascular and extravascular extracellular compartments) phases. Magnetic resonance cholangiopancreatography (MRCP) images can be obtained to better evaluate the biliary tree. Patient cooperation with breath-holding instructions is required to achieve high-quality images.

## Contrast Agents

Gadolinium contrast agents have strong paramagnetic effects that shorten predominately the T1 relaxation times of tissues, leading to increased signal intensity (enhancement) on T1-weighted images.[3] The 2 main categories of contrast agents used for liver MR imaging are (1) extracellular and (2) hepatocyte-specific. Extracellular contrast agents are more widely used, providing information on the pattern and degree of enhancement analogous to iodinated contrast agents for CT. After intravenous injection, they circulate the vascular system and are distributed into extracellular spaces before undergoing renal excretion. Hepatocyte-specific contrast agents provide this extracellular dynamic information plus unique additional delayed phase information. On delayed images, tumors of hepatocellular origin with functioning hepatocytes and biliary excretion take up and retain hepatocyte-specific contrast to some degree, whereas other lesions generally do not. This allows for better characterization of focal liver lesions and potentially increases the detection of small lesions that would otherwise be missed.[2]

Hepatocyte-specific contrast agents currently approved for clinical use by the Food and Drug Administration are gadobenate dimeglumine (MultiHance; Bracco Diagnostics Inc, Princeton, NJ) and gadoxetate disodium (Eovist; Bayer Health-Care, Wayne, NJ; marketed as Primovist in Europe). In a patient with normal liver and renal function, gadoxetate disodium has a much greater percentage of biliary excretion (50%) than gadobenate dimeglumine (3%–5%).[4] Therefore, more intense liver enhancement and earlier hepatocyte-phase imaging is achieved with gadoxetate disodium (usually within 20 minutes) than gadobenate dimeglumine (usually performed after 60–90-minute delay).[2,3] T2-weighted and diffusion-weighted images can be obtained after injection of gadoxetate disodium to improve time efficiency.

The FDA-approved, manufacturer-recommended dose of gadoxetate disodium (0.025 mmol/kg) is only one-fourth that of gadobenate dimeglumine and extracellular contrast agents (0.1 mmol/kg), resulting in a relatively weaker T1 shortening effect.[2] A smaller volume of contrast (prefilled 10-mL syringe) is typically administered. If injected at a rate of 2 mL/s, it may take less time to deliver the contrast bolus than it does to complete a single high-quality data acquisition.[4] Consequently, it can be challenging to capture peak arterial phase enhancement. Shortened scanning times or reduced injection rates of 1 mL/s have been proposed to overcome this temporal mismatch.[4] Additional methods to avoid missing peak arterial phase include using a bolus timing technique, such as automated bolus detection algorithm or fluoroscopic triggering, or obtaining multiple consecutive arterial phase data sets with higher temporal but lower spatial resolution.[4,5]

## Diffusion-Weighted Imaging

Diffusion-weighted imaging (DWI), a technique that derives image contrast from differences in random motion of water molecules, has become a standard part of abdominal MR imaging protocols in recent years. The underlying principle is that different biologic tissues exhibit varying levels of restricted water diffusion, dependent on such factors as tissue cellularity and cell membrane integrity.[6] The ability to depict areas of high

**Table 1**
**Example of comprehensive liver MR imaging protocol**

| Protocol Step | Sequence |
|---|---|
| Precontrast images | T2-weighted single-shot fast SE<br>T1-weighted in and opposed phase GRE<br>Diffusion-weighted imaging<br>T2-weighted FS fast SE<br>3D T1-weighted FS spoiled GRE<br>T2-weighted MRCP (optional) |
| Postcontrast images | Dynamic 3D T1-weighted FS spoiled GRE (in hepatic arterial, portal venous, and equilibrium phases)<br>Delayed hepatocyte phase (if applicable) |

*Abbreviations:* FS, fat-suppressed; GRE, gradient echo; MRCP, MR cholangiopancreatography; SE, spin echo; 3D, three-dimensional.

cellularity can be helpful in hepatic lesion detection and characterization in a noninvasive manner. DWI does not rely on intravenous gadolinium; therefore, its use is particularly attractive in patients with poor renal function who cannot receive contrast because of the potential risk of nephrogenic systemic fibrosis.[7]

In general, DWI uses a fast single-shot echo-planar imaging-based sequence. Images at our institution are obtained at 3 different b-values (ranging from low to high) to calculate an apparent diffusion coefficient (ADC) map. Low b-value (ie, 50 s/mm$^2$) or "black blood" diffusion images result in improved lesion detection owing to suppression of bright signal from vessels or periportal tissue and lack of motion blurring compared with standard T2-weighted turbo spin-echo (TSE) and single-shot TSE images.[8–10] In our experience, subtle or small additional lesions easily overlooked on conventional MR images may be much more conspicuous on low b-value diffusion images. Higher b-value (ie, 500 and 800 s/mm$^2$) images provide more diffusion information and help with lesion characterization. Common benign liver lesions generally have higher ADC values than malignant lesions. This may allow for quick differentiation of a hepatic cyst or hemangioma from a solid hepatocellular mass or metastasis. However, overlap exists between ADC values of solid benign hepatocellular lesions, such as focal nodular hyperplasia (FNH) or hepatocellular adenoma (HCA), and those of malignant lesions.[7,10–15] Thus, information provided by DWI needs to be interpreted in conjunction with lesion morphology and signal characteristics on other sequences.

## FOCAL LIVER LESIONS
### Hemangioma

Hemangioma is the most common benign liver tumor, with a reported prevalence as high as 20%.[16–18] Most hemangiomas (60%–80%) are diagnosed in adults between 30 and 50 years of age.[19] There is a clear female predominance (2:1 to 5:1 ratio).[20] In most cases, hemangiomas are discovered incidentally and are of no clinical consequence. Accurate diagnosis is critical to avoid unnecessary further workup, including biopsy.

The gross and histologic features of hemangiomas lend to their characteristic appearance at MR imaging. Hemangiomas consist of numerous vascular channels, each lined with a single layer of epithelial cells and separated by fibrous septae.[21] They are usually well defined, often round or mildly lobulated. Due to the long T2 relaxation time of their blood-filled spaces, hemangiomas demonstrate T2 hyperintense signal classically described as "light bulb bright" or isointense to cerebral spinal fluid (CSF).[16] They are often slightly less T2 hyperintense than simple cysts or CSF on single-shot TSE images. Nevertheless, this T2 hyperintense signal is one of the most reliable findings in diagnosing hemangiomas.[22] They appear hypointense to adjacent liver on T1-weighted images. Following contrast, a pattern of discontinuous peripheral nodular enhancement with progressive, centripetal filling on more delayed images is characteristic (**Fig. 1**).[23]

Incomplete filling by contrast is common in hemangiomas larger than 3 cm due to central scarring. This is especially true for "giant" hemangiomas, a term generally reserved for lesions larger than 5 cm, which may also enhance asymmetrically because of regions of thrombosis.[24] In giant hemangiomas, irregular or "flame-shaped" discontinuous peripheral enhancement may dominate or coexist with the typical nodular enhancement pattern seen in smaller hemangiomas.[21] They also may look more complex on T2-weighted images, sometimes with a multiloculated appearance resulting from a network of hypointense septae or with a central T2 hyperintense cleft, which may be from cystic degeneration or liquefaction (**Fig. 2**).[20,21]

Conversely, some small (<2 cm) hemangiomas show rapid complete filling on the arterial-phase images. They are typically high signal intensity on T2-weighted images. These small lesions, referred to as "flash-filling" hemangiomas, are often associated with adjacent arterioportal shunting, most commonly seen as a wedge-shaped subcapsular area of transient hyperenhancement during the arterial phase (**Fig. 3**).[22,23] Segmental or lobar perfusional variants also can be seen in association with larger hemangiomas.

Most hemangiomas remain stable in size on follow-up imaging.[17] Larger lesions can sometimes be associated with symptoms related to mass-effect on adjacent structures. Other complications have occasionally been reported, most often with giant hemangiomas. These include intratumoral hemorrhage, inflammatory changes, or consumptive coagulopathy (Kasabach-Merritt syndrome).[24] Such complicated lesions may require aggressive management, such as arterial embolization or resection.

Rarely, hemangiomatous lesions can diffusely replace the liver parenchyma. In contrast to the sharp borders of classic hemangiomas, boundaries of so-called "hemangiomatosis" are ill defined. This pattern has been observed adjacent to giant hemangiomas (see **Fig. 2B**), and in some cases, can be a manifestation of

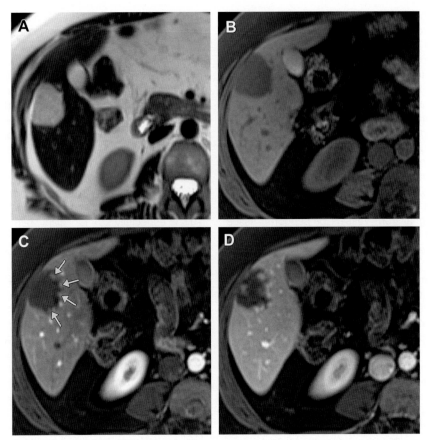

**Fig. 1.** Typical hemangioma. (*A*, *B*) A well-circumscribed mass demonstrates uniform T2 hyperintense and T1 hypointense signal. (*C*) Characteristic discontinuous peripheral nodular enhancement is seen during arterial phase (*arrows*). (*D*) Subsequent postcontrast images show progressive centripetal filling of the hemangioma.

systemic diseases, such as hereditary hemorrhagic telangiectasia.[25]

"Sclerosed" hemangiomas have predominately fibrosed and obliterated vascular spaces and may represent the end stage of hemangioma involution.[20] The typical imaging features of a hemangioma are altered or lost, making a prospective diagnosis challenging (**Fig. 4**). Hemangiomas can be especially difficult to diagnose in the setting of cirrhosis, where they are less common than in the general population and may sclerose. Doyle and colleagues[17] described features suggestive of sclerosed hemangiomas in a series of 10 lesions: geographic margins, volume loss with capsular retraction, adjacent wedge-shaped perfusional variant, nodular regions of internal enhancement (not necessarily in the periphery of the lesion), and presence of other more typical hemangiomas within the liver. All sclerosed hemangiomas in this series were T2 hyperintense to a variable degree; however, certain malignant lesions can also be T2 hyperintense. These include hypervascular metastases from a primary neuroendocrine tumor (pancreatic islet cell, carcinoid, or pheochromocytoma), breast cancer, renal cell carcinoma, thyroid cancer, melanoma, or sarcoma, in addition to cystic-appearing metastases from mucinous gastrointestinal malignancies.[22,26] Capsular retraction is not specific for "sclerosed" hemangioma; it also can be a feature of peripheral cholangiocarcinoma, epithelioid hemangioendothelioma, and liver metastasis.[20] Prior imaging should be evaluated to determine if the lesion had a more typical appearance of hemangioma previously.

Some hypervascular tumors or treated metastases can mimic peripheral nodular enhancement or show prolonged contrast enhancement (**Fig. 5**). The presence of an early complete (rather than discontinuous) rim of peripheral enhancement or "washout" of contrast on delayed images can help differentiate these metastatic lesions from hemangiomas.[22,26]

As gadoxetate disodium–enhanced MR imaging is increasingly used, it is important to recognize certain pitfalls that may arise with hemangiomas.

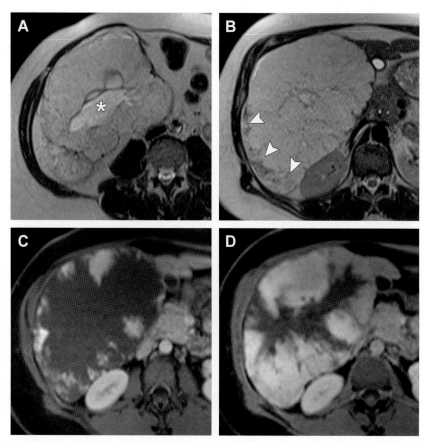

**Fig. 2.** Giant hemangioma. (*A*) Large T2 hyperintense mass with a central T2 hyperintense cleft (*asterisk*) from cystic degeneration or liquefaction. (*B*) Note the more ill-defined "hemangiomatosis" adjacent to its posterior border (*arrowheads*), a pattern that can be seen adjacent to giant hemangiomas. (*C, D*) Postcontrast images demonstrate characteristic peripheral discontinuous "flame-shaped" pattern of enhancement with progressive but incomplete centripetal filling on delayed images.

On 20-minute delayed hepatocyte-phase images, hemangiomas appear hypointense relative to the liver because they lack hepatocytes. However, the gradual process of contrast uptake by hepatocytes and removal from vascular spaces begins even earlier. Hemangiomas may appear hypointense relative to the increasingly bright background liver parenchyma as early as the equilibrium phase. With flash-filling hemangiomas, a resulting "pseudowashout" appearance can mimic hypervascular metastases (**Fig. 6**).[27] Furthermore, some small hemangiomas lack the typical enhancement pattern and can be firmly diagnosed only on delayed images when they appear isointense to blood pool. With gadoxetate disodium, delayed fill-in of these small atypical hemangiomas could be masked, making the diagnosis more difficult.[28] The typical high signal on T2-weighted images may be helpful in these cases. We try to use conventional gadolinium agents instead of gadoxetate disodium-

enhanced MR imaging for the characterization of hemangiomas.

## Focal Nodular Hyperplasia

FNH is the second most common benign liver tumor, with an estimated prevalence of 3% to 8%.[29] Most often found in young and middle-aged women, FNH can be seen across all age groups and also occurs in men.[30] A clear female predominance (8:1 ratio) suggests a role for endogenous or exogenous estrogens in its pathogenesis. Some investigators suggest a link between oral contraceptives and FNH because of reports of size regression following their withdrawal[29,31,32]; however, their potential influence is controversial. In one study of 216 women with FNH, Mathieu and colleagues[33] suggested that (1) neither size nor number of FNHs were influenced by oral contraceptives and (2) size changes during follow-up were rare and did not seem to depend on their use.

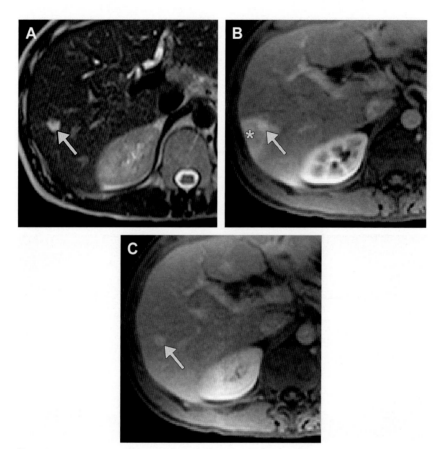

**Fig. 3.** Flash-filling hemangioma with associated perfusional variant. (*A*) A small well-defined T2 hyperintense liver lesion is present (*arrow*). (*B*) During arterial phase, this shows rapid complete filling by contrast (*arrow*). Note the adjacent wedge-shaped subcapsular region of transient hyperenhancement (*asterisk*). (*C*) The hemangioma (*arrow*) retains contrast on more delayed images, its signal intensity following that of blood pool.

FNH is usually a well-circumscribed, nonencapsulated mass less than 5 cm in diameter found in an otherwise healthy liver. The pathogenesis is not fully understood, but it is generally considered a hyperplastic response to a congenital or acquired vascular anomaly. Histologically, multiple small nodules composed of normal hepatocytes are clustered about a central scar of fibrous connective tissue. Characteristic pathologic findings include an enlarged feeding artery, numerous capillaries, and malformed biliary ductules. Generally, these lesions do not contain portal veins.[29]

FNH has been called a "stealth lesion" for being invisible on noncontrast CT; it is also isointense or nearly isointense to adjacent liver parenchyma on many MR imaging sequences (**Fig. 7**). FNH is typically homogeneous in signal intensity and appears isointense to slightly hypointense on T1-weighted images and isointense to slightly hyperintense on T2-weighted images.[30] A stellate central scar of T2 hyperintense signal (related to vascular channels, bile ductules, or edema) may be present, especially in lesions larger than 3 cm (**Fig. 8**).[29,30,34] Because its vascular supply is predominately arterial, FNH typically shows intense uniform enhancement during arterial phase.[34] The lesion usually fades to become isointense or slightly hyperintense to the liver on portal venous and equilibrium phases; if present, the central scar shows delayed enhancement. These typical features allow for a confident diagnosis based on imaging alone.

Because there is no evidence to support malignant potential of FNHs, and their associated complication rate is extremely low, management is conservative.[29] Only a minority of lesions require biopsy. Atypical findings that can be misleading include (1) heterogeneous T1 and T2 signal intensity, (2) hyperintense signal on precontrast T1-weighted images, and (3) hypointense signal relative to the liver during hepatic venous and equilibrium phases suggesting "washout."[29] Occasionally, FNH may exhibit a pseudocapsule

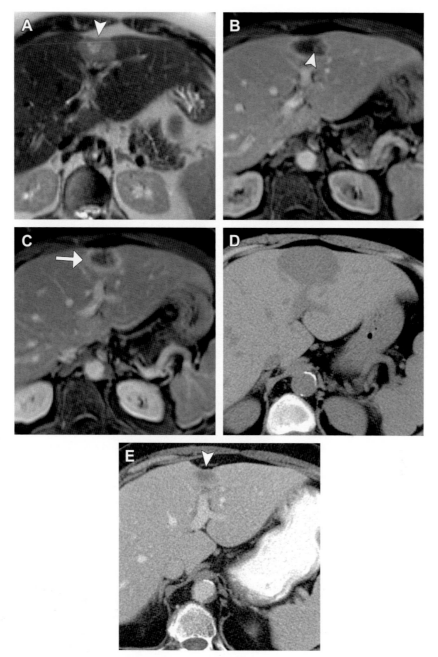

**Fig. 4.** Sclerosing hemangioma (*A*) Heterogeneous, mildly T2 hyperintense mass with overlying capsular retraction (*arrowhead*). (*B*) Portal venous phase image demonstrates a continuous rim of enhancement with some internal nodular foci of enhancement (*arrowhead*). (*C*) Equilibrium phase image shows progressively thick rim of peripheral enhancement (*arrow*). Biopsy performed at this time was consistent with a hemangioma. (*D*) Noncontrast CT image from an outside institution 2 years prior shows that the mass was previously larger. (*E*) One year later, it continued to decrease in size with progressive capsular retraction (*arrowhead*).

related to compression of adjacent liver parenchyma, perilesional vessels, or an inflammatory reaction.[29,35] Rare instances of fat accumulation within FNH have been reported in the literature, a finding usually suggestive of HCA or hepatocellular carcinoma (HCC).[30,36] Fat within FNH may be more commonly seen with diffuse hepatic steatosis but the lesion will often have other features typical of FNH. FNH is most commonly solitary; these atypical features have been more

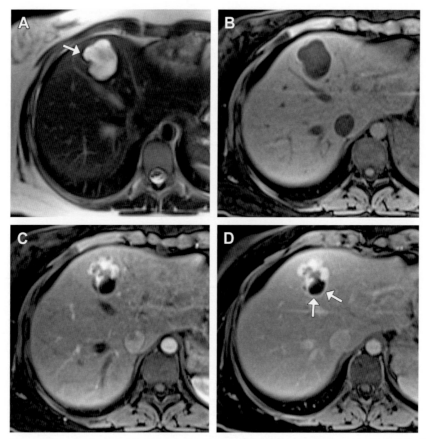

Fig. 5. Potential pitfall: solitary sarcoma metastasis mimicking hepatic hemangioma. (A) Slightly lobulated T2 hyperintense mass in segment 4a has circumscribed margins (arrow). (B) It is uniformly T1 hypointense. (C) Irregular peripheral nodular enhancement is seen during arterial phase. (D) Equilibrium phase shows no progressive filling; however, note the thin continuous rim of enhancement along its posterior wall (arrows). This mass grew on short-term follow-up imaging. Biopsy confirmed a metastasis in this patient with a history of rhabdomyosarcoma.

commonly reported in the setting of multiple FNH lesions.[35]

Small FNH lesions often lack a visible central scar and this should not be misconstrued as an atypical feature. In one study, 42 (80%) of 49 FNH lesions 3 cm in size or smaller lacked a central scar.[37] Conversely, central scars may be seen in other lesions, including fibrolamellar carcinoma and HCC.[38] One must always relate the imaging findings with the clinical context. By definition, a diagnosis of FNH should not be made in a cirrhotic liver.[39] Because fibrolamellar carcinoma also occurs in young adults without underlying liver disease, other features must be used to distinguish it from FNH. The central scar of fibrolamellar carcinoma is usually hypointense on all sequences and does not enhance, owing to collagen and/or coarse calcification.[40] Rarely, it appears T2 hyperintense with delayed enhancement due to increased vascularity, mimicking the central scar of FNH.[40,41] Confounding the issue, the central scar in FNH can show atypical features, such as low T2 signal intensity or only mild enhancement during the equilibrium phase.[29,35] Clues useful for distinguishing fibrolamellar carcinoma from FNH include large size (>10 cm), tumor heterogeneity, large scar (width >2 cm), calcification, invasion of adjacent vessels, lymphadenopathy, and extrahepatic metastases.[38] In addition, fibrolamellar carcinoma is relatively rare compared with FNH.

Due to overlapping patient populations and imaging features, a common diagnostic challenge is to distinguish atypical FNH from HCA, an important distinction that may alter patient management. The hepatocyte-specific contrast agent gadoxetate disodium can be useful in such cases. FNH contains densely packed functioning hepatocytes and abnormal blind-ending bile ductules, resulting in contrast retention and delayed biliary excretion. FNH often shows vivid enhancement

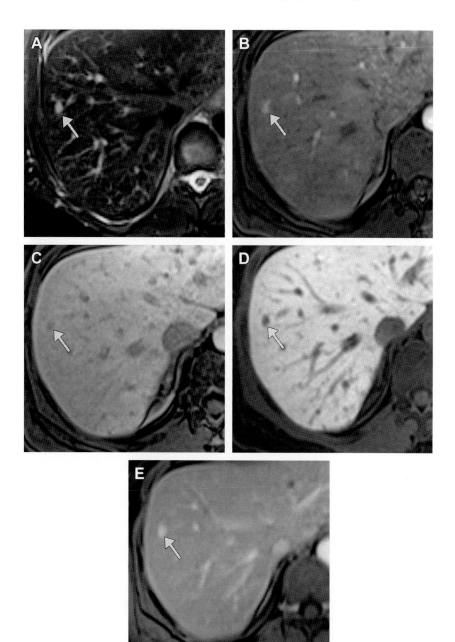

**Fig. 6.** Potential pitfall: pseudowashout of a flash-filling hemangioma with gadoxetate disodium-enhanced MR imaging. (*A*) T2-weighted fat-suppressed image shows a small circumscribed T2 hyperintense lesion (*arrow*). (*B*) Gadoxetate disodium–enhanced MR imaging reveals uniform arterial hyperenhancement (*arrow*). (*C*) The lesion becomes hypointense relative to the increasingly bright liver parenchyma during equilibrium phase, simulating washout (*arrow*). (*D*) It is uniformly hypointense to liver on hepatocyte phase (*arrow*), as expected for a hemangioma. (*E*) Same patient examined with an extracellular contrast agent displays the more familiar appearance of hemangioma retaining contrast on delayed images (*arrow*).

on delayed hepatocyte-phase images, although the degree can vary.[2,4] In a study by van Kessel and colleagues,[42] 19 (73%) of 26 cases of FNH were hyperintense or at least isointense to liver on delayed images, 23% were predominately hypointense with a hyperintense rim, and only 1 case was hypointense without an enhancing rim. The central scar does not typically retain contrast

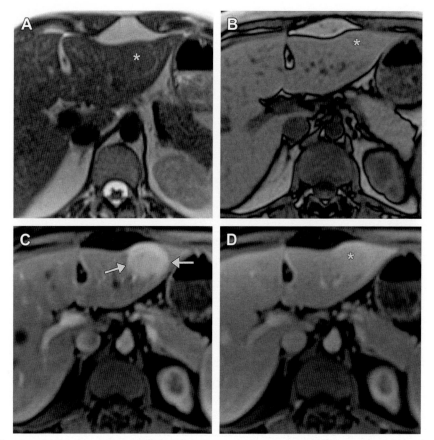

**Fig. 7.** FNH as "stealth" lesion. (*A*) There is a slight contour bulge of the lateral left hepatic lobe due to an underlying T2 isointense mass (*asterisk*). (*B*) The mass is isointense to liver on opposed-phase T1-weighted imaging (*asterisk*), unlike a fat-containing lesion. (*C*) It demonstrates uniform arterial hyperenhancement (*arrows*). (*D*) It then fades to become nearly isointense to liver during portal venous phase (*asterisk*).

on delayed images using gadoxetate disodium, and together with radiating fibrous septae, it may result in a characteristic spoke-wheel appearance.[4,43] Conversely, HCAs are usually hypointense to liver on hepatocyte phase images because, although they have functioning hepatocytes, they lack bile ductules.[37] However, HCAs can occasionally appear isointense or even hyperintense to liver with the underlying mechanism of transport poorly understood.[4]

### Hepatocellular Adenoma

HCA is a less common benign primary neoplasm of the liver. Though most often encountered in women of childbearing age taking oral contraceptives, it can occur in other women as well as men. In recent years, HCA has been categorized into 3 distinct subtypes based on genetic and pathologic features: (1) inflammatory, (2) hepatocyte nuclear factor 1-alpha (HNF-1α) inactivated, and (3) β-catenin-activated lesions. Some exhibit both β-catenin-activation and inflammatory features.[44]

Unclassified HCAs are a small group that lack specific morphologic or immunophenotypical features.[45]

Inflammatory HCA is the most common subtype (40%–50%) and includes lesions formerly known as "telangiectatic" FNH or HCA. It occurs most frequently in young women on oral contraceptives and in obese patients. Histopathology reveals intense polymorphous inflammatory infiltrates, marked sinusoidal dilatation, and abnormal thick-walled arteries.[46] HNF-1α–inactivated HCA is the second most common subtype (30%–35%), resulting from biallelic inactivation of the HNF-1α tumor suppressor gene. This also inactivates liver fatty acid–binding protein, leading to intralesional fat deposition. This subtype occurs exclusively in women, most of whom (>90%) take oral contraceptives; some are also associated with maturity-onset diabetes of the young (MODY) type 3 and familial hepatic adenomatosis.[46] The β-catenin mutated HCA subtype (10%–15%) occurs with sustained activation of the β-catenin

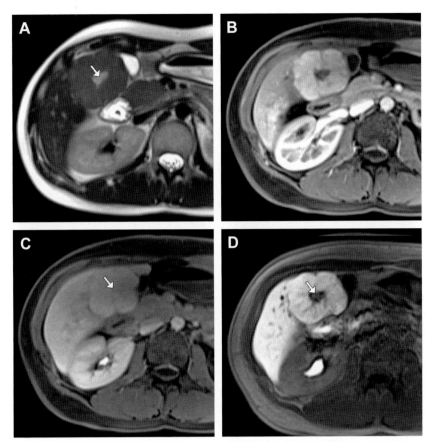

**Fig. 8.** FNH with central scar; gadoxetate disodium–enhanced MR imaging. (*A*) Slightly T2 hyperintense mass has a focal T2 bright central scar (*arrow*). (*B*) The mass demonstrates uniform arterial hyperenhancement. (*C*) There is delayed enhancement of the central scar during equilibrium phase (*arrow*). (*D*) On 20-minute delayed hepatocyte phase images, the mass retains contrast while its central scar does not (*arrow*).

gene, resulting in uncontrolled hepatocyte formation; it occurs more frequently in men and is associated with anabolic steroid use, glycogen storage disease, and familial adenomatosis polyposis.[46]

HCAs are reported to be solitary in most cases (70%–80%), but it is not uncommon for a patient to have 2 or 3 lesions at imaging.[47] Some have found that HCAs are more often multiple in the setting of hepatic steatosis.[48] Presence of more than 10 lesions is rare, originally defined as "liver adenomatosis" by Flejou and colleagues[49] in 1985 as a distinct entity occurring in men and women without risk factors for HCA. It had been suggested that the lesions in adenomatosis are not steroid dependent and are more likely to lead to impaired liver function, hemorrhage, and possibly malignant degeneration.[50] However, more recent evidence suggests adenomatosis is not a specific entity, as once thought, and that lesion size and subtype, not overall number, are important to consider for possible complications.[51]

HCAs are usually well defined, sometimes with a capsule (17%–30%), and can range in size from smaller than 1 cm to larger than 15 cm.[47,52,53] Most patients are asymptomatic at the time of discovery, but some present with abdominal pain, hemorrhage, abnormal liver function tests, or seldom with a palpable mass.[51] The overall rate of hemorrhage is 20% to 25%; larger size (>5 cm) and subcapsular location are risk factors for rupture and bleeding.[46,54] Of the different subtypes, inflammatory HCAs may be more prone to bleed owing to sinusoidal dilatation, peliotic areas, and abnormal arteries.[46]

According to a meta-analysis by Stoot and colleagues,[55] the rate of malignant transformation of HCA to HCC is 4.2%; this occurs more commonly in lesions larger than 5 cm and in men.[53,54] The β-catenin-activated subtype carries the highest risk of malignant transformation; however, some inflammatory HCAs regardless of β-catenin status may also develop HCC.[45] HNF-1α–inactivated HCAs carry the lowest risk of malignant transformation.[45] Thus, recognition of subtype may be relevant with regard to how patients are managed.

As a group, HCA has a variable appearance at imaging; yet, investigators have shown that specific MR imaging patterns may allow for pathologic subtype characterization. Diffuse intralesional fat deposition on chemical shift imaging is characteristic of HNF-1α–inactivated HCA; this finding alone is 86.7% sensitive and 100% specific for HCA subtype characterization (**Fig. 9**).[44] Intralesional fat is seen much less often with inflammatory HCAs, but when it does occur it is usually focal or patchy and heterogeneous rather than uniformly diffuse.[44,45,56] Owing to typical findings of sinusoidal dilatation at histopathology, distinguishing features of inflammatory HCAs include (1) marked T2 hyperintensity, especially in the periphery of the lesion, and (2) strong arterial phase enhancement that persists on more delayed images. Together, these 2 findings are 85.2% sensitive and 87.5% specific for diagnosis (**Fig. 10**).[44] van Aalten and colleagues[56] observed a characteristic "atoll sign" in nearly half (43%) of inflammatory HCAs in their series but not with other subtypes. This refers to a lesion with a peripheral ringlike band of T2 hyperintense signal and a central portion that is isointense to the liver, thus resembling a coral atoll (**Fig. 11**). van Aalten and colleagues[56] suggested that findings of vaguely defined scars or poorly defined T2 hyperintense areas within a lesion might be related to β-catenin-activation (**Fig. 12**), but larger sample sizes are needed to confirm this association. For now, biopsy remains the best option for diagnosing this subtype at greatest risk for malignant transformation.

Imaging features of HCA may overlap with other lesions. In young, otherwise healthy patients, the differential diagnosis commonly includes FNH. Lesion heterogeneity in this population is more suggestive of HCA, particularly if there is variable T1 signal intensity related to hemorrhage or fat content.[52,57] Central scars characteristic of FNH are rarely seen in HCA.[53] Intralesional fat is much more commonly seen in HCA. Nonetheless, it may be difficult to distinguish some HCAs from atypical FNHs, and gadoxetate disodium–enhanced MR imaging may prove helpful in this setting. Distinguishing HCA from HCC is of even greater importance. Both may contain intralesional fat (up to 40% of HCC).[52] Both typically show arterial hyperenhancement. Occasionally, HCA will demonstrate washout or presence of a capsule, other shared features with HCC. Clinical history, including patient demographics and any risk factors for HCC, as well as the background appearance of the liver, including cirrhotic morphology, should provide clues to the correct diagnosis.

Proposed management strategies for HCA rely on cross-sectional imaging for diagnosis and subtype characterization, as well as clinical history and lesion size to determine the need for biopsy or surgical resection. For simplification, HCAs can be initially characterized at MR imaging as (1) diffusely steatotic or (2) either heterogeneous or nonsteatotic. If the patient is taking oral contraceptives or steroids, repeat imaging is recommended 3 to 6 months after discontinuation.[46] Stable and regressing HCAs may be monitored with continued follow-up. Growing lesions warrant further evaluation based on patient sex and lesion size. Surgical resection is advocated for large HCAs (>5 cm) and any HCAs found in men or patients with glycogen storage disease due to an association with β-catenin-activated subtype and increased HCC risk.[46] Females with small (<5 cm) heterogeneous HCAs may warrant percutaneous biopsy to search for β-catenin mutation.[46] Females with small (<5 cm) diffusely steatotic HCAs are at low risk for malignancy, but may benefit from genetic counseling regarding family history of HCA, adenomatosis, and/or MODY type 3.[46,51]

## PYOGENIC LIVER ABSCESS

Pyogenic liver abscesses (PLAs) are localized collections of pus resulting from bacterial infection with destruction of the liver parenchyma and stroma.[58,59] PLAs account for 80% of liver abscesses of all varieties in the United States and Western countries.[60] They may develop as a result of ascending cholangitis (due to benign or malignant biliary obstruction or complication of biliary procedures), hematogenous spread of gastrointestinal infection via the portal vein, diffuse septicemia via the hepatic artery, intrahepatic rupture of cholecystitis, or superinfection of necrotic tissue.[58,61]

With advances in antimicrobial therapy and surgical and/or medical management, biliary tract pathology has surpassed portal seeding from appendicitis and diverticulitis as the most common source of PLA.[62,63] Meddings and colleagues[64] observed the incidence of PLA (3.6 per 100,000) in the United States to be rising and attributed this to an aging population and growing prevalence of hepatobiliary disease, biliary intervention, diabetes, and liver transplantation, all known risk factors for PLA. Diabetes is also implicated in many of the so-called cryptogenic cases of PLAs.[65]

PLAs resulting from hematogenous spread of infection usually manifest as one or a few

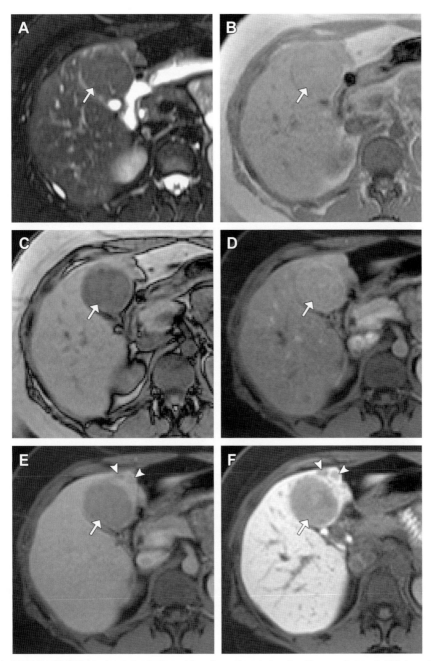

**Fig. 9.** HCA (HNF-1α–inactivated or steatotic subtype); gadoxetate disodium–enhanced MR imaging. (*A*) T2-weighted fat-suppressed image demonstrates a uniformly isointense hepatic mass (*arrow*). (*B*) The mass is isointense to liver on in-phase T1-weighted imaging (*arrow*). (*C*) Diffuse signal dropout of the mass on opposed-phase T1-weighted imaging indicates intracellular fat (*arrow*). (*D*) The mass uniformly enhances to a slightly greater degree than adjacent liver during arterial phase (*arrow*). (*E*) The mass becomes hypointense relative to liver during portal venous phase ("washout") (*arrow*); subtle small adjacent lesions also become apparent (*arrowheads*). (*F*) The dominant mass (*arrow*) and small adjacent lesions (*arrowheads*) all remain hypointense to liver during hepatocyte phase, with the small lesions best seen on this series. Multiple HCAs were confirmed at resection.

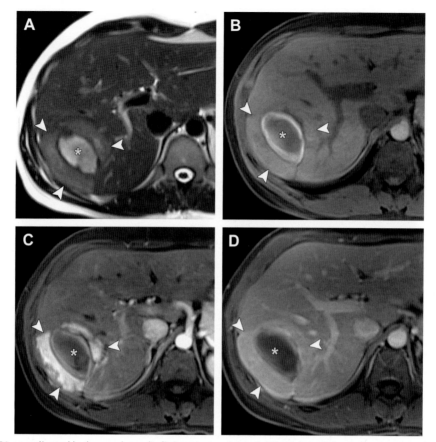

**Fig. 10.** HCA complicated by hemorrhage (inflammatory subtype). (*A*) Slightly T2 hyperintense mass (*arrowheads*) in the posterior right lobe contains a central ovoid region of bright signal surrounded by a thin T2 hypointense rim (*asterisk*). (*B*) The mass itself is isointense to liver on T1-weighted fat-suppressed images (*arrowheads*), whereas the central region is partially T1 hyperintense compatible with blood products (*asterisk*). (*C, D*) Postcontrast images demonstrate strong arterial hyperenhancement of the mass (*arrowheads*) that persists on delayed images without washout. The central region does not enhance, in keeping with hemorrhage (*asterisk*). Surgical pathology revealed inflammatory HCA, which is suggested by its T2 signal intensity and enhancement pattern; inflammatory HCA is the subtype most prone to hemorrhage.

large lesions, with preference for the right lobe due to its size and propensity to receive most of the portal blood flow.[58,66] PLAs of biliary origin tend to be greater in number and smaller in size[58]; those smaller than 2 cm may be classified as microabscesses.[61] Solitary abscesses are more likely than multiple abscesses to be polymicrobial.[63] Common causative organisms are *Streptococcus* species, *Escherichia coli*, and *Klebsiella*, with *Klebsiella* accounting for the highest percentage of cases in large recent Asian case studies.[60,63,64,67,68]

Most patients have fevers at the time of presentation, as many as 99% in one case series by Wong and colleagues.[67] Patients also commonly experience chills and right upper quadrant pain.[60,65] However, the presenting symptoms of PLA can be highly variable. Clinically occult or "cold" abscesses manifest with nonspecific symptoms, such as weight loss or vague abdominal pain.[61]

PLAs can have a variable appearance at MR imaging, but are generally sharply marginated and T2 hyperintense and T1 hypointense. Microabscesses are more difficult to appreciate on precontrast T1-weighted images but become more conspicuous after contrast due to central nonenhancement.[58] Intense early wall enhancement is characteristic, usually between 2 and 5 mm in thickness and relatively uniform (**Fig. 13**).[69] This wall enhancement persists on delayed images, with little to no perceptible change in thickness.[69] Internal septations are occasionally seen (**Fig. 14**). A focal cluster of microabscesses separated by enhancing septae suggests the early stage of coalescence into a larger abscess cavity.[58] This

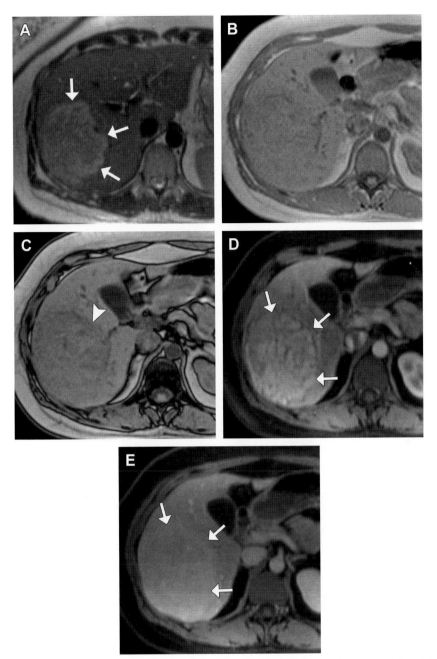

**Fig. 11.** HCA (inflammatory subtype): "atoll sign." (*A*) Large right hepatic mass exhibits a peripheral ringlike band of T2 hyperintense signal (*arrows*) and less pronounced mildly T2 hyperintense signal centrally, with overall appearance likened to a coral atoll. (*B*) The mass is nearly isointense to liver on in-phase T1-weighted imaging. (*C*) There is subtle signal loss on opposed-phase T1-weighted imaging suggesting intracellular fat (*arrowhead*), although not as pronounced or diffuse as described with HNF-1α–inactivated subtype. (*D, E*) Postcontrast images demonstrate arterial hyperenhancement that persists on delayed imaging (*arrows*). Inflammatory HCA was found at resection.

so-called "cluster sign" favors a diagnosis of PLA over other types of liver abscesses.[70]

Perilesional edema manifested by mild increased T2 signal and/or perilesional enhancement differences is not uncommon, especially with larger abscesses. Patterns include (1) adjacent wedge-shaped transient arterial hyperenhancement alone or (2) adjacent wedge-shaped or circumferential surrounding edema with associated hyperenhancement during arterial and

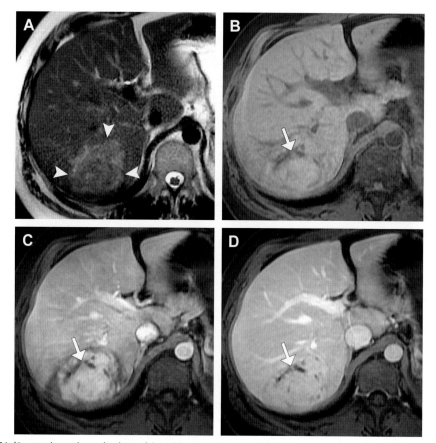

**Fig. 12.** HCA (β-catenin-activated subtype) in a 31-year-old male. (*A*) Heterogeneous, mildly T2 hyperintense mass in the posterior right lobe has a peripheral band of mildly T2 hyperintense signal (*arrowheads*). (*B*) Precontrast fat-suppressed T1-weighted image demonstrates an eccentric poorly defined T1 hypointense scar (*arrow*). (*C*) The mass exhibits heterogeneous arterial hyperenhancement and slightly more uniform enhancement during portal venous phase (*D*) with exception of the nonenhancing eccentric scar (*arrows*). HCA with β-catenin mutation was found at resection. This subtype occurs more frequently in men. It has been suggested that vaguely defined scars or poorly defined T2 hyperintense areas within a lesion might relate to β-catenin activation, but this is not definitive and biopsy remains the best option for diagnosing this subtype.

delayed phases.[69] Perilesional edema also has been described as highly suggestive of abscess formation at CT.[71] Proposed etiologies include adjacent sinusoidal dilatation or inflammatory response.[58]

DWI is very helpful in making the diagnosis of PLA. Due to the high viscosity and cellularity of pus, abscess cavities demonstrate restricted diffusion (see **Figs. 13** and **14**).[59] This allows for quick differentiation of PLAs from benign cysts that lack restricted diffusion. Some investigators also have suggested that DWI can potentially help differentiate PLAs from certain cystic or necrotic primary or metastatic liver neoplasms, as abscess cavities may demonstrate overall greater restricted diffusion (lower ADC values).[7,59]

Prompt diagnosis and treatment of PLA is necessary for a good outcome. Identifying a potential source, such as diverticulitis, biliary disease, or appendicitis, is critical and may require additional imaging. Broad-spectrum antibiotics should be initiated and subsequently modified once sensitivities become available. Antibiotics alone can be effective for some patients with small (<3 cm) abscesses[62]; however, most PLAs require drainage and/or treatment of underlying biliary obstruction if present.[58] Image-guided percutaneous catheter drainage has replaced surgical intervention as the most common approach.[62,72]

## HEPATIC CYSTS

Simple hepatic cysts are common benign liver lesions that are typically incidentally discovered. They are usually round or ovoid with smooth margins and range in size from a few millimeters to

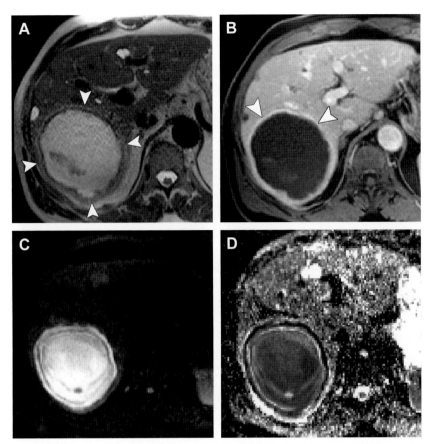

**Fig. 13.** Pyogenic liver abscess. (*A*) Large rounded predominately T2 hyperintense mass in the posterior right lobe has a rim of mild increased T2 signal that may in part relate to surrounding edema (*arrowheads*). (*B*) Postcontrast images show relatively uniform wall enhancement (*arrowheads*). (*C*) Contents are markedly hyperintense on the high b-value (800 s/mm²) diffusion-weighted image. (*D*) Pronounced low signal on the corresponding ADC map indicates restricted diffusion, typical of abscess.

several centimeters. On MR imaging, simple cysts are markedly T2 hyperintense and T1 hypointense (isointense to fluid), have very thin or imperceptible walls, and do not enhance following contrast.[73,74]

## CILIATED HEPATIC FOREGUT CYST

Ciliated hepatic foregut cyst (CHFC), a term first used by Wheeler and Edmondson in 1984,[75] is an uncommon solitary benign hepatic cyst that appears histologically similar to bronchogenic and esophageal duplication cysts. It is thought to arise due to abnormal budding of the embryologic foregut. Characteristically, it is lined by a pseudostratified, ciliated, mucin-secreting, columnar epithelium, with bands of smooth muscle in the cyst wall and an outer fibrous capsule.[75]

CHFCs are likely underdiagnosed but important to not confuse with malignancy. Most often, a CHFC is found within or in close proximity to the medial left hepatic lobe (segment 4).[76]

Subcapsular location is also characteristic[77]; in some cases, the cyst wall extends slightly beyond the contour of the liver.[78] It is typically unilocular with an average size of 3.6 cm (range of 1.1–13.0 cm).[76] Most cases are diagnosed in the fifth or sixth decade, with a slight male predominance (1.1:1.0 ratio).[76,79]

The true prevalence of CHFC is difficult to establish, as most are asymptomatic and discovered incidentally.[80] Some believe they do not cause symptoms unless they become infected or large enough to compress adjacent organs.[78] Rare cases of very large CHFCs resulting in obstructive jaundice[80,81] and portal hypertension[82] due to mass-effect on the biliary tree and portal vein, respectively, have been reported. Malignant transformation is another rare complication; at least 4 cases of squamous cell carcinoma arising in CHFC have been reported in the literature.[83–86]

The diagnosis may be difficult at CT, as the fluid may be complicated and of greater density than

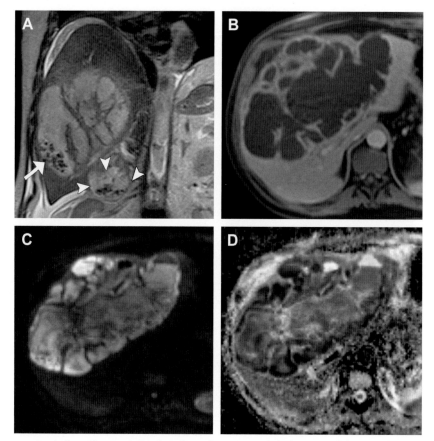

**Fig. 14.** Large pyogenic liver abscess due to intrahepatic rupture of cholecystitis. (*A*) Coronal T2-weighted image shows a large multiloculated T2 hyperintense hepatic mass containing several tiny spilled gallstones (*arrow*). Gallstones are also seen in the adjacent gallbladder (*arrowheads*). (*B*) Postcontrast image during equilibrium phase shows diffuse enhancement of its outer wall and several internal septae. (*C*) The mass exhibits restricted diffusion, with bright signal on the high b-value (800 s/mm$^2$) diffusion-weighted image and low signal on the corresponding ADC map (*D*).

simple fluid, potentially mimicking a solid and/or hypovascular or necrotic mass.[77,87] MR imaging better demonstrates their cystic nature and proteinaceous fluid content (**Fig. 15**). They are well-defined, T2 hyperintense, and mostly unilocular lesions. Variable signal intensity on T1-weighted images, ranging from hypointense to hyperintense signal, reflects differences in protein concentration.[78] Rarely, they may be associated with a fluid-fluid level.[79] Contrast-enhanced images easily confirm their cystic nature by demonstrating only thin wall enhancement.[78] Primary differential considerations include simple or complicated (infected or hemorrhagic) cysts and biliary cystadenomas. CHFCs should be diagnosed based on their classic subcapsular location in the medial segment of the left hepatic lobe.

CHFCs generally have a benign course. Surgical excision is recommended for symptomatic and/or large lesions producing mass-effect.[82,84]

Because case reports of malignant transformation with poor outcomes have been described, some have recommended surgical excision or enucleation of CHFCs regardless of size.[76] Current data may be limited by small sample sizes. Regardless, careful attention can be made at imaging for any irregular wall thickness or solid component that might suggest the rare development of carcinoma.

## BILE DUCT HAMARTOMAS

Bile duct hamartomas (BDH), also known as biliary hamartomas and von Meyenburg complexes, are benign liver lesions that result from ductal plate malformations involving the small interlobular bile ducts.[88] They consist of focally disordered collections of bile ducts surrounded by abundant fibrous stroma[89] and are considered part of a spectrum of fibropolycystic liver disease that also includes

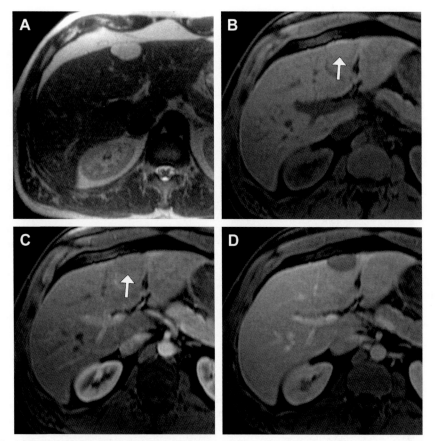

**Fig. 15.** Ciliated hepatic foregut cyst. (*A*) Typical subcapsular T2 hyperintense cystic lesion in segment 4 extends slightly beyond the contour of the liver. (*B*) On precontrast fat-suppressed T1-weighted imaging, this appears iso-intense to liver due to proteinaceous fluid content (*arrow*). (*C*) The lesion remains nearly isointense to adjacent liver parenchyma during arterial phase (*arrow*). (*D*) It becomes hypointense to liver during the portal venous phase but should not be mistaken for a solid enhancing lesion with "washout."

congenital hepatic fibrosis, autosomal dominant polycystic liver disease, and Caroli disease.[90]

BDHs can vary in number from as few as 1 or 2 small (≤10 mm) cystic liver lesions to numerous scattered small lesions of near uniform or varying size (**Fig. 16**).[89] Initial case reports warned of potential confusion with metastases, especially in patients with known extrahepatic malignancy[91,92]; however, MR imaging readily distinguishes BDHs from solid lesions.[90] They are well-defined T2 hyperintense cystic lesions that lack communication with the biliary tree and may exhibit lobulated

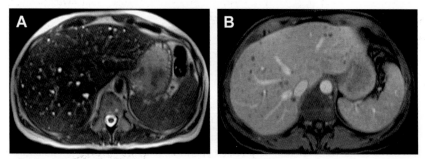

**Fig. 16.** Multiple bile duct hamartomas. (*A*) Numerous subcentimeter T2 hyperintense cystic foci are scattered throughout the liver. (*B*) The lesions appear hypointense to liver on postcontrast images and should not to be mistaken for hypoenhancing solid lesions or metastases.

margins, thin septations, and a characteristic thin rim of enhancement related to adjacent compressed liver parenchyma and inflammation (**Fig. 17**).[90,92] Identification of a 1-mm to 2-mm "mural nodule" owing to conjunctive septae within at least one lesion has been proposed to increase diagnostic specificity of BDH.[88] Overall, these cyst wall features may help in the differentiation from simple cysts, although this distinction is usually not needed, as most BDHs are of no clinical significance.[90] Lack of restricted diffusion helps distinguish them from microabscesses.

More recently, Martin and colleagues[90] described less common large cystic and complicated variants they collectively named "giant BDH." This term applies to lesions larger than 2 cm, although they can be much larger (>10 cm) and develop complications, such as hemorrhage and right upper quadrant pain.[90] A clue to diagnosis is that they coexist with smaller typical BDHs and have less internal complexity than biliary cystadenomas (BCAs).

## BILIARY CYSTADENOMA

BCA is a rare cystic neoplasm that is generally found in middle-aged women but can occur at any age and occasionally in men. It is histologically similar to mucinous cystic neoplasm of the pancreas.[93,94] Many believe that all BCAs are premalignant. Lesions are subdivided at pathology based on the presence or absence of ovarian stroma, found only in women and considered a favorable prognostic indicator.[93] Typical gross pathology features include a characteristic multilocular appearance[95] and presence of a fibrous capsule.[93]

Most BCAs are intrahepatic (85%), but they also may arise from the common duct or rarely the gallbladder.[93] They are usually large lesions, with a mean size of 12 cm in one larger series (ranging from 3 to 40 cm).[93] Often slow growing, they may present with nonspecific symptoms, such as abdominal pain.[93,95,96] Some patients present with jaundice from associated biliary

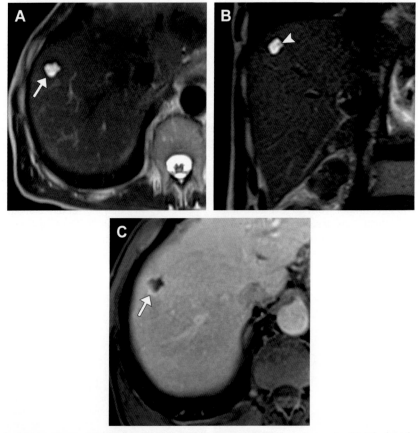

**Fig. 17.** Bile duct hamartoma. (*A*) Small well-defined T2 hyperintense lesion (*arrow*) with lobulated margins has a suggestion of a few thin internal septations. (*B*) Coronal T2-weighted image demonstrates a tiny mural nodule owing to conjunctive septae (*arrowhead*), a finding proposed to increase diagnostic specificity of BDH. (*C*) Post-contrast image shows a characteristic thin rim of enhancement (*arrow*).

obstruction.[96,97] Occasionally, they are asymptomatic and discovered incidentally.

On imaging studies, BCAs usually appear as large, well-defined multilobulated intrahepatic cystic masses with internal septae (**Fig. 18**). Infrequently, they appear unilocular at imaging. BCAs are typically T2 hyperintense and show variable T1 signal intensity due to proteinaceous content or blood products (**Fig. 19**).[93,98] Fluid-fluid levels occasionally result.[97,98] Frahm and colleagues[99] reported a more unusual case of BCA with multiple intracystic masses on T2-weighted images representing large blood clots floating in hemorrhagic cystic fluid. Compared with CT, MR imaging can better evaluate the relationship of the mass to the bile ducts and also can help detect the unusual case of intraductal tumoral extension.[97] MR imaging also can better demonstrate enhancement of the capsule, septae, and any mural nodules.[100] Mural or septal nodularity increases the likelihood of malignancy.[93,95,101]

It can be difficult to differentiate BCA and its malignant counterpart biliary cystadenocarcinoma (BCAC) preoperatively, but this is usually unnecessary because both require complete surgical excision. Subtotal excision or treatments reserved for simple cysts (ie, aspiration, drainage, or marsupialization) result in near universal recurrence and occasional malignant transformation.[96] The differential diagnosis includes other lesions that appear septated or multilobulated. Liver abscesses usually have thicker walls at MR imaging[98] and are associated with clinical and/or laboratory signs of infection. Hydatid cysts occur in endemic regions and are characterized by the development of daughter cysts in their periphery.[61] A cystic metastasis or rare cystic HCC may appear similar, but underlying primary malignancy or cirrhosis are usually known. Embryonal sarcoma of the liver is an unusual tumor that predominantly affects children but can affect adults as well; it can mimic a complicated cystic lesion such as BCA owing to

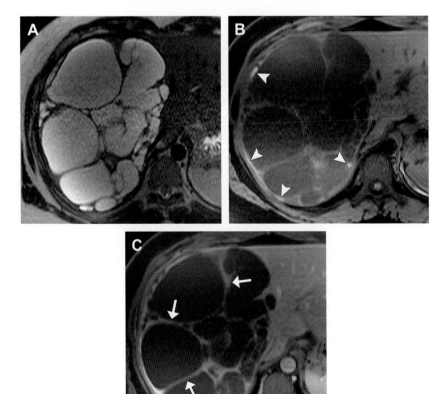

**Fig. 18.** Biliary cystadenoma. (*A*) Large T2 hyperintense cystic mass has multiple thick septations resulting in a multilocular appearance. (*B*) Small peripheral foci of T1 hyperintense signal on precontrast images reflect hemorrhage or proteinaceous material (*arrowheads*). (*C*) Postcontrast images demonstrate enhancement of the septae (*arrows*) and outer capsule. Multiloculated biliary cystadenoma was confirmed at resection.

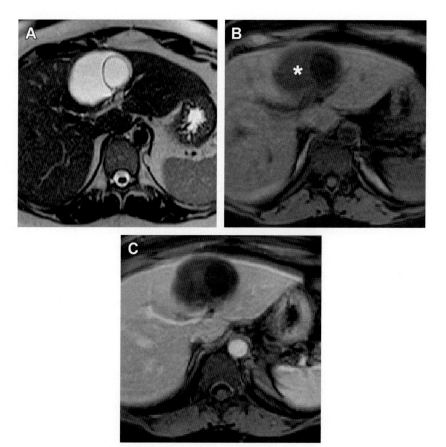

**Fig. 19.** Mucinous biliary cystadenoma. (*A*) T2 hyperintense cystic lesion contains a smaller eccentric internal cystic component or daughter cyst. (*B*) The larger component is of slightly greater T1 signal intensity reflecting protein-aceous material (*asterisk*). (*C*) Postcontrast imaging demonstrates no enhancing components. Mucinous biliary cystadenoma was found at surgery.

its misleading T2-hyperintense signal created by abundant myxoid stroma.[102,103]

## SUMMARY

Focal liver lesions are commonly encountered during routine imaging studies. MR imaging plays an important role in the workup of the otherwise indeterminate lesion, and often can be definitive in characterization. It is important to consider the characteristic MR imaging features of benign focal hepatic lesions so as to avoid biopsy, surgery, and extensive workups. Advances in MR imaging technology and in some cases, a better understanding of the lesion itself, have allowed for improved lesion diagnosis.

## REFERENCES

1. American College of Radiology. ACR Appropriateness Criteria®: liver lesion — initial characterization. Available at: http://www.acr.org/Quality-Safety/Appropriateness-Criteria/Diagnostic/∼/media/ACR/Documents/AppCriteria/Diagnostic/LiverLesionInitial Characterization.pdf. Accessed July 6, 2013.
2. Fidler J, Hough D. Hepatocyte-specific magnetic resonance imaging contrast agents. Hepatology 2011;53(2):678–82.
3. Seale MK, Catalano OA, Saini S, et al. Hepatobiliary-specific MR contrast agents: role in imaging the liver and biliary tree. Radiographics 2009; 29(6):1725–48.
4. Ringe KI, Husarik DB, Sirlin CB, et al. Gadoxetate disodium-enhanced MRI of the liver: part 1, protocol optimization and lesion appearance in the noncirrhotic liver. AJR Am J Roentgenol 2010;195(1): 13–28.
5. Tanimoto A, Lee JM, Murakami T, et al. Consensus report of the 2nd International Forum for Liver MRI. Eur Radiol 2009;19(Suppl 5):S975–89.
6. Koh DM, Collins DJ. Diffusion-weighted MRI in the body: applications and challenges in oncology. AJR Am J Roentgenol 2007;188(6):1622–35.
7. Taouli B, Koh DM. Diffusion-weighted MR imaging of the liver. Radiology 2010;254(1):47–66.

8. Okada Y, Ohtomo K, Kiryu S, et al. Breath-hold T2-weighted MRI of hepatic tumors: value of echo planar imaging with diffusion-sensitizing gradient. J Comput Assist Tomogr 1998;22(3):364–71.

9. Hussain SM, De Becker J, Hop WC, et al. Can a single-shot black-blood T2-weighted spin-echo echo-planar imaging sequence with sensitivity encoding replace the respiratory-triggered turbo spin-echo sequence for the liver? An optimization and feasibility study. J Magn Reson Imaging 2005;21(3):219–29.

10. Parikh T, Drew SJ, Lee VS, et al. Focal liver lesion detection and characterization with diffusion-weighted MR imaging: comparison with standard breath-hold T2-weighted imaging. Radiology 2008;246(3):812–22.

11. Taouli B, Vilgrain V, Dumont E, et al. Evaluation of liver diffusion isotropy and characterization of focal hepatic lesions with two single-shot echo-planar MR imaging sequences: prospective study in 66 patients. Radiology 2003;226(1):71–8.

12. Bruegel M, Holzapfel K, Gaa J, et al. Characterization of focal liver lesions by ADC measurements using a respiratory triggered diffusion-weighted single-shot echo-planar MR imaging technique. Eur Radiol 2008;18(3):477–85.

13. Miller FH, Hammond N, Siddiqi AJ, et al. Utility of diffusion-weighted MRI in distinguishing benign and malignant hepatic lesions. J Magn Reson Imaging 2010;32(1):138–47.

14. Agnello F, Ronot M, Valla DC, et al. High-b-value diffusion-weighted MR imaging of benign hepatocellular lesions: quantitative and qualitative analysis. Radiology 2012;262(2):511–9.

15. Cieszanowski A, Anysz-Grodzicka A, Szeszkowski W, et al. Characterization of focal liver lesions using quantitative techniques: comparison of apparent diffusion coefficient values and T2 relaxation times. Eur Radiol 2012;22(11):2514–24.

16. Caseiro-Alves F, Brito J, Araujo AE, et al. Liver haemangioma: common and uncommon findings and how to improve the differential diagnosis. Eur Radiol 2007;17(6):1544–54.

17. Doyle DJ, Khalili K, Guindi M, et al. Imaging features of sclerosed hemangioma. AJR Am J Roentgenol 2007;189(1):67–72.

18. Vilgrain V, Uzan F, Brancatelli G, et al. Prevalence of hepatic hemangioma in patients with focal nodular hyperplasia: MR imaging analysis. Radiology 2003;229(1):75–9.

19. Markovic MV, Petricusic L, Curic J, et al. Magnetic resonance imaging of chronic bleeding into a giant hepatic hemangioma. Eur J Radiol Extra 2011;77: e9–11.

20. Vilgrain V, Boulos L, Vullierme MP, et al. Imaging of atypical hemangiomas of the liver with pathologic correlation. Radiographics 2000;20(2):379–97.

21. Danet IM, Semelka RC, Braga L, et al. Giant hemangioma of the liver: MR imaging characteristics in 24 patients. Magn Reson Imaging 2003;21(2): 95–101.

22. Jang HJ, Kim TK, Lim HK, et al. Hepatic hemangioma: atypical appearances on CT, MR imaging, and sonography. AJR Am J Roentgenol 2003; 180(1):135–41.

23. Jeong MG, Yu JS, Kim KW. Hepatic cavernous hemangioma: temporal peritumoral enhancement during multiphase dynamic MR imaging. Radiology 2000;216(3):692–7.

24. Prasanna PM, Fredericks SE, Winn SS, et al. Best cases from the AFIP: giant cavernous hemangioma. Radiographics 2010;30(4):1139–44.

25. Jhaveri KS, Vlachou PA, Guindi M, et al. Association of hepatic hemangiomatosis with giant cavernous hemangioma in the adult population: prevalence, imaging appearance, and relevance. AJR Am J Roentgenol 2011;196(4):809–15.

26. Silva AC, Evans JM, McCullough AE, et al. MR imaging of hypervascular liver masses: a review of current techniques. Radiographics 2009;29(2): 385–402.

27. Doo KW, Lee CH, Choi JW, et al. "Pseudo washout" sign in high-flow hepatic hemangioma on gadoxetic acid contrast-enhanced MRI mimicking hypervascular tumor. AJR Am J Roentgenol 2009;193(6): W490–6.

28. Goshima S, Kanematsu M, Watanabe H, et al. Hepatic hemangioma and metastasis: differentiation with gadoxetate disodium-enhanced 3-T MRI. AJR Am J Roentgenol 2010;195(4):941–6.

29. Marin D, Brancatelli G, Federle MP, et al. Focal nodular hyperplasia: typical and atypical MRI findings with emphasis on the use of contrast media. Clin Radiol 2008;63(5):577–85.

30. Mortele KJ, Praet M, Van Vlierberghe H, et al. CT and MR imaging findings in focal nodular hyperplasia of the liver: radiologic-pathologic correlation. AJR Am J Roentgenol 2000;175(3):687–92.

31. Scalori A, Tavani A, Gallus S, et al. Oral contraceptives and the risk of focal nodular hyperplasia of the liver: a case-control study. Am J Obstet Gynecol 2002;186(2):195–7.

32. Scott LD, Katz AR, Duke JH, et al. Oral contraceptives, pregnancy, and focal nodular hyperplasia of the liver. JAMA 1984;251(11):1461–3.

33. Mathieu D, Kobeiter H, Maison P, et al. Oral contraceptive use and focal nodular hyperplasia of the liver. Gastroenterology 2000;118(3):560–4.

34. Buetow PC, Pantongrag-Brown L, Buck JL, et al. Focal nodular hyperplasia of the liver: radiologic-pathologic correlation. Radiographics 1996;16(2): 369–88.

35. Hussain SM, Terkivatan T, Zondervan PE, et al. Focal nodular hyperplasia: findings at state-of-the-art MR

imaging, US, CT, and pathologic analysis. Radiographics 2004;24(1):3–17 [discussion: 18–9].

36. Chaoui A, Mergo PJ, Lauwers GY. Unusual appearance of focal nodular hyperplasia with fatty change. AJR Am J Roentgenol 1998; 171(5):1433–4.

37. Grazioli L, Morana G, Federle MP, et al. Focal nodular hyperplasia: morphologic and functional information from MR imaging with gadobenate dimeglumine. Radiology 2001;221(3):731–9.

38. Blachar A, Federle MP, Ferris JV, et al. Radiologists' performance in the diagnosis of liver tumors with central scars by using specific CT criteria. Radiology 2002;223(2):532–9.

39. International Working Party. Terminology of nodular hepatocellular lesions. Hepatology 1995;22:11.

40. McLarney JK, Rucker PT, Bender GN, et al. Fibrolamellar carcinoma of the liver: radiologic-pathologic correlation. Radiographics 1999;19(2): 453–71.

41. Hamrick-Turner JE, Shipkey FH, Cranston PE. Fibrolamellar hepatocellular carcinoma: MR appearance mimicking focal nodular hyperplasia. J Comput Assist Tomogr 1994;18(2):301–4.

42. van Kessel CS, de Boer E, Kate FJ, et al. Focal nodular hyperplasia: hepatobiliary enhancement patterns on gadoxetic-acid contrast-enhanced MRI. Abdom Imaging 2013;38(3):490–501.

43. Karam AR, Shankar S, Surapaneni P, et al. Focal nodular hyperplasia: central scar enhancement pattern using gadoxetate disodium. J Magn Reson Imaging 2010;32(2):341–4.

44. Laumonier H, Bioulac-Sage P, Laurent C, et al. Hepatocellular adenomas: magnetic resonance imaging features as a function of molecular pathological classification. Hepatology 2008;48(3):808–18.

45. Ronot M, Bahrami S, Calderaro J, et al. Hepatocellular adenomas: accuracy of magnetic resonance imaging and liver biopsy in subtype classification. Hepatology 2011;53(4):1182–91.

46. Katabathina VS, Menias CO, Shanbhogue AK, et al. Genetics and imaging of hepatocellular adenomas: 2011 update. Radiographics 2011;31(6):1529–43.

47. Grazioli L, Federle MP, Brancatelli G, et al. Hepatic adenomas: imaging and pathologic findings. Radiographics 2001;21(4):877–92 [discussion: 892–4].

48. Furlan A, van der Windt DJ, Nalesnik MA, et al. Multiple hepatic adenomas associated with liver steatosis at CT and MRI: a case-control study. AJR Am J Roentgenol 2008;191(5):1430–5.

49. Flejou JF, Barge J, Menu Y, et al. Liver adenomatosis. An entity distinct from liver adenoma? Gastroenterology 1985;89(5):1132–8.

50. Grazioli L, Federle MP, Ichikawa T, et al. Liver adenomatosis: clinical, histopathologic, and imaging findings in 15 patients. Radiology 2000;216(2): 395–402.

51. Bioulac-Sage P, Laumonier H, Couchy G, et al. Hepatocellular adenoma management and phenotypic classification: the Bordeaux experience. Hepatology 2009;50(2):481–9.

52. Paulson EK, McClellan JS, Washington K, et al. Hepatic adenoma: MR characteristics and correlation with pathologic findings. AJR Am J Roentgenol 1994;163(1):113–6.

53. Brancatelli G, Federle MP, Vullierme MP, et al. CT and MR imaging evaluation of hepatic adenoma. J Comput Assist Tomogr 2006;30(5):745–50.

54. Dokmak S, Paradis V, Vilgrain V, et al. A single-center surgical experience of 122 patients with single and multiple hepatocellular adenomas. Gastroenterology 2009;137(5):1698–705.

55. Stoot JH, Coelen RJ, De Jong MC, et al. Malignant transformation of hepatocellular adenomas into hepatocellular carcinomas: a systematic review including more than 1600 adenoma cases. HPB (Oxford) 2010;12(8):509–22.

56. van Aalten SM, Thomeer MG, Terkivatan T, et al. Hepatocellular adenomas: correlation of MR imaging findings with pathologic subtype classification. Radiology 2011;261(1):172–81.

57. Chung KY, Mayo-Smith WW, Saini S, et al. Hepatocellular adenoma: MR imaging features with pathologic correlation. AJR Am J Roentgenol 1995; 165(2):303–8.

58. Mendez RJ, Schiebler ML, Outwater EK, et al. Hepatic abscesses: MR imaging findings. Radiology 1994;190(2):431–6.

59. Chan JH, Tsui EY, Luk SH, et al. Diffusion-weighted MR imaging of the liver: distinguishing hepatic abscess from cystic or necrotic tumor. Abdom Imaging 2001;26(2):161–5.

60. Tian LT, Yao K, Zhang XY, et al. Liver abscesses in adult patients with and without diabetes mellitus: an analysis of the clinical characteristics, features of the causative pathogens, outcomes and predictors of fatality: a report based on a large population, retrospective study in China. Clin Microbiol Infect 2012;18(9):E314–30.

61. Mortele KJ, Segatto E, Ros PR. The infected liver: radiologic-pathologic correlation. Radiographics 2004;24(4):937–55.

62. Mezhir JJ, Fong Y, Jacks LM, et al. Current management of pyogenic liver abscess: surgery is now second-line treatment. J Am Coll Surg 2010; 210(6):975–83.

63. Branum GD, Tyson GS, Branum MA, et al. Hepatic abscess. Changes in etiology, diagnosis, and management. Ann Surg 1990;212(6):655–62.

64. Meddings L, Myers RP, Hubbard J, et al. A population-based study of pyogenic liver abscesses in the United States: incidence, mortality, and temporal trends. Am J Gastroenterol 2010; 105(1):117–24.

65. Foo NP, Chen KT, Lin HJ, et al. Characteristics of pyogenic liver abscess patients with and without diabetes mellitus. Am J Gastroenterol 2010; 105(2):328–35.

66. Law ST, Li KK. Is hepatic neoplasm-related pyogenic liver abscess a distinct clinical entity? World J Gastroenterol 2012;18(10):1110–6.

67. Wong WM, Wong BC, Hui CK, et al. Pyogenic liver abscess: retrospective analysis of 80 cases over a 10-year period. J Gastroenterol Hepatol 2002; 17(9):1001–7.

68. Pang TC, Fung T, Samra J, et al. Pyogenic liver abscess: an audit of 10 years' experience. World J Gastroenterol 2011;17(12):1622–30.

69. Balci NC, Semelka RC, Noone TC, et al. Pyogenic hepatic abscesses: MRI findings on T1- and T2-weighted and serial gadolinium-enhanced gradient-echo images. J Magn Reson Imaging 1999;9(2):285–90.

70. Jeffrey RB Jr, Tolentino CS, Chang FC, et al. CT of small pyogenic hepatic abscesses: the cluster sign. AJR Am J Roentgenol 1988;151(3):487–9.

71. Mathieu D, Vasile N, Fagniez PL, et al. Dynamic CT features of hepatic abscesses. Radiology 1985; 154(3):749–52.

72. Rajak CL, Gupta S, Jain S, et al. Percutaneous treatment of liver abscesses: needle aspiration versus catheter drainage. AJR Am J Roentgenol 1998;170(4):1035–9.

73. Elsayes KM, Narra VR, Yin Y, et al. Focal hepatic lesions: diagnostic value of enhancement pattern approach with contrast-enhanced 3D gradient-echo MR imaging. Radiographics 2005;25(5): 1299–320.

74. Horton KM, Bluemke DA, Hruban RH, et al. CT and MR imaging of benign hepatic and biliary tumors. Radiographics 1999;19(2):431–51.

75. Wheeler DA, Edmondson HA. Ciliated hepatic foregut cyst. Am J Surg Pathol 1984;8(6):467–70.

76. Sharma S, Dean AG, Corn A, et al. Ciliated hepatic foregut cyst: an increasingly diagnosed condition. Hepatobiliary Pancreat Dis Int 2008;7(6):581–9.

77. Kadoya M, Matsui O, Nakanuma Y, et al. Ciliated hepatic foregut cyst: radiologic features. Radiology 1990;175(2):475–7.

78. Shoenut JP, Semelka RC, Levi C, et al. Ciliated hepatic foregut cysts: US, CT, and contrast-enhanced MR imaging. Abdom Imaging 1994; 19(2):150–2.

79. Rodriguez E, Soler R, Fernandez P. MR imagings of ciliated hepatic foregut cyst: an unusual cause of fluid-fluid level within a focal hepatic lesion (2005.4b). Eur Radiol 2005;15(7):1499–501.

80. Vick DJ, Goodman ZD, Deavers MT, et al. Ciliated hepatic foregut cyst: a study of six cases and review of the literature. Am J Surg Pathol 1999; 23(6):671–7.

81. Dardik H, Glotzer P, Silver C. Congenital hepatic cyst causing jaundice: report of a case and analogies with respiratory malformations. Ann Surg 1964;159:585–92.

82. Harty MP, Hebra A, Ruchelli ED, et al. Ciliated hepatic foregut cyst causing portal hypertension in an adolescent. AJR Am J Roentgenol 1998; 170(3):688–90.

83. Vick DJ, Goodman ZD, Ishak KG. Squamous cell carcinoma arising in a ciliated hepatic foregut cyst. Arch Pathol Lab Med 1999;123(11):1115–7.

84. de Lajarte-Thirouard AS, Rioux-Leclercq N, Boudjema K, et al. Squamous cell carcinoma arising in a hepatic forgut cyst. Pathol Res Pract 2002;198(10):697–700.

85. Furlanetto A, Dei Tos AP. Squamous cell carcinoma arising in a ciliated hepatic foregut cyst. Virchows Arch 2002;441(3):296–8.

86. Zhang X, Wang Z, Dong Y. Squamous cell carcinoma arising in a ciliated hepatic foregut cyst: case report and literature review. Pathol Res Pract 2009;205(7):498–501.

87. Kimura A, Makuuchi M, Takayasu K, et al. Ciliated hepatic foregut cyst with solid tumor appearance on CT. J Comput Assist Tomogr 1990;14(6):1016–8.

88. Tohme-Noun C, Cazals D, Noun R, et al. Multiple biliary hamartomas: magnetic resonance features with histopathologic correlation. Eur Radiol 2008; 18(3):493–9.

89. Lev-Toaff AS, Bach AM, Wechsler RJ, et al. The radiologic and pathologic spectrum of biliary hamartomas. AJR Am J Roentgenol 1995;165(2):309–13.

90. Martin DR, Kalb B, Sarmiento JM, et al. Giant and complicated variants of cystic bile duct hamartomas of the liver: MRI findings and pathological correlations. J Magn Reson Imaging 2010;31(4):903–11.

91. Zheng RQ, Zhang B, Kudo M, et al. Imaging findings of biliary hamartomas. World J Gastroenterol 2005;11(40):6354–9.

92. Semelka RC, Hussain SM, Marcos HB, et al. Biliary hamartomas: solitary and multiple lesions shown on current MR techniques including gadolinium enhancement. J Magn Reson Imaging 1999; 10(2):196–201.

93. Buetow PC, Buck JL, Pantongrag-Brown L, et al. Biliary cystadenoma and cystadenocarcinoma: clinical-imaging-pathologic correlations with emphasis on the importance of ovarian stroma. Radiology 1995;196(3):805–10.

94. Ishak KG, Willis GW, Cummins SD, et al. Biliary cystadenoma and cystadenocarcinoma: report of 14 cases and review of the literature. Cancer 1977;39(1):322–38.

95. Korobkin M, Stephens DH, Lee JK, et al. Biliary cystadenoma and cystadenocarcinoma: CT and sonographic findings. AJR Am J Roentgenol 1989;153(3):507–11.

96. Thomas KT, Welch D, Trueblood A, et al. Effective treatment of biliary cystadenoma. Ann Surg 2005; 241(5):769–73 [discussion: 773–5].

97. Baudin G, Novellas S, Buratti MS, et al. Atypical MRI features of a biliary cystadenoma revealed by jaundice. Clin Imaging 2006;30(6):413–5.

98. Lewin M, Mourra N, Honigman I, et al. Assessment of MRI and MRCP in diagnosis of biliary cystadenoma and cystadenocarcinoma. Eur Radiol 2006; 16(2):407–13.

99. Frahm C, Zimmermann A, Heller M, et al. Uncommon presentation of a giant biliary cystadenoma: correlation between MRI and pathologic findings. J Magn Reson Imaging 2001;14(5): 649–52.

100. Williams DM, Vitellas KM, Sheafor D. Biliary cystadenocarcinoma: seven year follow-up and the role of MRI and MRCP. Magn Reson Imaging 2001;19(9):1203–8.

101. Choi BI, Lim JH, Han MC, et al. Biliary cystadenoma and cystadenocarcinoma: CT and sonographic findings. Radiology 1989;171(1):57–61.

102. Buetow PC, Buck JL, Pantongrag-Brown L, et al. Undifferentiated (embryonal) sarcoma of the liver: pathologic basis of imaging findings in 28 cases. Radiology 1997;203(3):779–83.

103. Tsukada A, Ishizaki Y, Nobukawa B, et al. Embryonal sarcoma of the liver in an adult mimicking complicated hepatic cyst: MRI findings. J Magn Reson Imaging 2010;31(6):1477–80.

# Hepatocellular Carcinoma and Other Hepatic Malignancies: MR Imaging

Christopher G. Roth, MD[a],*, Donald G. Mitchell, MD[b]

## KEYWORDS

- Hepatocellular carcinoma • Liver metastases • Cholangiocarcinoma • Fibrolamellar carcinoma
- Hepatoblastoma • Epithelioid hemangioendothelioma • Embryonal sarcoma • Hepatic lymphoma

## KEY POINTS

- Magnetic resonance imaging is the most accurate noninvasive diagnostic method to evaluate liver lesions.
- Categorizing malignant liver lesions based on solid versus cystic nature and solid lesion vascularity provides a useful diagnostic algorithm.
- Hepatocellular carcinoma is the most common primary hepatic malignancy, usually occurring in the setting of chronic liver disease, representing the end point of the carcinogenic pathway and featuring an array of distinctive imaging features.
- Metastases are the most common secondary malignant liver lesions and malignant liver lesions overall and generally conform to the vascularity algorithmic approach.

## INTRODUCTION

Characterizing liver lesions is a common endeavor in clinical practice. Although the ultimate goal is to assign a definitive diagnosis, the first step is generally to differentiate benign from malignant lesions. Malignant lesion management depends on the diagnosis, whereas benign lesions are managed expectantly. Malignant lesion management ranges from surveillance or local ablative treatment in the case of small hepatocellular carcinoma (HCC) lesions to surgical resection in a variety of clinical scenarios to nonsurgical treatments, such as intra-arterial chemotherapy for multiple malignant lesions. Therefore, accurate diagnosis is important. However, malignant liver lesions often feature distinctive characteristics facilitating accurate diagnosis.

There are several malignant liver lesions, but liver metastases and HCC outnumber the rest (**Table 1**). The 2 most common malignant liver lesions generally harbor clues to the diagnosis. Metastases (the most common hepatic malignancy[1]) usually present in a multifocal distribution with known primary malignancy outside the liver, whereas HCC (the most common primary hepatic malignancy) usually arises in the setting of cirrhosis. Beyond these clues, lesion-specific magnetic resonance (MR) imaging features generally present the most accurate diagnostic information short of histopathologic analysis. In a study analyzing the ability of MR imaging to characterize 96 lesions that are indeterminate on computed tomography (CT), MR imaging definitively characterized 58% of these with 99% accuracy.[2] Because of its diagnostic accuracy and technical

[a] Department of Radiology, TJUH, Methodist, Thomas Jefferson University, 2301 South Broad Street, Philadelphia, PA 19148, USA; [b] Department of Radiology, Thomas Jefferson University, 1094 Main Building, 132 South 10th Street, Philadelphia, PA 19107, USA
* Corresponding author.
E-mail address: christopher.roth@jefferson.edu

Radiol Clin N Am 52 (2014) 683–707
http://dx.doi.org/10.1016/j.rcl.2014.02.015
0033-8389/14/$ – see front matter © 2014 Elsevier Inc. All rights reserved.

| Table 1 | |
| --- | --- |
| **Malignant liver tumors** | |
| Epithelial tumors | HCC |
| | Intrahepatic cholangiocarcinoma |
| | Bile duct cystadenocarcinoma |
| | Combined HCC and cholangiocarcinoma |
| | Hepatoblastoma |
| | Undifferentiated carcinoma |
| Nonepithelial tumors | Epithelioid hemangioendothelioma |
| | Angiosarcoma |
| | Embryonal sarcoma |
| | Rhabdomyosarcoma |
| | Others |
| Miscellaneous tumors | Solitary fibrous tumor |
| | Teratoma |
| | Yolk sac tumor |
| | Carcinosarcoma |
| | Kaposi sarcoma |
| | Rhabdoid tumor |
| | Others |
| Hematopoietic and lymphoid tumors | Non-Hodgkin lymphoma |
| Secondary tumors | Carcinoma > lymphoma > sarcoma |

Data from Hirohashi S, Ishak KG, Kojiro M, et al. Pathology and genetics of tumors of the digestive system. In: Hamilton SR, Aaltonen LA, editors. World Health Organization classification of tumors. Lyon (France): IARC Press; 2000. p. 203–17.

| Table 2 | |
| --- | --- |
| **Malignant liver lesions by vascularity** | |
| **Hypovascular Lesions** | **Hypervascular Lesions** |
| Intrahepatic cholangiocarcinoma | Hepatocellular carcinoma |
| Lymphoma | Sarcomas |
| **Hypovascular Metastases** | **Hypervascular Metastases** |
| Colorectal carcinoma | Renal cell carcinoma |
| Pancreatic adenocarcinoma | Neuroendocrine tumors |
| Gastric carcinoma | Breast carcinoma |
| Lung carcinoma | Melanoma |
| Genitourinary (prostate, bladder) | Carcinoid tumor |

advancements ensuring superior and more reproducible image quality, MR imaging has gained an increasingly central role in evaluating liver lesions. Familiarity with MR imaging features is therefore increasingly important and certain general principles provide a useful framework.

Although many MR imaging features deserve attention, enhancement is usually the most important. Most malignant (and solid benign) liver lesions are either hypovascular or hypervascular; the remaining lesions are isovascular (**Table 2**). In addition, this lesional enhancement scheme is universally referenced and important to understand. Hypervascular liver lesions enhance avidly (more than normal liver), whereas hypovascular liver lesions enhance less than normal liver on arterial-phase images. Malignant lesions typically show relative hypointensity to liver on portal-phase and delayed postcontrast images. A constellation of additional imaging features help to further characterize liver lesions (**Table 3**). In addition, a small minority of malignant lesions are cystic, necessitating the ability to discriminate solid from cystic lesions. Appreciating these features requires an understanding of MR imaging technique and the usefulness of the various MR sequences.

## NORMAL ANATOMY AND IMAGING TECHNIQUE

The normal liver appearance serves as the background against which to describe the appearance of liver lesions. For example, most malignant liver lesions are hyperintense to the low signal of normal liver on T2-weighted imaging (T2WI), with the opposite appearance on T1-weighted imaging (T1WI), because of the higher content of bound water of hepatic parenchyma. Although a complete description of the liver imaging protocol is beyond the scope of this article, a brief review and systematic approach facilitates the discussion of lesion differential diagnosis. Sequences generally stratify into 2 major categories: T1 weighted and T2 weighted (**Table 4**). Because the liver receives approximately three-quarters of its blood supply from the portal system and the remainder from the hepatic artery, peak hepatic enhancement occurs during the portal phase and only mild enhancement is perceptible during the arterial phase. On delayed images, malignant lesions usually appear hypointense. This effect is magnified with hepatobiliary (HB) agents such as gadoxetate disodium, with which the normal liver retains contrast, accentuating the relative hypointensity of most liver lesions (typically imaged 20 minutes after injection: the hepatocyte or hepatobiliary phase [HP]).

T1WI sequences provide additional diagnostic information in characterizing liver lesions. Although out-of-phase (OOP) and in-phase images are usually acquired simultaneously, these

**Table 3**
**Malignant liver lesion features**

|  | Scar | Capsule | Calcium | Fat | Blood | Cystic |
|---|---|---|---|---|---|---|
| HCC | X | X | — | X | X | X |
| FLC | X | — | X | — | — | — |
| IC | X | — | X | — | — | — |
| Metastases | — | — | X | — | X | X |
| Angiosarcoma | — | — | — | — | X | — |
| Biliary cystadenocarcinoma | — | X | — | — | — | X |

*Abbreviations:* FLC, fibrolamellar carcinoma; IC, intrahepatic cholangiocarcinoma.

T1-weighted images are usually displayed as 2 separate sequences, and each possesses unique attributes. In addition to their inherent T1 contrast, OOP images add sensitivity to microscopic fat, which is occasionally present in HCC. T1-weighted in-phase images display susceptibility artifact as increased blooming compared with their counterpart OOP images, depicting hemosiderin in chronic hemorrhage or iron in hemochromatosis, for example. The T1-weighted fat-suppressed precontrast sequence optimally displays paramagnetic substances including gadolinium, melanin, and methemoglobin.

Moderately T2-weighted images (echo time [TE] approximately 80 milliseconds) maximize tissue contrast for water bound to macromolecules, which generally exists in higher concentration in malignant lesions compared with normal liver tissue. As a result, these lesions appear bright on moderately T2-weighted images. However, signal of hepatic lesions decays at higher TE, and lesion conspicuity fades on heavily T2-weighted images (TE approximately 180–200 milliseconds). Heavily T2-weighted images better show free water molecules, which are present in cerebrospinal fluid, bile, and cysts, and cystic or necrotic change in malignant lesions. Diffusion-weighted images typically combine T2 weighting with diffusion weighting, maximizing contrast between the high

bound water content and diffusion restriction of most malignant liver lesions relative to liver parenchyma.[3]

## IMAGING FINDINGS AND PATHOLOGY
### Primary Lesions

#### Hepatocellular carcinoma
HCC is the most common primary malignant tumor and is derived from hepatocytes. The most common causes are chronic viral infection (hepatitis B and C), aflatoxin $B_1$ ingestion, and chronic alcohol abuse. HCC usually develops in the setting of cirrhosis along a predictable carcinogenetic pathway (**Fig. 1**). The common denominator is chronic inflammation inducing regeneration, which is the substrate for carcinogenesis; 70% to 99% of HCC lesions develop in the setting of macronodular cirrhosis.[4] Although most HCCs associated with chronic hepatitis B virus (HBV) infection occur in cirrhosis (70%–80%), HBV is carcinogenic independently of cirrhosis, which is not true of chronic hepatitis C virus (HCV) infection.[5]

The annual incidence of HCC is more than 1 million worldwide, and approximately 20,000 in the United States.[6] HCC affects men 2 to 4 times as frequently as women and rarely develops before the age of 40 years, peaking in incidence around 70 years of age. Regardless of the cause,

**Table 4**
**MR imaging protocol scheme**

| T1-weighted Sequences | | T2-weighted Sequences | |
|---|---|---|---|
| Pulse Sequence | Utility | Pulse Sequence | Utility |
| Out of phase | Microscopic fat | Steady state | Solid tissue/fluid |
| In phase | Susceptibility | Heavily weighted | Free water |
| Precontrast | Paramagnetism | Moderately weighted | Bound water |
| Dynamic | Solid tissue | MRCP | Water only |
| Delayed | Extracellular | Diffusion weighted | Hypercellular |

*Abbreviation:* MRCP, magnetic resonance cholangiopancreatography.

80% to 90% of patients are cirrhotic, with the 5-year cumulative HCC risk in cirrhosis ranging between 5% and 30%, depending on the cause and stage of cirrhosis.[7] Nonspecific clinical signs (hepatomegaly, ascites, fever, and jaundice) overlap with signs of cirrhosis, which is usually present. Laboratory value derangements, specifically increased liver function tests (aspartate aminotransferase, alanine aminotransferase, AP, and GGT), reflect underlying liver disease and/or HCC. However, although alpha fetoprotein (AFP) levels increase in the absence of HCC, a significantly increased AFP level of more than 500 ng/mL or a continuously increasing AFP level strongly suggests HCC.

The American Association for the Study of Liver Diseases recommends surveillance for patients at high risk for HCC.[8] However, the evidence to support surveillance is mixed. In a randomized controlled trial including approximately 19,000 patients with HBV, serial AFP assessment and ultrasonography (US) surveillance every 6 months resulted in a 37% reduction in mortality from HCC.[9] Nonetheless, other studies have shown less or no benefit and the evidence for surveillance is collectively modest. Surveillance generally varies by institution and serial AFP and US tends to be the norm. However, some institutions substitute MR imaging for US. US is useful for screening, but lacks specificity, especially in the setting of cirrhosis.[10] As a result, when not used as the primary surveillance modality, MR imaging has a major problem-solving role in a subset of patients with abnormal or equivocal US or CT findings.

Although HCC generally features classic imaging findings, the appearance varies depending on the stage of development, with more advanced HCCs showing a greater degree of heterogeneity and variability. The American College of Radiology (ACR) Liver Imaging Reporting and Data System (LI-RADS)[11] defines major imaging features, such as arterial-phase hyperenhancement, portal or delayed phase hypoenhancement (washout appearance), capsule appearance, venous invasion, and threshold growth (at least 50% increase in diameter within 6 months). In addition, LI-RADS enumerates several ancillary features that favor HCC, such as mild to moderate T2 hyperintensity, restricted diffusion, mosaic architecture, nodule-in-nodule appearance, intralesional fat, blood products, and other features that are discussed in greater detail in the ACR LI-RADS Web site (http://www.acr.org/Quality-Safety/Resources/LIRADS).

The multitude of HCC imaging features requires careful review of multiple imaging sequences, especially in the case of large, advanced HCCs.

With continued growth and development, HCCs tend to show increasing hemorrhage and necrosis and the propensity to invade portal and hepatic veins. Although smaller, less advanced HCCs show the solitary growth pattern, and additional growth patterns observed in advanced HCC include multifocal and infiltrative patterns. When not complicated by coagulative necrosis, hemorrhage, or intralesional fat, advanced HCCs tend to be T1 hypointense and T2 hyperintense. However, early HCCs are commonly T1 hyperintense and T2 hypointense or isointense. The characteristic T2 mosaic signal intensity pattern reflects multiple tumoral growth centers interspersed with foci of necrosis and noncancerous regenerative tissue (Figs. 2 and 3).[12] Foci of hemorrhage show the reverse signal characteristics and intralesional fat usually manifests with OOP signal loss (and less likely signal loss on fat-saturated sequences) (see Fig. 3; Fig. 4). An outer fibrous capsule measuring 0.5 to 3 mm in thickness generally appears uniformly hypointense with delayed enhancement (Fig. 5). With increased thickness, a concentric capsular appearance with inner uniformly hypointense fibrous and outer T2-hyperintense vascular rings is occasionally observed.[13] Venous invasion simulates the signal and enhancement characteristics of the parent tumor; bland tumor thrombus appears as a uniformly hypointense, nonenhancing filling defect on steady-state and postcontrast images (Fig. 6). The peripheral hepatic tissue typically shows T2 hyperintensity reflecting edematous change[14] and arterial compensatory hyperenhancement. The tumor shows arterial hyperenhancement, which is homogeneous, multinodular, or heterogeneous with portal and delayed washout. With hepatobiliary agents, most HCC lesions show prominent hypointensity against the hyperintense parenchymal background because of the absence of functional hepatocytes. Well-differentiated HCCs rarely show hypointensity on delayed HP images. Diffusion-weighted images usually show hyperintensity with corresponding hypointensity on the apparent diffusion coefficient (ADC) map images reflecting hypercellularity and restricted diffusion (see Fig. 5).

Given the poor prognosis (overall 1-year survival rate of 47%[15]) combined with the progressive nature of the underlying chronic liver disease, liver transplantation (LT) has become the recommended treatment of patients presenting with early-stage HCC. The United Network for Organ Sharing (UNOS) was established to facilitate the equitable allocation of donor livers, historically guided by the Milan Criteria (MC). The MC restrict donor livers to patients with either 1 lesion smaller than 5 cm or up to 3 lesions smaller than 3 cm with no

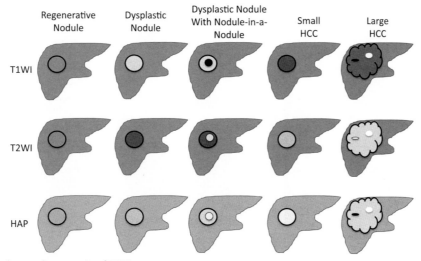

Fig. 1. Stepwise carcinogenesis of HCC.

extrahepatic manifestations and no vascular invasion.[16] Whether the MC are too restrictive has been the subject of debate, and more lenient criteria, such as the UCSF (University of California, San Francisco) Criteria (1 tumor ≤ 6.5 cm or ≤3 tumors ≤4.5 cm and total diameter ≤8 cm[17]), have been proposed with promising results.[18] In addition to observing these criteria (typically institutionally dependent), awareness of the extrahepatic patterns of spread has important implications for patient management. In addition to direct portal and hepatic venous invasion, HCC has a propensity for lymphatic and distant metastatic spread, especially when exceeding 5 cm.[19] Extrahepatic HCC has been reported to have a survival rate of approximately 25% and median survival period of 7 months.[20] Most common extrahepatic metastatic destinations are the lungs,

followed by regional lymph nodes (perihepatic, peripancreatic, and retroperitoneal), regional spread along the diaphragm, adrenal glands, and bones (Fig. 7).[21]

HCC percutaneous ablative techniques have been developed to prolong transplant candidacy in patients with chronic liver disease and small HCCs; radiofrequency ablation (RFA) has superseded other percutaneous methods. In patients with advanced HCC (without vascular invasion or extrahepatic spread), transarterial chemotherapy is the only treatment that has proved to extend life expectancy.[22–25] Regardless of the treatment modality, the best indicator of successful ablation is absent enhancement on postcontrast images. Whether from hemorrhagic necrosis or lipiodol after chemoembolization, the ablation cavity occasionally appears T1 hyperintense and

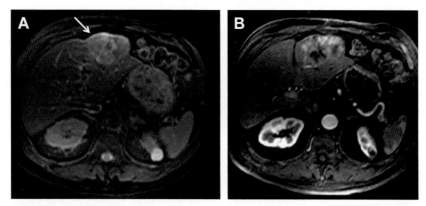

Fig. 2. HCC mosaic appearance. (A) Axial fat-suppressed T2-weighted image reveals a heterogeneously moderately hyperintense lesion bulging the liver capsule (arrow) showing the mosaic appearance with multiple internal foci of varying signal intensity. (B) Axial arterial-phase postcontrast image also shows a mosaic enhancement pattern.

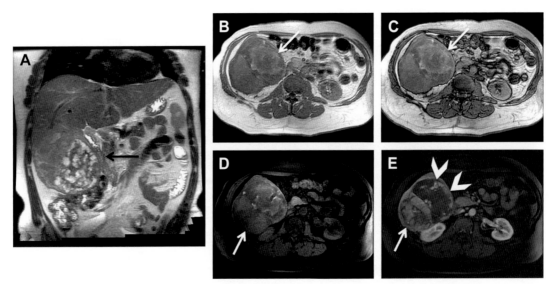

**Fig. 3.** Hemorrhagic HCC. (*A*) Coronal T2-weighted image shows a large, complex HCC extends inferiorly from the liver (*arrow*) with near fluid hyperintensity. (*B*) Axial in-phase T1-weighted image shows mild central hyperintensity in the anterior component (*arrow*). (*C*) Axial OOP T1-weighted image shows no signal loss, excluding intracellular fat (*arrow*). (*D*) Axial fat-suppressed T1-weighted image shows hyperintensity (*arrow*), confirming paramagnetism and excluding macroscopic fat. (*E*) Axial arterial-phase postcontrast axial image shows avid enhancement in the solid component (*arrow*) and minimal, peripheral enhancement surrounding the hemorrhage (*arrowheads*).

subtracted images better show the presence or absence of enhancement in this instance.[26] Although a thin, smooth rim of hyperemic reactive tissue persists around the ablated cavity for several months,[27] nodular or masslike internal or perilesional enhancement suggests residual or recurrent tumor (**Fig. 8**). Lack of hyperintensity on diffusion-weighted imaging (DWI) and evidence of regression of restricted diffusion on ADC maps corroborates successful tumor ablation.[28]

Early HCCs are smaller, well differentiated, and typically show more homogeneous imaging features (**Fig. 9**). HCCs less than 2 cm usually show intense arterial enhancement, rapid washout, and T2 hyperintensity.[29] Small HCC lesion variability is a function of the carcinogenic pathway (see

**Fig. 1**); as nodules degenerate from dysplastic to neoplastic, imaging features evolve. As a result, familiarity with cirrhotic nodule imaging features is an integral part of understanding and correctly identifying HCC imaging appearance.

The premalignant dysplastic nodule is defined as a cluster of dysplastic hepatocytes lacking the histologic criteria for malignancy. Dysplastic nodules also usually lack arterial hyperenhancement (except for a small minority of high-grade lesions) because their main blood supply is the portal venous system, in contradistinction to most HCCs.[30,31] Dysplastic nodules generally show enhancement commensurate with the normal liver as a function of their common blood supply. In addition, dysplastic nodule T2 signal is usually

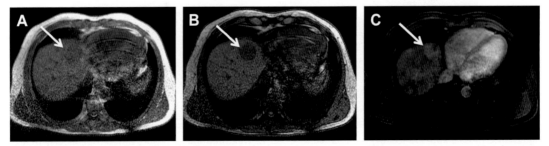

**Fig. 4.** HCC with intralesional fat. (*A*) Axial in-phase T1-weighted image shows a faintly hypointense lesion near the liver dome (*arrow*). (*B*) Corresponding axial OOP image shows prominent signal loss indicating intracellular fat (*arrow*). (*C*) Axial arterial-phase postcontrast image shows hypervascularity (*arrow*).

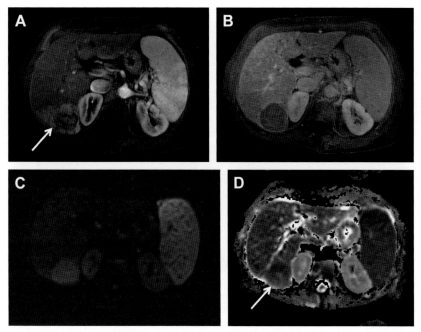

**Fig. 5.** HCC capsule. (*A*) Axial arterial-phase postcontrast image shows a heterogeneously hypervascular lesion (*arrow*) with adjacent perilesional enhancement. (*B*) Axial delayed postcontrast image showing lesional washout with a late enhancing capsule. (*C*) Axial diffusion-weighted image shows lesional hyperintensity. (*D*) Corresponding apparent diffusion coefficient (ADC) map reveals hypointensity (*arrow*) indicating diffusion restriction.

hypointense and virtually never hyperintense (in contradistinction to HCC).[32,33] Dysplastic nodules usually show T1 and T2 signal isointensity to normal liver. Occasional dysplastic nodular T1 hyperintensity has been attributed to intralesional accumulation of lipid, protein, and/or copper.[34,35]

Regenerative nodules (RNs) have the T1 and T2 signal of normal liver, but may be depicted as high T1 signal, low T2 signal, and delayed postcontrast hypointensity against the background of reticular fibrosis. RNs develop in response to parenchymal damage caused by chronic inflammation and ensuing fibrosis (see **Fig. 1**) and represent island of histologically normal hepatocytes, usually surrounded by bridging bands of reticular fibrosis. As such, RNs lack unpaired arterial blood supply and usually show no abnormal hyperarterial enhancement. Hypervascular nodules are occasionally diagnosed histologically as RNs, without dysplasia, and are likely benign hyperplastic nodules, similar to focal nodular hyperplasia. However, most RNs show signal intensity and enhancement characteristics that are identical to those of normal hepatic parenchyma.[36] Siderotic

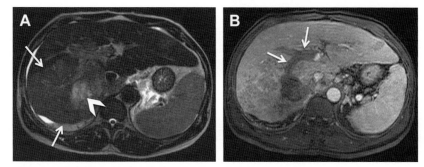

**Fig. 6.** HCC with venous invasion. (*A*) Axial T2-weighted image reveals a large, mildly hyperintense lesion (*arrows*) with a cystic/necrotic focus (*arrowhead*). (*B*) Axial portal-phase postcontrast image shows heterogeneous washout with extensive thrombus throughout the visualized right portal vein (*arrows*).

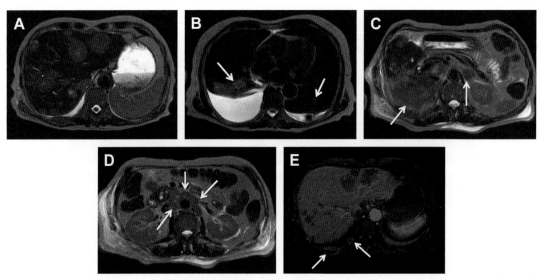

Fig. 7. HCC metastatic spread. (*A*) Axial T2-weighted image shows multifocal hyperintense HCC lesions. (*B*) Axial T2-weighted image reveals bilateral pleural effusions and large right and small left lower lobe metastases (*arrows*). (*C*) Axial T2-weighted image shows bilateral adrenal metastases (*arrows*). (*D*) Axial T2-weighted image shows metastatic retroperitoneal lymphadenopathy (*arrows*). (*E*) The axial T1-weighted fat-suppressed postcontrast image shows multiple washed out multifocal HCC lesions and 2 rib lesions (*arrows*).

RNs also enhance isointensely and show uniform hypointensity and susceptibility artifact because of the iron deposition (**Fig. 10**).

In summary, evaluating the liver for possible HCC requires not just an understanding of HCC imaging features but also an appreciation of the liver nodule carcinogenic pathway and the imaging appearances of its precursors. The sine qua non is generally arterial hyperenhancement and ancillary features include diffusion restriction, washout and hypointensity on HP imaging, mosaic enhancement pattern, delayed capsular

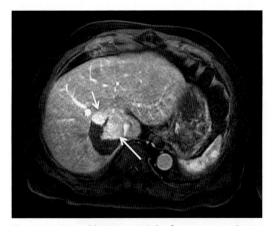

Fig. 8. HCC ablation. Axial fat-suppressed T1-weighted postcontrast image shows gross peripheral, nodular enhancement (*arrows*) in a previously ablated HCC, indicating residual or recurrent tumor.

enhancement, T2 hyperintensity, intralesional fat and/or hemorrhage, and occasionally vascular invasion.

### Fibrolamellar carcinoma

Fibrolamellar carcinoma (FLC) represents a malignant hepatocellular tumor with clinical, histopathologic, and imaging features distinct from HCC. Although several HCC cytologic variants exist (**Table 5**), FLC is distinguished from other hepatocellular malignancies by the younger age at presentation (adolescents and young adults), lack of known risk factors or association with cirrhosis and chronic liver disease, absence of serum tumor markers, and better prognosis and chance for surgical cure.

The imaging diagnosis of FLC relies on a combination of clinical and imaging factors. First, FLC peaks during the second and third decades of life without gender predilection. The appearance of a large, solitary, lobulated, heterogeneously hypervascular mass in a young patient without chronic liver disease or cirrhosis suggests the possibility of FLC (**Fig. 11**). Uniformly hypointense radial septa and central scar (approximately 70% of cases[37]) showing at most mild delayed enhancement further supports the diagnosis of FLC. FLCs are generally T1 hypointense and T2 hyperintense and usually show lobulated borders, and intratumoral calcification is observed in 35% to 55% of cases. Capsular retraction and vascular invasion or encasement are rare findings

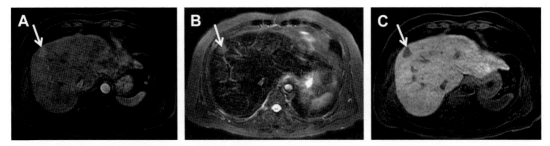

**Fig. 9.** Small HCC. (*A*) Axial fat-suppressed T1-weighted arterial-phase postcontrast image shows a uniformly hypervascular lesion (*arrow*). (*B*) Axial inversion recovery image shows uniform hyperintensity (*arrow*). (*C*) Axial fat-suppressed T1-weighted delayed hepatobiliary-phase image confirms lack of functional hepatocytes (*arrow*).

(approximately 10% and 5%, respectively) and are more common in cholangiocarcinoma and HCC.[38]

### Intrahepatic cholangiocarcinoma

Cholangiocarcinoma, a malignant tumor composed of cells of biliary ductal origin, arises anywhere along the intrahepatic or extrahepatic biliary tree. There are 3 anatomic categories of cholangiocarcinoma: (1) extrahepatic (common bile duct), (2) at or near the hepatic ductal (hilar) confluence (Klatskin tumor), and (3) intrahepatic (or peripheral). The intrahepatic cholangiocarcinoma (IHC) is the second most common primary hepatic malignancy, constituting approximately 10% to 20% of all primary malignancies.[39–41]

Chronic biliary inflammation confers a risk of developing cholangiocarcinoma and several specific risk factors have been identified (**Table 6**). Although most of these risk factors are more prevalent in the Eastern world, primary sclerosing cholangitis is among the most common risk factors in Western countries.

Three cholangiocarcinoma growth patterns have been observed and codified by the Liver Cancer Study Group of Japan: (1) mass forming, (2) periductal infiltrating, and (3) intraductal.[42] IHC typically shows the mass-forming growth pattern as a homogeneous, intraparenchymal mass with well-defined borders and (occasionally) peripheral biliary dilatation. Although central T2

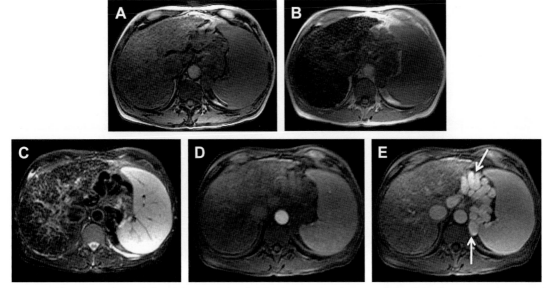

**Fig. 10.** Siderotic nodules. (*A*) Axial T1-weighted OOP image showing grossly nodular liver parenchyma and splenomegaly. (*B*) Axial T1-weighted in-phase image reveals marked nodular signal loss, or susceptibility, induced by iron distributed throughout the siderotic nodules. (*C*) Axial T2-weighted fat-suppressed image also reveals marked hypointensity of the many siderotic nodules. Serpiginous signal voids correspond with varices. (*D*) Axial fat-suppressed T1-weighted arterial-phase image shows uniform enhancement without abnormal hypervascularity. (*E*) Axial T1-weighted portal-phase image shows even nodular enhancement with enhancing interdigitating fibrotic bands. Massive gastrohepatic varices (*arrows*) indicate portal hypertension.

**Table 5**
Selected hepatocellular cytologic/pathologic variants

| Variant | Features |
| --- | --- |
| Pleomorphic cell | Common in poorly differentiated tumors |
| Clear cell | Abundant glycogen (OOP signal loss) |
| Sarcomatous change | Central necrosis and hemorrhage |
| Fatty change | Diffuse fatty change in small tumors |
| Sclerosing | Intense fibrosis Hypervascular with progressive enhancement Capsular retraction |
| Fibrolamellar | Not associated with cirrhosis Hypointense delayed-enhancing central scar Hypointense delayed-enhancing radial septa |

hypointensity reflecting desmoplasia is an occasional finding, T2 hyperintensity is the rule with commensurate T1 hypointensity. In addition, a distinctive enhancement pattern with minimal to moderate thin peripheral enhancement with gradual centripetal progression to hyperenhancement on delayed images also helps to narrow the differential diagnosis (**Fig. 12**).[43] With hepatobiliary contrast agents, prominent hypointensity on delayed images reflects the lack of functional hepatocytes.[44] An additional diagnostic clue is the presence of capsular retraction (**Fig. 13**), reflecting fibrosis, which is a common feature of cholangiocarcinoma. Although vascular encasement commonly occurs, macroscopically visible tumor thrombus is rarely detected.

IHC rarely shows a periductal-infiltrating growth pattern, extending along and narrowing the involved biliary radicle with exuberant wall thickening and a branching or spiculated morphology (**Fig. 14**). Ductal narrowing or obliteration with upstream dilatation often assists in identifying the primary lesion. The intraductal growth pattern is also rarely shown by IHC, generally manifesting with an intraductal papillary mass with proximal biliary dilatation.

*Biliary cystadenocarcinoma*
Biliary cystadenocarcinoma (BCC) and its benign counterpart biliary cystadenoma (BC) are tumors arising from hepatobiliary epithelium proximal to the hepatic hilum. These cystic lesions are lined by epithelium with papillary infoldings usually

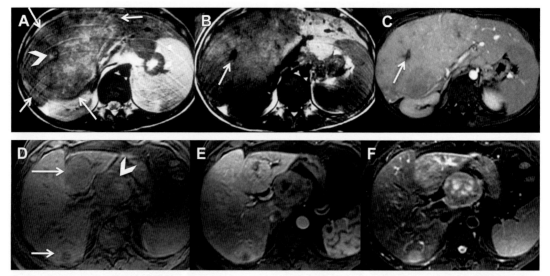

**Fig. 11.** FLC. (*A*) Axial T2-weighted image from a study performed decades ago (attesting to the rarity of FLC) shows a large, heterogeneously hyperintense lesion in the right lobe (*arrows*) with a central scar (*arrowhead*). (*B*) The corresponding axial T1-weighted image shows the central scar to better advantage (*arrow*). (*C*) The T1-weighted postcontrast image shows mildly heterogeneous enhancement and the nonenhancing central scar (*arrow*). Note the normal appearance of the spared lateral segment. (*D*) Axial T1-weighted precontrast image performed 15 years later in a patient with normal liver morphology shows 2 hypointense lesions (*arrows*) and periportal lymphadenopathy (*arrowhead*). (*E*) Arterial-phase postcontrast T1-weighted image shows heterogeneous arterial enhancement. (*F*) Axial T2-weighted image shows heterogeneous lesional hyperintensity.

**Table 6**
**Risk factors for cholangiocarcinoma**

| | |
|---|---|
| Liver flukes | *Clonorchis sinensis* |
| | *Opisthorchis viverini* |
| Hepatolithiasis (recurrent pyogenic cholangitis) | |
| Primary sclerosing cholangitis | |
| Viral infections | Human immunodeficiency virus |
| | HBV |
| | HCV |
| | Epstein-Barr virus |
| Anatomic anomalies | Anomalous pancreaticobiliary junction |
| | Choledochal cyst |
| Malformation (fibrocystic liver diseases; eg, Caroli disease) | |
| Environmental and occupational toxins | Thorotrast |
| | Dioxin |
| | Polyvinyl chloride |
| Biliary-enteric drainage procedures | |
| Excessive alcohol consumption | |

*Data from* Chung YE, Kim MJ, Park YN, et al. Varying appearances of cholangiocarcinoma: Radiologic-pathologic correlation. Radiographics 2009;29:683–700.

secreting fluid, which is more commonly mucous than serous. BCCs are rare tumors (estimated incidence: BC, 1 in 20,000–100,000 and BCC, 1 in 10 million) presenting with an average age of between 50 and 60 years of age.[45,46] Although BCs are lined by columnar epithelium with ovarianlike stroma and are essentially limited to women, BCCs generally lack ovarian stroma, although they seem to favor women as well.[47] Although BCCs are thought to undergo malignant transformation from BCs, the details are not understood and malignant change either focally or multifocally involves the epithelial lining.

BCs and BCCs are usually multiloculated and well-circumscribed lesions ranging in size from a few centimeters to more than 20 cm, often with a fibrous capsule (**Fig. 15**). Cystic contents are usually mucinous, T1 hypointense, and T2 hyperintense, and occasional fluid-fluid levels indicate hemorrhage. Septal and mural calcifications are occasionally present (**Fig. 16**). Enhancement of the peripheral capsule and variable septation and mural nodularity helps to differentiate these lesions from other hepatic cystic lesions. Chief diagnostic differential considerations include biliary cystic hamartomas (more common septated cystic masses), hemorrhagic and infected hepatic cysts, pyogenic abscesses, cystic metastases, and hydatid cysts. BC and BCC are diagnoses of exclusion, but lesion-specific imaging features

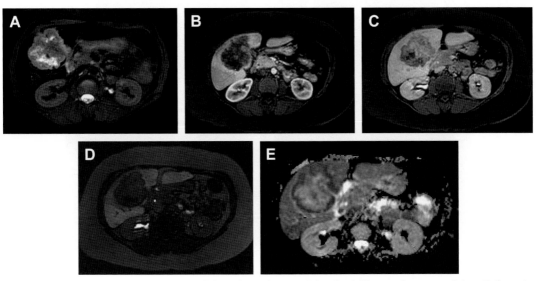

**Fig. 12.** Intrahepatic cholangiocarcinoma. (*A*) Moderately T2-weighted axial image shows a peripherally hyperintense lesion with central hypointensity. (*B*) The arterial-phase postcontrast fat-suppressed T1-weighted image shows early peripheral enhancement. (*C*) The delayed postcontrast fat-suppressed T1-weighted image shows the centripetally progressive enhancement pattern. (*D*) The 20 minute–delayed hepatobiliary T1-weighted image shows lack of contrast uptake and nonhepatocellular composition. (*E*) The ADC map image shows peripheral hypointensity and diffusion restriction corresponding with the hypercellular zone with relative hyperintensity and facilitated diffusion in the necrotic center.

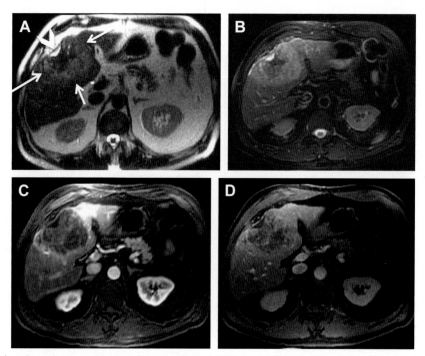

**Fig. 13.** Cholangiocarcinoma with capsular retraction. (*A*) The axial heavily T2-weighted image shows a mildly hyperintense lesion (*arrows*) with central hypointensity with marked focal indentation of the liver surface (*arrowhead*) corresponding with capsular retraction. (*B*) The moderately T2-weighted fat-suppressed image shows the peripheral hyperintensity and central hypointensity pattern to better advantage and also shows the capsular retraction. (*C*) The arterial-phase postcontrast fat-suppressed T1-weighted image reveals early peripheral enhancement. (*D*) The delayed postcontrast fat-suppressed T1-weighted image shows the delayed centripetal enhancement pattern.

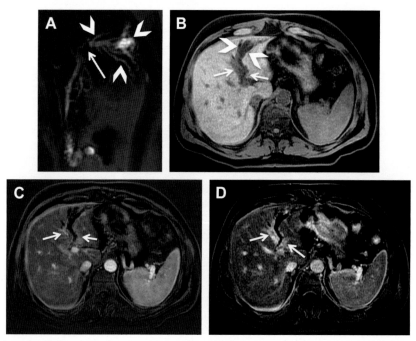

**Fig. 14.** Intrahepatic cholangiocarcinoma with periductal-infiltrating growth pattern. (*A*) The two-dimensional radial MR cholangiopancreatography image shows high-grade segmental narrowing of the left hepatic bile duct (*arrow*) with upstream biliary dilatation (*arrowheads*). (*B*) The corresponding T1-weighted fat-suppressed image shows ill-defined, confluent periportal hypointensity (*arrows*) with tubular fluid hypointensity (*arrowheads*) corresponding with biliary dilatation. (*C*) T1-weighted portal-phase subtracted postcontrast image shows mild lesional enhancement (*arrows*). (*D*) The corresponding T1-weighted delayed subtracted postcontrast image shows progressive enhancement (*arrows*).

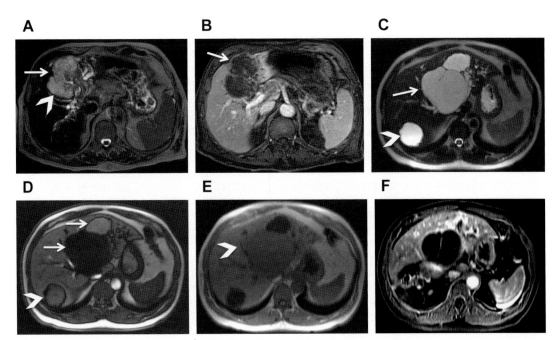

**Fig. 15.** Biliary cystadenocarcinoma. (*A*) Axial heavily T2-weighted image shows a large, moderately hyperintense lesion centered in the medial segment (*arrow*) with associated intrahepatic biliary dilatation. The hypointense fibrous capsule is visible along the posterior margin (*arrowhead*). (*B*) The T1-weighted postcontrast image shows nodular septal enhancement corresponding with solid, neoplastic tissue. The enhancing fibrous capsule is best visualized along the ventral margin (*arrow*). (*C*) A heavily T2-weighted image in a different patient reveals a large, biloculated and septated cystic lesion in the left lobe (*arrow*) with mild irregular thickening of the septa. (*D, E*) The in-phase image shows variable locular signal intensity with T1 hypointensity (*arrows*) and mild hyper-intensity of the larger locule (*arrowhead*) indicating proteinaceous contents. (*F*) The fat-suppressed postcontrast T1-weighted image shows capsular and septal enhancement.

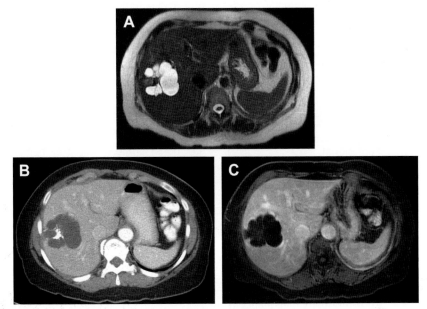

**Fig. 16.** Biliary cystadenocarcinoma with calcification. (*A*) The heavily T2-weighted axial image reveals a complex cystic lesion in the anterior segment with an eccentric hypointensity. (*B*) The MR hypointensity corresponds with calcification as seen on the axial contrast-enhanced CT image. (*C*) The delayed postcontrast T1-weighted image shows peripheral enhancement of the fibrous capsule and internal septal enhancement.

help to eliminate other cystic lesions from consideration (**Table 7**). Because of the impossibility of excluding malignancy (after infection has been excluded) and the inaccuracy of diagnostic methods (a recent study showed 30% combined sensitivity of CT, US, and fine-needle aspiration) these lesions are generally resected surgically.[48]

## Hepatoblastoma

Hepatoblastoma is the most common pediatric malignant liver tumor, composed of embryonal cells with divergent differentiation patterns, ranging from embryonal cells to fetal hepatocytes to osteoid material to fibrous connective tissue to striated muscle. Hepatoblastoma stratifies into 2 broad histologic types: the epithelial and the mixed epithelial and mesenchymal types (**Table 8**). Epithelial forms are often the well-differentiated fetal variety (approximately 31% of tumors), although nearly half also contain an embryonal epithelial component that resembles embryonal or small, round cell neoplasms. In addition to fetal and embryonal epithelial elements, mixed tumors include primitive and differentiated mesenchymal tissues.[49]

The median age of occurrence is 1 year and 90% of hepatoblastomas present before the age of 5 years, with a slight male predilection (1.5:1 to 2:1).[50] These tumors are most commonly detected in the setting of an enlarging abdomen and anorexia and weight loss are common accompanying signs. Abdominal pain, nausea and vomiting, and (especially) jaundice less frequently occur. Approximately 5% are associated with any of

**Table 7**
**Differential diagnosis in biliary cystadenocarcinoma (and BC)**

| Lesion | Discriminating Feature(s) |
|---|---|
| Hemorrhagic or infected hepatic cyst | No enhancement Perilesional enhancement Clinical signs of infection |
| Pyogenic abscess | Cluster sign Perilesional enhancement Secondary signs (diaphragmatic elevation, right pleural effusion) Clinical signs of infection |
| Cystic metastasis | Multiplicity Known primary malignancy |
| Hydatid cyst | Daughter cysts Scolices Characteristic demographics |

**Table 8**
**Histologic classification of hepatoblastoma**

| Epithelial Type (%) | Mixed Epithelial and Mesenchymal Type (%) |
|---|---|
| Fetal pattern (31) Embryonal and fetal pattern (19) | Mesenchymal tissue limited to osteoid, cartilaginous, and fibrous tissue (19) |
| Macrotrabecular pattern (3) Small cell undifferentiated pattern (3) | Teratoid with other tissues including striated muscle, melanin, and squamous epithelium (25) |

several clinical syndromes, malformations, and other conditions, including Gardner syndrome, familial adenomatous polyposis, and Beckwith-Wiedemann syndrome. Although nonspecific anemia frequently accompanies this neoplasm, AFP is the primary diagnostic and surveillance laboratory parameter, and it is increased in up to 90% of patients.[51]

Eighty percent of hepatoblastomas are solitary, involving the right lobe in 58% of cases. Hepatoblastomas range in size from a few centimeters to more than 15 cm and generally show lobulated borders (**Fig. 17**). The histologic composition affects the imaging appearance to some extent, with epithelial neoplasms more homogeneous and mixed tumors showing a greater degree of heterogeneity. Like most tumors, hepatoblastoma is usually T1 hypointense and T2 hyperintense; fibrous septa appear hypointense on both T1WI ad T2WI and show progressive enhancement. Hemorrhage and calcification also occasionally complicate the imaging appearance and tumors have a propensity for portal and hepatic venous invasion. Its relative hypovascularity differentiates hepatoblastoma from its chief diagnostic differential consideration, infantile hemangioendothelioma, which is typically hypervascular, although a hypervascular rim is occasionally present in hepatoblastoma.[52] Other differentiating features of infantile hemangioendothelioma with respect to hepatoblastoma include younger patient population, finer calcifications (typically chunky in hepatoblastoma), and rare AFP increase. Mesenchymal hamartoma of the liver (MHL) affects the same age group and is distinguished by its predominantly cystic nature and lack of AFP increase. Although AFP levels are often increased with HCC, which shares the predilection for venous invasion, the respective age groups are virtually mutually exclusive (HCC generally more than 5 years of

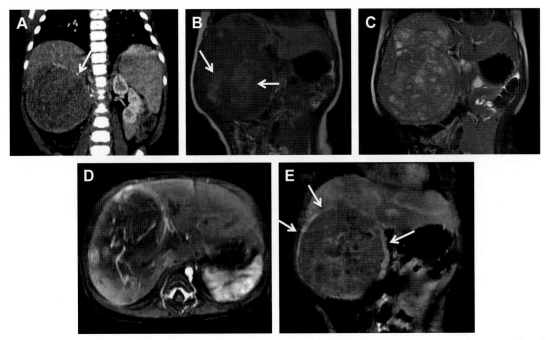

**Fig. 17.** Hepatoblastoma in a 14-month-old infant. (*A*) The coronally reformatted CT image shows peripheral calcification (*arrow*) in a hypovascular liver mass. (*B*) Coronal T1-weighted MR image shows hyperintense hemorrhage (*arrow*) in the large otherwise hypointense liver mass. (*C*) Coronal T2-weighted MR image shows the large mass with lobulated borders with internal heterogeneity at least partially caused by hemorrhage. (*D*) Arterial-phase postcontrast image shows the lesional hypovascularity. (*E*) The delayed coronal postcontrast image shows the enhancing capsule (*arrows*), which is an occasional hepatoblastoma feature. (*Courtesy of* Victor HO, MD, Philadelphia, PA.)

age) and enhancement characteristics are disparate (HCC is hypervascular).

Although 40% to 60% of hepatoblastomas are unresectable when diagnosed, surgical resection is the mainstay of treatment. Neoadjuvant chemotherapy increases the respectability rate to up to 85% and the overall survival rate is reportedly 65% to 70%.[53]

## Epithelioid hemangioendothelioma

Epithelioid hemangioendothelioma (EH) is a rare tumor of variable malignant potential composed of epithelioid or spindle cells growing along vessels or forming new vessels. Compared with other vascular tumors, EH has aggressiveness intermediate between benign infantile hemangioendothelioma and highly aggressive angiosarcoma. EH affects a wide age range (12–86 years of age) with a mean onset of 47 years.[54,55] Although right upper quadrant pain, hepatomegaly, and weight loss are occasional presenting complaints, many EHs are discovered incidentally and tumor markers are not increased.[56]

Two dichotomous imaging patterns represent opposite extremes of disease progression. The early-stage multifocal form manifests with multiple, peripheral nodular foci of variable size from a few millimeters to up to several centimeters (**Fig. 18**). With enlargement and coalescence, the advanced-stage diffuse pattern develops. The concentric zonal or targetoid appearance reflects the histologic growth pattern with an avascular, stomal central region with peripheral neoplastic cells extending along hepatic sinusoids.[57] Although the central hypocellular region may be complicated by hemorrhage, necrosis, or calcification, it generally shows relative T1 hypointensity and T2 hyperintensity. Peripheral enhancement is accordingly generally restricted to the outer, cellular zone. Along with the characteristic peripheral distribution, capsular retraction is observed in 25% of cases.[58,59]

When multifocal, metastatic disease and multifocal HCC constitute the differential diagnostic considerations. Lack of the associated findings (primary malignancy in metastatic disease and chronic liver disease in HCC) argue against these alternatives. EH also potentially simulates angiosarcoma, which is differentiated by its rapidly progressive clinical course.

## Sarcomas

Primary hepatic sarcomas are rare tumors, constituting less than 1% of all hepatic malignancies.[60]

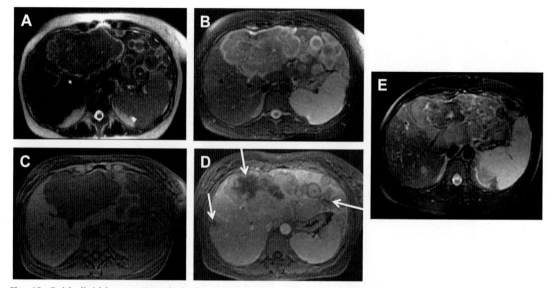

**Fig. 18.** Epithelioid hemangioendothelioma. (*A*) Axial heavily T2-weighted image shows multifocal coalescing targetoid lesions with peripheral hyperintensity surrounding central hypointensity. (*B*) Axial moderately T2-weighted fat-suppressed image shows the lesions to better advantage because of improved tissue contrast. (*C*) Axial precontrast T1-weighted image reveals lesional hypointensity. (*D*) Axial postcontrast T1-weighted image shows peripheral enhancement and central avascularity best seen in the dominant lesions (*arrows*). (*E*) Axial T2-weighted fat-suppressed image 2 years later shows progression with increased coalescence resulting in an infiltrative pattern.

More common lesions include angiosarcoma, embryonal sarcoma, epithelioid hemangioendothelioma, fibrosarcoma, leiomyosarcoma, and malignant fibrous histiosarcoma, and rhabdomyosarcoma in the pediatric population. Angiosarcoma represents the highly aggressive vascular neoplastic counterpart to the more indolent EH, and approximately 200 cases are diagnosed annually.[61] Although most (75%) have no known cause, the remainder have been linked to environmental carcinogens: Thorotrast administration (angiography contrast agent used from 1930s–1950s), vinyl chloride, and organic arsenic exposure. Hemochromatosis and androgenic-anabolic steroid use have also been implicated as causal agents.[62] Angiosarcoma peaks in the seventh decade and strongly favors men, with a ratio of approximately 4:1.[63,64] Multiple imaging appearances have been reported: multiple nodules, dominant masses, and diffuse infiltration.[65] Notwithstanding the pattern, the lesions typically show heterogeneous T1 hypointensity and T2 hyperintensity and occasionally show hemorrhage or fluid-fluid levels. Temporal enhancement is protean with virtually equal rates of hypovascular, isovascular, and hypervascular enhancement patterns (compared with liver) and most show progressive enhancement over time.[66] Most patients have metastatic lesions at the time of diagnosis

and the most common site is the lung followed by the spleen. Resection is the only hope of cure and prognosis is dismal, with most patients dying within 6 months of diagnosis.

Embryonal sarcoma (ES) mostly, but not exclusively, affects the pediatric population, usually in the 6 to 10-year-old age range, but adult cases have been reported.[67] ES accounts for approximately 6% of all primary pediatric hepatic tumors, ranking fourth or fifth in overall prevalence among pediatric liver tumors.[68] Tumor markers, such as AFP, are not increased. Although usually asymptomatic in children, adults often complain of right upper quadrant pain, abdominal mass, anorexia, and intermittent fever.[69]

ESs are generally large, well-demarcated tumors, usually between 10 and 20 cm, composed of spindle-shaped and stellate undifferentiated sarcomatous cells packed in whorls or sheets and scattered in a myxoid ground substance. The myxomatous stroma explains the characteristic appearance of ESs, which has been confused with cystic lesions, including hydatid disease.[70] Although more heterogeneous, signal intensity approximates fluid and enhancement is minimal, except in the hypointense, enhancing septa (**Fig. 19**). Although not substantiated in the literature, relative diffusion restriction (hyperintense on diffusion-weighted images and hypointense on

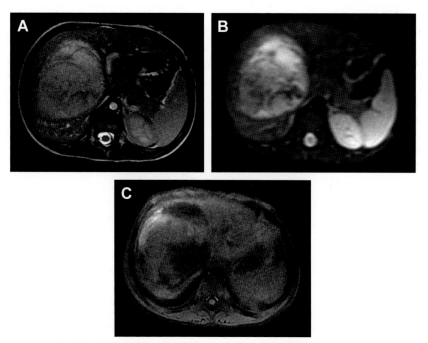

**Fig. 19.** ES in a 4-year-old child. (*A*) Axial T2-weighted image reveals a large hyperintense lesion in the right lobe. (*B*) The corresponding axial diffusion-weighted image shows higher intensity compared with the T2-weighted image, suggesting hypercellularity. (*C*) Delayed postcontrast image confirms enhancement and the presence of solid tissue. (*Courtesy of* Victor HO, MD, Philadelphia, PA.)

ADC maps) compared with fluid theoretically distinguishes ES from cystic causes. ES has historically portended a dismal prognosis with most patients dying within a year. More recently, long-term survival has improved with combined surgical resection and chemotherapy; a pediatric study reported a 20-year survival rate of 71%.[71]

Hepatobiliary rhabdomyosarcoma (HR) arises anywhere along the biliary tract, almost exclusively in children (usually less than 5 years of age). Although rare, it represents 1% of pediatric liver tumors and constitutes the most common pediatric biliary neoplasm. Of the rhabdomyosarcoma histologic varieties, only the embryonal subtype arises from biliary epithelium. Because of the biliary origin, jaundice is a common presenting sign and may be accompanied by abdominal distention, fever, hepatomegaly, or nausea and vomiting. Although AFP levels are normal, conjugated bilirubin and alkaline phosphatase are generally increased. Up to 30% have metastasized at the time of diagnosis.[72]

HRs are generally large tumors measuring between 8 and 20 cm[73,74] with polypoid or botryoidal projections into the biliary ductal lumen. Although potentially arising anywhere along the biliary tree, most tumors arise in proximity to the porta hepatis. Growth along the biliary tree with multiple irregular filling defects and biliary dilatation are the most characteristic imaging findings. Fluid-intensity foci corresponding with cystic spaces are commonly present in HRs and enhancement characteristics are highly variable.

Complete surgical resection is usually not possible (approximately 20%–40% of cases). However, multimodal therapy (surgery, radiation, and chemotherapy) offers favorable outcomes to patients with local disease, with up to 78% survival.[75]

## Lymphoma

Hepatic lymphoma encompasses 2 forms: primary and secondary. Primary hepatic lymphoma (PHL) is defined as an extranodal intrahepatic lymphoma with at least most of the disease confined to the liver. PHL constitutes 0.016% of all cases of non-Hodgkin lymphoma (NHL)[76] and usually shows the diffuse large B-cell type. In contrast, secondary hepatic lymphoma (SHL) occurs in up to 20% of patients with Hodgkin lymphoma and up to 50% of patients with NHL.[77]

PHL has been reported more commonly to manifest with a solitary, well-defined lesion, but multiplicity is common. SHL has more protean imaging characteristics with a greater propensity for multifocality and diffusely infiltrative disease.[78] Individual PHL and SHL lesions show similar imaging characteristics and tend to be hypointense on T1WI with variability on T2WI (from hypointense to moderately hyperintense). Although generally showing minimal enhancement, evidence suggests a direct relationship between the degree of T2 hyperintensity and the degree of enhancement, theorizing that T2 hyperintensity reflects a large extracellular space with feeding vessels delivering more contrast during the arterial phase (**Fig. 20**).[79] Rim enhancement is another occasional characteristic feature.[33] The chief diagnostic differential considerations are metastatic disease and infectious and inflammatory causes, including sarcoidosis.

*Metastases*

In the Western world, metastases outnumber primary hepatic tumors by a 40:1 ratio.[80,81] Autopsy studies have shown that 40% of patients with extrahepatic cancer have hepatic metastases.[82] The rich arterial and portal venous blood supply delivers a potentially abundant supply of circulating neoplastic cells. After tumor cells are deposited in the hepatic sinusoids, they induce angiogenesis through the native sinusoidal endothelium, enhancing the likelihood of survival.[83] Most metastases from abdominal organs reach the liver through the portal venous system; metastases from other primary sites usually gain access through the systemic circulation. Lymphatic spread is uncommon and peritoneal spread is

rare. Although cirrhosis confers an increased risk of HCC, it exerts a protective effect against metastases.[84,85]

Most liver metastases are carcinomas with lymphoma a distant second, followed by sarcomas. In order of prevalence by primary site in the Western world, the range for carcinomas is:

Upper gastrointestinal tract (stomach, gallbladder, pancreas): 44% to 78%
Colon: 56% to 58%
Breast: 52% to 53%
Lung: 42% to 43%
Esophagus: 30% to 32%
Genitourinary organs: 24% to 38%

Between 20% and 50% of lymphoma cases involve the liver, and a minority of sarcomas metastasize to the liver.

In two-thirds of cases, metastases induce clinically evident manifestations, mostly referable to liver involvement and include hepatomegaly, ascites, abdominal fullness, right upper quadrant pain, jaundice, anorexia, and weight loss. Liver function tests are increased in approximately three-quarters of patients and, with the exception of carcinoembryonic antigen in colon carcinoma, tumor markers are not increased.

Although accurate alternatives to MR imaging exist to evaluate the liver for metastases, they

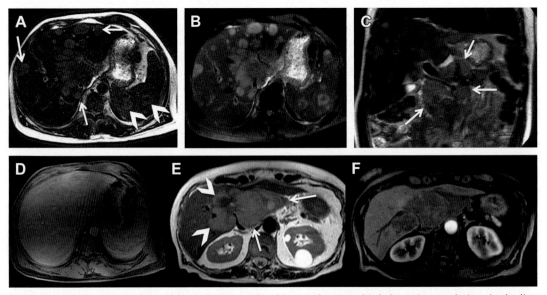

**Fig. 20.** Hepatic lymphoma. (*A*) Axial heavily T2-weighted image shows multiple hyperintense lesions in the liver (*arrows*) and spleen (*arrowheads*). (*B*) Axial fat-suppressed moderately T2-weighted image shows greater tissue contrast, rendering these lesions more conspicuous. (*C*) Coronal T2-weighted image shows extensive periportal lymphadenopathy (*arrows*) in addition to the numerous liver lesions. (*D*) Postcontrast image shows mild lesional enhancement. (*E*) Axial T2-weighted image in a different patient shows marked periportal lymphadenopathy (*arrows*) and a few central parenchymal lesions (*arrowheads*) with mild hyperintensity. (*F*) Axial postcontrast image in the same patient shows minimal enhancement.

lack the convenience and noninvasiveness of MR imaging. Intraoperative ultrasonography has proved sensitivity for identifying liver lesions, but lacks the specificity in discriminating between benign and malignant and increases intraoperative time.[86] Likewise, CT arterial portography (CTAP) requires common femoral artery access in an angiography suite and direct cannulation of the proper hepatic artery, as opposed to a simple intravenous injection of contrast.[87] Multiple studies have shown comparable performance between MR imaging and CTAP and superior performance compared with routine contrast-enhanced CT.[88-91] A recent meta-analysis compared the sensitivities of MR imaging and CT for detecting colorectal liver metastases and showed better per-patient and per-lesion sensitivity for MR imaging.[92]

Despite the evidence that all liver metastases, regardless of the primary tumor, induce arterialization with developing tumor vasculature,[93] a convenient classification scheme stratifies lesions into hypervascular and hypovascular categories. Metastases enhancing more than normal liver parenchyma during the arterial phase are hypervascular and those enhancing less are hypovascular, generally in accordance with the primary tumor.

Hypervascular metastases include renal cell carcinoma, neuroendocrine tumors, melanoma, breast carcinoma, carcinoid, and thyroid carcinoma, and most other metastases are hypovascular. Regardless of relative vascularity, metastases typically follow a predictable enhancement pattern temporally with an arterial-phase peripheral ring followed by peripheral washout and centripetally progressive enhancement (**Fig. 21**). Although the arterial rim enhancement is a useful diagnostic sign (reflecting peritumoral desmoplastic reaction, inflammatory cell accumulation, and/or vascular proliferation),[94] it lacks specificity; abscesses and inflammatory pseudotumors also feature this finding.

On unenhanced images, most metastases appear T1 hypointense and moderately T2 hyperintense. Liquefactive necrosis increases the T2 hyperintensity of metastases (specifically, neuroendocrine tumors, sarcomas, and melanoma), conferring hyperintensity even on heavily weighted, long-TE T2WI, whereas other metastases generally lose signal.[95] Cystic and hyperplastic neoplasms also frequently show pronounced T2 hyperintensity. On T2WI, 25% of metastases, most notably colorectal metastases, show a peripheral hyperintense rim of viable tissue

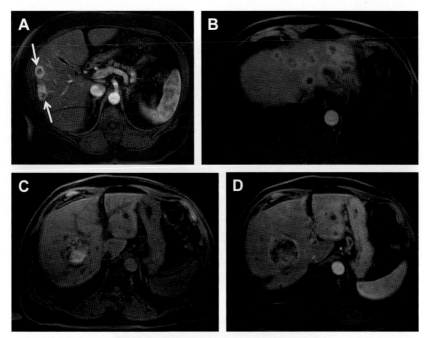

**Fig. 21.** Metastatic enhancement pattern. (*A*) The axial fat-suppressed T1-weighted arterial-phase postcontrast image shows renal cell carcinoma metastatic lesions (*arrows*) showcasing ring enhancement. (*B*) The axial fat-suppressed T1-weighted arterial-phase postcontrast image in a different patient with metastatic ocular melanoma shows multiple ring-enhancing liver metastases. (*C*) An axial fat-suppressed T1-weighted precontrast image in the same patient shows a hyperintense, melanotic metastasis. (*D*) The corresponding arterial-phase postcontrast T1-weighted fat-suppressed image shows metastatic ring enhancement.

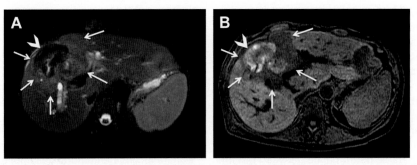

**Fig. 22.** Colorectal metastases. (*A*) Axial T2-weighted fat-suppressed image reveals a large mildly hyperintense lesion (*arrows*) with central hypointense coagulative necrosis (*arrowhead*). (*B*) Axial fat-suppressed T1-weighted image inverts the lesional appearance with peripheral hypointensity (*arrows*) and central hyperintensity (*arrowhead*).

surrounding central hypointensity (mucin, coagulative necrosis, and/or fibrin) (**Fig. 22**).[96] Another characteristic finding is the so-called doughnut sign, referring to the necrotic center surrounded by peripheral viable tumor cells with relative central T1 hypointensity/T2 hyperintensity and relative peripheral T1 hyperintensity/T2 hypointensity (**Fig. 23**).[96,97]

A subset of liver metastases shows T1 hyperintensity for a variety of reasons (**Fig. 24**). T1 hyperintensity either indicates the presence of a paramagnetic substance or fat. The most common multifocal fat-containing tumor is HCC, which

generally shows signal loss on OOP images (discussed earlier). Paramagnetic substances such as melanin, extracellular methemoglobin, and protein also induce T1 hyperintensity in selected metastases.[98] Melanoma metastases are often (uniformly) T1 hyperintense (and T2 hypointense) because of their melanotic content (and/or occasional hemorrhage). Coagulative necrosis, generally developing in the hypoxic center of large metastases, contains T1-hyperintense extracellular methemoglobin and fails to enhance.

DWI represents a recent supplement to the traditional MR imaging approach to detecting liver

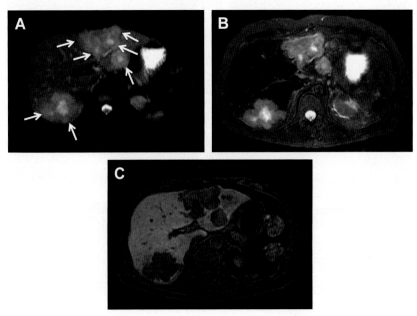

**Fig. 23.** The doughnut sign. (*A*) Axial fat-suppressed T2-weighted image shows multiple metastases (*arrows*) with moderate peripheral hyperintensity and marked cystic central hyperintensity. (*B*) Axial short tau inversion recovery image obtained after Eovist administration shows the lesions to better advantage with greater tissue contrast. (*C*) Hepatobiliary-phase postcontrast image confirms nonhepatocellular cause as hypointensity against the relatively hyperintense background.

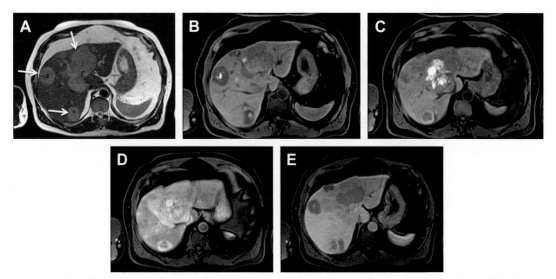

**Fig. 24.** T1-hyperintense metastases. (*A*) Axial T2-weighted image shows multiple mildly hyperintense liver lesions (*arrows*). (*B*, *C*) The axial T1-weighted fat-suppressed images show lesional hyperintensity corresponding with melanin in patient with uveal melanoma metastatic disease. (*D*) The arterial-phase postcontrast fat-suppressed T1-weighted image reveals characteristic hypervascularity. (*E*) The delayed postcontrast fat-suppressed T1-weighted image shows lesional washout, typical of metastases and most malignant lesions.

metastases. Most liver metastases restrict diffusion and appear hyperintense on DWI (and dark on ADC maps). DWI has achieved better performance in detecting liver metastases compared with T2WI[99,100] and comparable performance compared with dynamic contrast-enhanced imaging[101] in comparative studies. With its superior tissue contrast and continued MR hardware improvements improving DWI quality and guaranteeing reproducibility, DWI is becoming a mainstay in liver imaging for metastases (and the evaluation of the other tumors and nonneoplastic indications).

Liver-specific contrast agents are another recent development in hepatic MR imaging, and HP-phase imaging is becoming the MR imaging gold standard for imaging metastases. Although minimal enhancement on 20 minute–delayed images is occasionally observed in metastases, possibly because of slow clearance from the interstitial space related to desmoplasia, the hypointensity compared with uniformly hyperintense normal liver is striking.[102] In a recent study, HP imaging achieved a sensitivity of 95% for detecting colorectal liver metastases (compared with 63% for multiphasic CT) and an overall detection of 92% for metastases of less than 1 cm.[103] Vogl and colleagues[104] reported that 56% more metastatic lesions are visible with HP contrast agents compared with extracellular agents. The supporting evidence strongly recommends the use of HB contrast agents and delayed HP imaging for metastases.

## SUMMARY

MR imaging has become the mainstay for the noninvasive evaluation of liver lesions. The first step is to differentiate benign from malignant lesions, which relies on a combination of lesion assessment, background liver assessment, and clinical parameters. Washout generally indicates malignancy, along with other imaging features, such as vascular invasion and diffusion restriction. Cirrhosis increases the risk of HCC, the most common primary hepatic malignancy, and presents a constellation of pre-HCC nodular lesions, but protects against metastatic disease. Although cirrhosis favors HCC, metastases prevail over all other malignant liver lesions in noncirrhotic livers, and multiplicity and presence of a primary malignancy generally signals the diagnosis. Without a known primary malignancy, several imaging findings help to classify lesions (hypervascular vs hypovascular) and potentially suggest the organ of origin, but imaging features generally overlap.

In the adult population, non-HCC primary malignancies are uncommon, with IHCs the next most common lesions and other malignant lesions, such as BCC, sarcomas, and primary lymphoma, are exceedingly rare. Although generally not pathognomonic, the imaging features of these primary neoplasms are usually distinct enough from HCC to suggest an alternative diagnosis. In the pediatric population, the most common primary hepatic malignancies, hepatoblastoma and HCC, have mutually exclusive age group involvement (hepatoblastoma less than 5 years of age). In addition, the imaging features of these two lesions are distinctly different, with hepatoblastoma hypovascularity compared with HCC hypervascularity and the propensity of hepatoblastoma to calcify. Less common pediatric hepatic malignancies (ES and biliary rhabdomyosarcoma) also have unique imaging features and familiarity increases the likelihood of correct diagnosis.

In summary, MR imaging is the gold standard for the noninvasive evaluation of liver lesions. Using the array of imaging sequences (T1WI, T2WI, dynamic contrast-enhanced imaging, DWI, and HP imaging) confers optimal performance in detecting and characterizing liver tumors.

## REFERENCES

1. Parker SL, Tong T, Bolden S, et al. Cancer statistics. CA Cancer J Clin 1997;47:5–27.
2. Elsayes KM, Leyendecker JR, Menias CO, et al. MRI characterization of 124 CT-indeterminate focal hepatic lesions: evaluation of clinical utility. HPB (Oxford) 2007;9(3):208–15.
3. Hussain SM, Semelka RC. Liver masses. Magn Reson Imaging Clin N Am 2005;13(2):255–75.
4. El-Serag HB, Mason AC. Rising incidence of hepatocellular carcinoma in the United States. N Engl J Med 1999;340:745–50.
5. El-Serag HB. Hepatocellular carcinoma. N Engl J Med 2011;365:1118–27.
6. Ferlay J, Bray F, Pisani P, et al. GLOBOCAN 2000: cancer incidence, mortality and prevalence worldwide, version 1.0. International Agency for Research on Cancer cancerbase no. 5. Lyon (France): IARC; 2001.
7. Fattovich G, Stroffolini T, Zagni I, et al. Hepatocellular carcinoma in cirrhosis: incidence and risk factors. Gastroenterology 2004;127(Suppl 1):S35–50.
8. Bruix J, Sherman M. Management of hepatocellular carcinoma. Hepatology 2005;42:1208–36.
9. Zhang BH, Yang BH, Tang ZY. Randomized controlled trial of screening for hepatocellular carcinoma. J Cancer Res Clin Oncol 2004;130: 417–22.
10. Colli A, Fraguelli M, Casazza G, et al. Accuracy of ultrasonography, spiral CT, magnetic resonance, and alpha-fetoprotein in diagnosing hepatocellular carcinoma: a systematic review. Am J Gastroenterol 2006;101(3):513–23.
11. American College of Radiology. Liver imaging reporting and data system version 2013.1. Available at: http://www.acr.org/Quality-Safety/Resources/LIRADS/. Accessed May 11, 2013.
12. Choi BI, Lee GK, Kim ST, et al. Mosaic pattern of encapsulated hepatocellular carcinoma: correlation of magnetic resonance imaging and pathology. Gastrointest Radiol 1990;15:238–40.
13. Kadoya M, Matsui O, Takashima T, et al. Hepatocellular carcinoma: correlation of MR imaging and histopathologic findings. Radiology 1992;183: 819–25.
14. Ito K. Hepatocellular carcinoma: conventional MRI findings including gadolinium-enhanced dynamic imaging. Eur J Radiol 2006;58:186–99.
15. Altekruse SF, McGlynn KA, Reichman ME. Hepatocellular carcinoma incidence, mortality and survival trend in the United States from 1975 to 2005. J Clin Oncol 2009;27:1485–91.
16. Mazzaferro V, Regalia E, Doci R, et al. Liver transplantation for the treatment of small hepatocellular carcinomas in patients with cirrhosis. N Engl J Med 1996;334(11):693–9.
17. Yao FY, Ferrell L, Bass NM, et al. Liver transplantation for hepatocellular carcinoma: expansion of the tumor size limits does not adversely impact survival. Hepatology 2001;33(6):1394–403.
18. Patel SS, Arrington AK, McKenzie S, et al. Milan criteria and UCSF criteria: a preliminary comparative study of liver transplantation outcomes in the United States. Int J Hepatol 2012;2012:253517. http://dx.doi.org/10.1155/2012/253517.
19. Yuki K, Hirohashi S, Sakamoto M, et al. Growth and spread of hepatocellular carcinoma. Cancer 1990; 66:2174–9.
20. Natsuizaka M, Omura T, Akaike T, et al. Clinical features of hepatocellular carcinoma with extrahepatic metastases. J Gastroenterol Hepatol 2005;20: 1781–7.
21. Sneag DB, Krajewski K, Giardino A, et al. Extrahepatic spread of hepatocellular carcinoma: spectrum of imaging findings. AJR Am J Roentgenol 2011;197:W658–64.
22. Lo CM, Ngan H, Tso WK, et al. Randomized controlled trial of transarterial lipiodol chemoembolization for unresectable hepatocellular carcinoma. Hepatology 2002;35(5):1164–71.
23. Bruix J, Sala M, Llovet JM. Chemoembolization for hepatocellular carcinoma. Gastroenterology 2004; 127(5 Suppl 1):S179–88.
24. Llovet JM, Bruix J. Systematic review of randomized trials for unresectable hepatocellular carcinoma: chemoembolization improves survival. Hepatology 2003;37(2):429–42.
25. Llovet JM, Real MI, Montana X, et al. Arterial embolisation or chemoembolisation versus symptomatic treatment in patients with unresectable hepatocellular carcinoma: a randomised controlled trial. Lancet 2002;359(9319):1734–9.
26. Willatt JM, Hussain HK, Adusumilli S, et al. MR imaging of hepatocellular carcinoma in the cirrhotic liver: challenges and controversies. Radiology 2008;247(2):311–30.

27. Goldberg SN, Gazelle GS, Compton CC, et al. Treatment of intrahepatic malignancy with radiofrequency ablation: radiologic-pathologic correlation. Cancer 2000;88(11):2452–63.

28. Lu TL, Becce F, Bize P, et al. Assessment of liver tumor response by high-field (3T) MRI after radiofrequency ablation: short- and mid-term evolution of diffusion parameters within the ablation zone. Eur J Radiol 2012;81(9):e944–50.

29. Krinsky GA, Lee VS. MR imaging of cirrhotic nodules. Abdom Imaging 2000;25:471–82.

30. Matsui O, Kadoya M, Kameyama T, et al. Benign and malignant nodules in cirrhotic livers: distinction based on blood supply. Radiology 1991;178: 493–7.

31. Lee HM, Lu DS, Krasny RM, et al. Hepatic lesion characterization in cirrhosis: significance of arterial phase hypervascularity on dual-phase helical CT. AJR Am J Roentgenol 1997;169:125–30.

32. Hussain SM, Zondervan PE, Ijzermans JN, et al. Benign versus malignant hepatic nodules: MR imaging findings with pathologic correlation. Radiographics 2002;22:1023–39.

33. Elsayes KM, Narra VR, Yin Y, et al. Focal hepatic lesions: diagnostic value of enhancement pattern approach with contrast-enhanced 3D gradient-echo MR imaging. Radiographics 2005;25: 1299–320.

34. Earls JP, Theise ND, Weinreb JC, et al. Dysplastic nodules and hepatocellular carcinoma: thin-section MR imaging of explanted cirrhotic livers with pathologic correlation. Radiology 1996;201: 207–14.

35. Quaia E, De Paoli L, Pizzolato R, et al. Predictors of dysplastic nodule diagnosis in patients with liver cirrhosis on unenhanced and gadobenate dimeglumine-enhanced MRI with dynamic and hepatobiliary phase. AJR Am J Roentgenol 2013; 200(3):553–62.

36. Jeong YY, Yim NY, Heoung KK. Hepatocellular carcinoma in the cirrhotic liver with helical CT and MRI: imaging spectrum and pitfalls of cirrhosis-related nodules. AJR Am J Roentgenol 2005;185:1024–32.

37. Ichikawa T, Federle MP, Grazioli L, et al. Fibrolamellar hepatocellular carcinoma: imaging and pathologic findings in 31 recent cases. Radiology 1999;213:352–61.

38. McLarney JK, Rucker PT, Bender GN, et al. Fibrolamellar carcinoma of the liver: radiologic-pathologic correlation. Radiographics 1999;19: 453–71.

39. Khan SA, Thomas HC, Davidson BR, et al. Cholangiocarcinoma. Lancet 2005;366(9493):1303–14.

40. Lazaridis KN, Gores GJ. Cholangiocarcinoma. Gastroenterology 2005;128(6):1655–67.

41. Shaib Y, El-Serag HB. The epidemiology of cholangiocarcinoma. Semin Liver Dis 2004;24(2):115–25.

42. Liver Cancer Study Group of Japan. Classification of primary liver cancer. Tokyo: Kanehara; 1997.

43. Maetani Y, Itoh K, Watanabe C, et al. MR imaging of intrahepatic cholangiocarcinoma with pathologic correlation. AJR Am J Roentgenol 2001;176: 1499–507.

44. Péporté AR, Sommer WH, Nicolaou K, et al. Imaging features of intrahepatic cholangiocarcinoma in Gd-EOB-DTPA-enhanced MRI. Eur J Radiol 2013; 82:e101–6.

45. Ishak KG, Willis GW, Cummins SD, et al. Biliary cystadenoma and cystadenocarcinoma: report of 14 cases and review of the literature. Cancer 1977;39:322–38.

46. Wilkinson N. Hepatobiliary cystadenocarcinoma. Case Reports in Hepatology 2012;2012:298957. http://dx.doi.org/10.1155/2012/298957.

47. Edmundson HA. Tumors or the liver and intrahepatic bile ducts. In: Atlas of tumor pathology. Fascicle 25. Washington, DC: Armed Forces Institute of Pathology; 1958.

48. Teoh A, Ng SS, Lee KF, et al. Biliary cystadenoma and other complicated cystic lesions of the liver: diagnostic and therapeutic challenges. World J Surg 2006;30(8):1560–6.

49. Stocker JT. Hepatic tumors in children. Clin Liver Dis 2001;5(1):259–81.

50. Stocker JT, Schmidt D. Hepatoblastoma. In: Hamilton SR, Aatonen LA, editors. Pathology and genetics of tumours of the digestive system. Lyon (France): IARC Press; 2000. p. 184–9.

51. Meyers RL. Tumors of the liver in children. Surg Oncol 2007;16(3):195–203.

52. Dachman AH, Pakter RL, Ros PR, et al. Hepatoblastoma: radiologic-pathologic correlation in 50 cases. Radiology 1987;164(1):15–9.

53. Helmberger TK, Ros PR, Mergo PJ, et al. Pediatric liver neoplasms: a radiologic-pathologic correlation. Eur Radiol 1999;9(7):1339–47.

54. Ishak KG, Sesterhenn IA, Goodman ZD, et al. Epithelioid hemangioendothelioma of the liver: a clinicopathologic and follow-up study of 32 cases. Hum Pathol 1984;15:839–52.

55. Makhlouf HR, Ishak KG, Goodman ZD. Epithelioid hemangioendothelioma of the liver: a clinicopathologic study of 137 cases. Cancer 1999;85:562–82.

56. Chung EM, Lattin GE, Cube R, et al. From the archives of the AFIP: pediatric liver masses: radiology-pathologic correlation part 2. Malignant tumors. Radiographics 2011;31:483–507.

57. Buetow PC, Buck JL, Ros PR, et al. Malignant vascular tumors of the liver: radiologic-pathologic correlation. Radiographics 1994;14(1):153–66.

58. Miller WJ, Dodd GD III, Federle MP, et al. Epithelioid hemangioendothelioma of the liver: imaging findings with pathologic correlation. AJR Am J Roentgenol 1992;159:53–7.

59. Lyburn ID, Torreggiani WC, Harris AC, et al. Hepatic epithelioid hemangioendothelioma: sonographic, CT and MR imaging appearances. AJR Am J Roentgenol 2003;180:1359–64.

60. Weitz J, Klimstra DS, Cymes K, et al. Management of primary liver sarcomas. Cancer 2007;109: 1391–6.

61. Anon. Angiosarcoma of the liver: a growing problem? Br Med J (Clin Res Ed) 1981;282:504–5.

62. Falk H, Herbert J, Crowley S, et al. Epidemiology of hepatic angiosarcoma in the United States: 1964-1974. Environ Health Perspect 1981;41:107–13.

63. Locker GY, Doroshow JH, Zwelling LA, et al. The clinical features of hepatic angiosarcoma: a report of four cases and a review of the English literature. Medicine 1979;58:48–64.

64. Falk H, Thomas LB, Popper H, et al. Hepatic angiosarcoma associated with androgenic-anabolic steroids. Lancet 1979;2:1120–3.

65. Koyama T, Fletcher JG, Johnson CD, et al. Primary hepatic angiosarcoma: findings at CT and MR imaging. Radiology 2002;222:667–73.

66. Peterson MS, Baron RL, Rankin SC. Hepatic angiosarcoma: findings on multiphasic contrast-enhanced helical CT do not mimic hemangioma. AJR Am J Roentgenol 2000;175(1):165–70.

67. Stocker JT, Ishak KG. Undifferentiated (embryonal) sarcoma of the liver: report of 31 cases. Cancer 1978;42(1):336–48.

68. Weinberg AG, Finegold MJ. Primary hepatic tumors of childhood. Hum Pathol 1983;14:512–37.

69. Kim M, Tireno B, Slanetz PJ. Undifferentiated embryonal sarcoma of the liver. AJR Am J Roentgenol 2008;190:W261–2.

70. Faraj W, Mukherji D, Majzoub NE, et al. Primary undifferentiated embryonal sarcoma of the liver mistaken for hydatid disease. World J Surg Oncol 2010;8:58.

71. Bisogno G, Pilz T, Perilongo G, et al. Undifferentiated sarcoma of the liver in childhood: a curable disease. Cancer 2002;94:252–7.

72. Ruymann FB, Raney RB Jr, Crist WM, et al. Rhabdomyosarcoma of the biliary tree in childhood: a report from the Intergroup Rhabdomyosarcoma Study. Cancer 1985;56(3):575–81.

73. Donnelly LF, Bisset GS 3rd, Frush DP. Case 2: embryonal rhabdomyosarcoma of the biliary tree. Radiology 1998;208(3):621–3.

74. Roebuck DJ, Yang WT, Lam WW, et al. Hepatobiliary rhabdomyosarcoma in children: diagnostic radiology. Pediatr Radiol 1998;28(2):101–8.

75. Spunt SL, Lobe TE, Pappo AS, et al. Aggressive surgery is unwarranted for biliary tract rhabdomyosarcoma. J Pediatr Surg 2000;35(2):309–16.

76. Agmon-Levin N, Berger I, Shtalrid M, et al. Primary hepatic lymphoma: a case report and review of the literature. Age Ageing 2004;33:637–40.

77. Levy AD. Malignant liver tumors. Clin Liver Dis 2002;6:147–64.

78. Gazelle GS, Lee MJ, Hahn PF, et al. US, CT, and MRI of primary and secondary liver lymphoma. J Comput Assist Tomogr 1994;18(3):412–5.

79. Kelekis NL, Semelka RC, Siegelman ES, et al. Focal hepatic lymphoma: magnetic resonance demonstration using current techniques including gadolinium enhancement. Magn Reson Imaging 1997;15(6):625–36.

80. Berge T, Lundberg S. Cancer in Malmo 1958–69. Acta Pathol Microbiol Scand Suppl 1977;(S260): 140–9.

81. Pickren JW, Tsukada Y, Lane WW. Liver metastases: analysis of autopsy data. In: Weiss L, Gilbert HA, editors. Liver metastases. Boston: Hall Medical Publishers; 1982. p. 45–6.

82. Craig JR, Peters RL, Edmondson HA. Tumours of the liver and intrahepatic bile ducts. Washington, DC: AFIP; 1989. p. 147–202.

83. Terayama N, Terada T, Nakanuma Y. A morphometric and immunohistochemical study on angiogenesis of human metastatic carcinomas of the liver. Hepatology 1996;24:816–9.

84. Melato M, Laurino L, Mudi E, et al. Relationship between cirrhosis, liver cancer, and hepatic metastases. An autopsy study. Cancer 1989;64:455–9.

85. Uetsuji S, Yamamura M, Yamamichi K, et al. Absence of colorectal cancer metastasis to the cirrhotic liver. Am J Surg 1992;164:176–7.

86. Rummeny EJ, Marchal G. Liver imaging. Clinical applications and future perspectives. Acta Radiol 1997;38:626–30.

87. Nelson RC, Thompson GH, Chezmar JL, et al. CT during arterial portography: diagnostic pitfalls. Radiographics 1992;12:705–18.

88. Semelka RC, Cance WG, Marcos HB, et al. Liver metastases: comparison of current MR techniques and spiral CT during arterial portography for detection in 20 surgically staged cases. Radiology 1999; 213:86–91.

89. Soyer P, Levesque M, Caudron C, et al. MRI of liver metastases from colorectal cancer vs. CT during arterial portography. J Comput Assist Tomogr 1993;17:67–74.

90. Schima W, Kulinna C, Langenberger H, et al. Liver metastases of colorectal cancer: US, CT or MR? Cancer Imaging 2005;5A:S149–56.

91. Namasivayam S, Martin DR. Imaging of liver metastases. Cancer Imaging 2007;7:2–9.

92. Floriani I, Torri V, Rulli E, et al. Performance of imaging modalities in diagnosis of liver metastases from colorectal cancer: a systematic review and meta-analysis. J Magn Reson Imaging 2010;31:19–31.

93. Dezso K, Bugyik E, Papp V, et al. Development of arterial blood supply in experimental liver metastases. Am J Pathol 2009;175:835–43.

94. Semelka RC, Hussain SM, Marcos HB, et al. Perilesional enhancement of hepatic metastases: correlation between MR imaging and histopathologic findings–initial observations. Radiology 2000;215: 89–94.

95. Imam K, Bluemke DA. MR imaging in the evaluation of hepatic metastases. Magn Reson Imaging Clin N Am 2000;8:741–56.

96. Wittenberg J, Stark DD, Forman BH, et al. Differentiation of hepatic metastases from hepatic hemangiomas and cysts by using MR imaging. AJR Am J Roentgenol 1988;151:79–84.

97. Outwater E, Tomaszewski JE, Daly JM, et al. MRI appearance of hepatic colorectal metastases with pathologic correlation. Radiology 1991;180: 327–32.

98. Kelekis NL, Semelka RC, Woosley JT. Malignant lesions of the liver with high signal intensity on T1-weighted images. J Magn Reson Imaging 1996;6:291–4.

99. Andreana L, Burroughs AK. Treatment of early hepatocellular carcinoma: how to predict and prevent recurrence. Dig Liver Dis 2010;42(Suppl 3):S249–57.

100. Parikh T, Drew SJ, Lee VS, et al. Focal liver lesion detection and characterization with diffusion-weighted MR imaging: comparison with standard breath-hold T2-weighted imaging. Radiology 2008;246:812–22.

101. Hardie AD, Naik M, Hecht EM, et al. Diagnosis of liver metastases: value of diffusion-weighted MRI compared with gadolinium-enhanced MRI. Eur Radiol 2010;20(6):1431–41.

102. Kim A, Lee CH, Kim BH, et al. Gadoxetic acid-enhanced 3.0T MRI for the evaluation of hepatic metastasis from colorectal cancer: metastasis is not always seen as a "defect" on the hepatobiliary phase. Eur J Radiol 2012;81:3998–4004.

103. Muhi A, Ichikawa T, Motosugi U, et al. Diagnosis of colorectal hepatic metastases: comparison of contrast-enhanced CT, contrast-enhanced US, superparamagnetic iron oxide-enhanced MRI, and gadoxetic acid-enhanced MRI. J Magn Reson Imaging 2011;34:326–35.

104. Vogl TJ, Kummel S, Hammerstingl R, et al. Liver tumors: comparison of MR imaging with Gd-EOB-DTPA and Gd-DTPA. Radiology 1996;200:59–67.

# MR Imaging of Diffuse Liver Disease
## From Technique to Diagnosis

Thomas A. Hope, MD[a], Michael A. Ohliger, MD[a],
Aliya Qayyum, MD[b],*

## KEYWORDS

- Diffuse • Liver • Iron • Fat • MR imaging

## KEY POINTS

- Multiecho gradient-echo (GRE) techniques correct for the presence of both fat and water, resulting in more accurate quantification of both entities.
- Magnetic resonance (MR) elastography provides a robust technique for quantification of hepatic fibrosis, particularly in earlier stages not well evaluated with other techniques.
- Acute and chronic appearances of Budd-Chiari syndrome have distinct appearances caused by differences in collateral flow.
- Primary hemochromatosis has an injured reticuloendothelial system (RES) resulting in a different pattern of iron deposition than seen with secondary hemochromatosis (hemosiderosis).
- Chemotherapy-related diffuse liver disease includes hepatosteatosis and sinusoidal obstruction syndrome (SOS).

## INTRODUCTION

Over the past decade the role of MR imaging in the evaluation of diffuse liver disease has become common practice in clinical radiology. Although detection of focal liver lesions remains the mainstay of liver imaging, a growing cohort of patients are referred for evaluation of hepatosteatosis, iron deposition diseases, and cirrhosis. Additionally, knowledge of incidentally discovered diffuse diseases is important for abdominal imagers. This review begins with an overview of techniques used for fat and iron quantification as well as MR elastography. The second half focuses on specific hepatic diseases.

## TECHNIQUES

Percutaneous biopsy is often regarded as the gold standard for the evaluation of liver disease, but as

MR techniques mature, it is becoming apparent that the distribution of pathology is varied throughout the liver and that, MR imaging biomarkers may replace traditional pathology-based gold standards in the near future. This article describes the techniques currently used for evaluation of hepatic fat, iron, and stiffness.

### Iron Quantification

During the past decade, iron and fat quantification using multiple-echo sequences has replaced liver biopsies as a gold standard. This is intended to be a succinct overview of iron quantification and more in-depth reviews are available.[1] Iron, a paramagnetic ion, results in signal loss on MR imaging sequences due to its effects on T2 and T2*. The higher the iron content in a voxel, the faster the signal decreases as the echo time (TE) is increased. On GRE images, the rate at which

[a] Department of Radiology and Biomedical Imaging, University of California San Francisco, 505 Parnassus Avenue, San Francisco, CA 94143-0628, USA; [b] Department of Diagnostic Radiology, MD Anderson Cancer Center, 1515 Holcombe Blvd, Houston, TX 77030, USA
* Corresponding author.
E-mail address: aqayyum@mdanderson.org

Radiol Clin N Am 52 (2014) 709–724
http://dx.doi.org/10.1016/j.rcl.2014.02.016
0033-8389/14/$ – see front matter Published by Elsevier Inc.

signal falls is described by T2*, whereas on spin-echo acquisitions, the rate of signal decay is described by T2. Nonquantitative techniques for detecting the presence of iron include using a GRE acquisition with a long TE (ie, greater than 10 ms) and observing a loss of signal in the liver. Additionally, opposed-phase (OP) and in-phase (IP) acquisition can be used to see if there is loss of signal on the IP images, which are conventionally acquired at a later TE than the OP images. On some 3.0-T systems, the OP images may be acquired at a longer TE than the IP images. In this situation it is not possible to determine if the loss of signal is due to the presence of fat or iron. There are 2 quantitative techniques that are used to measure the presence of iron: the signal intensity ratio (SIR) and the relaxometry method.

### Signal intensity ratio

The SIR method compares the signal measured in the liver using multiple imaging parameters to a tissue in which iron is not deposited, typically skeletal muscle. To minimize changes in intensity due to relative changes in coil sensitivities, the body coil is used for the acquisition. The signal intensities are measured using multiple GRE sequences, and the most commonly used is that proposed by Gandon and colleagues[2] with the following parameters: 120/4/90°, 120/4/20°, 120/9/20°, 120/14/20°, and 120/21/20° (all represent TR/TE/flip angle). Values from regions of interest can then be entered into an online calculator (www.radio.univ-rennes1.fr) to obtain an estimate of the concentration of liver iron. This technique has a dynamic range of 3 to 375 μmol Fe/g. Although this technique is easy to implement, it requires 5 breath-holds and is limited by the interaction of hepatic fat content.

### Relaxometry

The second technique used is often termed, *relaxometry*. This technique acquires a series of echoes with increasing TEs and uses the rate of decay in signal intensity to calculate T2 or T2*. No comparison to other tissues is made as in the SIR method. If a spin-echo sequence is used for acquisition, T2 is measured, and if a GRE sequence is used, T2* is measured. T2 and T2* are inversely proportional to iron concentrations and, therefore, the inverse values are often reported, R2 and R2*, as described by the following equations.

$$R2 = \frac{1000}{T2} \text{ and } R2^* = \frac{100}{T2^*}$$

Although R2 measurements are more reproducible because they are less affected by magnetic field inhomogeneities, R2* measurements are more convenient because they can be obtained in a single breath-hold.

There is a Food and Drug Administration–approved relaxometry iron quantification sequence (FerriScan [St. Pierre method], Resonance Health, Claremont, Western Australia).[3] This method measures T2/R2 using 7 free-breathing T2-weighted sequences, which take more than 10 minutes to acquire. The data sets are then sent to a central analysis center where the images are processed and reports are sent back within 48 hours. The measured R2 correlates well with hepatic iron concentrations in milligrams of iron, *Fe*, per gram of dry weight using the following equation[3]:

$$[Fe] = \left(29.75 - \sqrt{900.7 - 2.283 \times R2}\right)^{1.424}$$

There are many factors that affect the measurement of signal decay. Most important is the magnetic field strength; the higher the magnet field the faster signal decays and, therefore, the higher the R2* measurements, so different calibrations must be set for each magnetic field strength used (1.5 T vs 3.0 T). The second important factor is the number and spacing of echoes acquired during the GRE sequence. The pulse sequences used today acquire multiple echoes, usually 6, after each excitation. The timing of the first echo should be acquired as quickly as possible (approximately 1 ms) to be sensitive to high levels of iron concentration. The last echo should be acquired by 15 ms, because later echoes may be corrupted by significant susceptibility artifact and noise. The spacing of the echoes between the first and last echo is controversial. Using the data from these multiple echoes, a decay curve can be fit to estimate the T2*. The simplest method to measure T2* is using a monoexponential function:

$$S = S_0 e^{\frac{-TE}{T2^*}}$$

Where the signal intensity, $S_0$, is the intensity expected at a TE of 0.

This estimate is limited by many assumptions and there are many monoexponential and biexponential models that have been proposed as well.[1]

The most commonly used T2* method is the Wood method.[4] This technique uses a GRE sequence with 17 echoes spaced between 0.8 and 4.8 ms. A single midhepatic slice is acquired during 1 breath-hold and the T2*/R2* is calculated using a monoexponential fit (as described previously) with a constant used to correct for noise in the system. The correlation between measured R2* and hepatic iron concentration is described by the following equation at 1.5 T:

$$[Fe] = 0.254 \times R2^* + 0.202$$

None of these techniques takes into account the presence of fat that significantly corrupts the calculated values.

## Fat Quantification

A short review of fat quantification techniques is provided, although more in-depth reviews are available.[5] All fat quantification techniques are based on the principle that fat and water resonate at different frequencies. Fat protons precess slower than water protons at a rate that depends on the field strength used. MR spectroscopy is often considered the gold standard for fat quantification. Because full spectra are available, water and fat are quantified by measuring the areas under the water and fat spectroscopic peaks, respectively. MR spectroscopy suffers from long imaging times and the need for specialized processing software.

The simplest approach for whole liver fat quantification is to compare images with and without chemical fat saturation. The fat fraction is then estimated by taking the difference between the images acquired with and without fat-saturation pulses.[6] This technique is limited primarily by inhomogeneities in the main magnetic field ($B_0$), which results in inconsistent fat saturation throughout the imaged volume.

More commonly, a 2-echo approach is performed whereby the presence of fat is visualized by taking advantage of the different frequencies at which fat protons process compared with water, often termed, *chemical shift–based methods*. The 2-echo techniques based on the Dixon method use 2 well-timed echoes, 1 during a time when fat and water signal are out of phase and 1 when they are IP, to create fat and water images (**Fig. 1**).[7] Although the Dixon technique was described in 1984, it was not until 1997 that quantification of hepatic fat was suggested.[8] The fat fraction is estimated based on measured signal intensity on the IP and OP images using the following equation:

$$\text{Fat fraction} = \frac{(\text{IP} - \text{OP})}{2 \times \text{IP}}$$

The 3 main failings of this technique are that its dynamic range is limited to 50% fat content; it does not take into account iron content; and it does not take into account that fat has multiple spectral peaks.

## Fat and Iron Quantification

Because the presence of fat and iron interferes with the quantification of each another, it is critical to include both in a model used to quantify either value. To make things more complex, fat is not represented by a single spectral peak but is composed of multiple peaks; therefore, there is never a true IP, and OP time point as is assumed with the 2-echo approach described previously. Recently, the term, *proton density fat fraction (PDFF)*, has been defined as the ratio of fat proton density to total proton density.[9] This term should

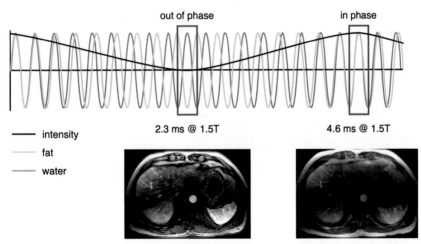

out of phase         in phase

—— intensity
―― fat
―― water

2.3 ms @ 1.5T        4.6 ms @ 1.5T

**Fig. 1.** Chemical shift–based method of fat and water separation. Diagrammatic representation of fat and water precession with water precessing at a higher frequency than fat. This results in periodic time points where fat and water signal are IP and out-of-phase. An image created from echoes collected while fat and water are IP creates an image where total intensity equals fat + water. Creating an image from echoes collected while fat and water are out-of-phase results in an image where total intensity equals water − fat. From these 2 echoes, a fat fraction can be calculated. Note that on the out-of-phase image, voxels that contain high amounts of fat (subcutaneous fat) and high amounts of water (spleen) have a high signal intensity.

only be used to describe a fat quantification technique that takes into account the multiple spectral peaks of fat and the presence of iron in addition to other corrections. These approaches are typically broken down into magnitude and complex methods depending on whether the analysis is performed on magnitude images or on the complex phase images. Although these techniques were initially developed for the quantification of hepatic fat, they result in a more accurate method of iron quantification as well if the correct imaging parameters are used.[10,11]

Magnitude-based techniques acquire multiple echoes and estimate the fat fraction based on the magnitude data measured.[12] These methods have a dynamic range of 0% to 50% fat concentration. The complex based techniques acquire multiple echos as well but use both the phase and magnitude data to recreate the fat estimation maps.[13] These techniques have a dynamic range from 0% to 100% fat concentration, although a fat fraction greater than 50% is rare, so the range may be of questionable relevance clinically. The complex techniques also need to correct for noise and eddy current issues that do not play a role in magnitude techniques. Currently there is 1 commercial product available to measure PDFF using complex based techniques, the IDEAL IQ sequence (GE Healthcare, Waukesha, Wisconsin)

(**Fig. 2**). Using either the magnitude or complex method, R2* maps and fat fraction maps are created, which allow a user to measure R2* or fat fraction within the liver using regions of interest.

## Elastography

The speed at which shear waves travel through a tissue depends on the stiffness of the tissue. In MR elastography, an external compression device is placed on the patient, typically over the right lobe of the liver that propagates waves through the patient along the transverse plane.[14] As these shear waves propagate through the tissue, liver parenchyma is displaced transiently in the superior and inferior direction by the shear wave (**Fig. 3**). By utilizing motion-encoding gradients similar to those used in phase-contrast imaging, these displacements along the z-axis can be measured. The acquisition is synchronized with the frequency of the external compressions, with varied phase offsets that permit measurement of the wavelength of shear waves as they are transmitted through the tissue. A single slice can be acquired in 1 breath-hold. Maps of wavelength are then created and converted into tissue stiffness, typically measured in kilopascals (**Fig. 4**). The stiffness maps, or elastograms, are displayed in both color and black and white. The color images are used for

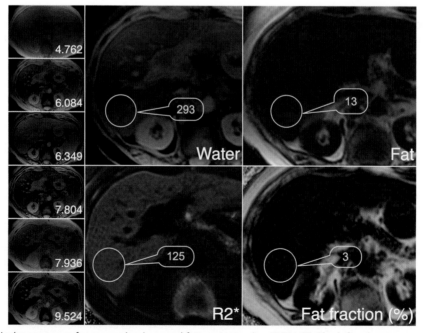

**Fig. 2.** Multiecho sequence for measuring iron and fat content using IDEAL IQ. The left column represents magnitude images reconstructed from the 6 different echos acquired during the acquisition. Complex phase data from each echo are then reconstructed to determine the fat and water content at each voxel. Additionally R2* values can be measured to determine hepatic iron content. In this case, the R2* measured 125, which equals to a T2* of 1/125 or 8 ms consistent with significant iron deposition.

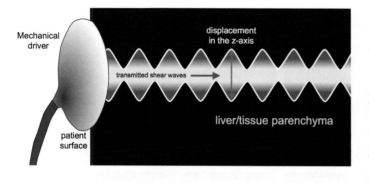

**Fig. 3.** MR elastography. An external mechanical driver is placed over the right lobe of the liver and compresses tissue with a specific frequency. This results in shear waves that are transmitted through the underlying liver. As the shear waves travel through the parenchyma, they result in displacement along the z-axis. This displacement is then measured using a motion-encoding gradient similar to that used in phase-contrast imaging placed along the z-axis. By timing this acquisition to the frequency of the mechanical driver and offsetting the acquisition by varying phases, the wavelength of the shear wave can be measured, which is then converted into tissue stiffness, measured in pascals.

visual interpretation: regions with high stiffness are depicted as red whereas those with low stiffness are depicted as blue. The actual stiffness can be measured on the gray-scale images using regions of interest within the liver, with the units as kilopascals.

Although elastography has been shown to be robust and reproducible, it can fail to produce adequate elastograms. The most common reason for failure is severe iron overload (**Fig. 5**). Typical MR elastography protocols use a GRE sequence that is sensitive to T2* and the typical TE used is approximately 20 ms. Therefore, in patients with high iron content, the T2* effect of the iron is such that there is little signal left for imaging with MR elastography.

## FIBROSIS AND CIRRHOSIS

Fibrosis forms in the setting of chronic inflammation. There are several grading schema used for pathologic staging of fibrosis; the most commonly used is METAVIR, which ranges from F0 to F4, with F4 describing bridging fibrosis seen with cirrhosis.

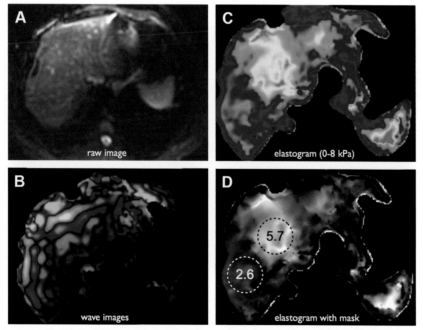

**Fig. 4.** MR elastography demonstrating focal fibrosis in segment 8. (*A*) Represents the magnitude image from the MR elastography acquisition that is predominantly T2 weighted. From these images, wave maps are created (*B*) depicting the shear waves as they propagate through the liver. (*C*) Shows the color elastogram image with areas that are blue showing normal pressures and red from severe fibrosis. (*D*) Shows normal pressures (2.6 kPa) in area of normal pressure and 5.7 kPa in area of marked fibrosis in segment 8.

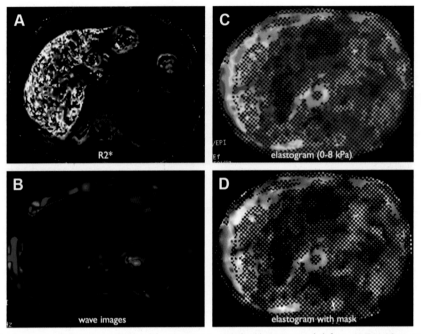

**Fig. 5.** MR elastography failure in patient with severe iron overload. R2* map (*A*) from IDEAL IQ acquisition demonstrates an R2* of over 400 (T2* less than 3) consistent with severe iron overload. Wave images (*B*) fail to generate in the hepatic parenchyma due to inadequate hepatic signal. Elastograms (*C, D*) demonstrate failure of the algorithm as shown by the hatched mask across the imaged slice.

Typical MR imaging (T2-weighted imaging and contrast-enhanced imaging) does not effectively evaluate for the presence of F0-F3 fibrosis and, therefore, misses the presence of clinically significant liver disease and cannot effectively distinguish the stages of fibrosis. Diffusion-weighted imaging (DWI) has been shown to correlate with the presence of early-stage fibrosis.[15] The theory is that the presence of increase interstitial fibrous tissue restricts the motion of water molecules, resulting in a decrease in the apparent diffusion coefficient (ADC). Unfortunately, DWI is limited because ADC measurements are not robust and, therefore, applying an ADC cutoff is impractical for the presence of fibrosis. The most robust technique available is MR elastography. Measurement cutoffs have been shown to be robust across sites and magnetic field strengths. Using a cutoff value of 2.93 kPa, MR elastography has been shown to have sensitivity and specificity of 98% and 99%, respectively, for detecting the presence of fibrosis.[16] In addition, MR elastography has been shown to more effectively measure fibrosis than DWI.[17] Specifically, MR elastography showed greater ability than DWI in discriminating stages F2 or greater, F3 or greater, and F4. Although stiffness values on MR elastography increased in relation to increasing severity of fibrosis, no consistent relationship was seen on DWI between ADC values and stage of fibrosis. MR imaging of

fibrosis also provides improved imaging of disease throughout the liver that can lead to over- or understaging on percutaneous biopsies (see **Fig. 4**).

Fibrosis eventually progresses to cirrhosis in the setting of chronic inflammation in the absence of intervention. Cirrhosis describes bridging fibrosis with marked architectural distortion and associated nodular regeneration. Pathologists usually characterize cirrhosis as either micronodular or macronodular depending on the size of the regenerative nodules, less than 3 mm for micronodular, and more than 3 mm for macronodular. The abnormal liver morphology is the most obvious sign of cirrhosis, which includes the nodular contour of the liver surface, caudate and left lateral lobe hypertrophy, and the notch sign along the posterior right lobe. Often, sequelae of portal hypertension are seen, including an enlarged main portal vein, splenomegaly, and the presence of varices. On MR imaging, the extensive fibrosis seen in the cirrhotic liver is T2 hyperintense and retains contrast on delayed imaging after the administration of extracellular contrast agents (**Fig. 6**). Using hepatobiliary agents, such as gadoxetate, the fibrosis is hypointense with respect to the adjacent liver. MR elastography has been shown more effective than the conventional anatomic features of cirrhosis on MR imaging.[18]

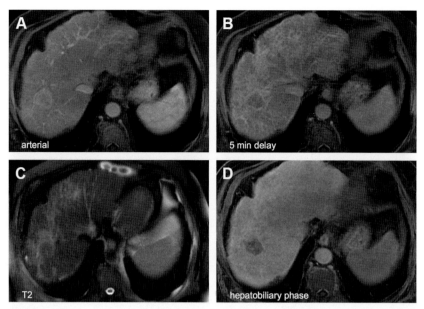

**Fig. 6.** Cirrhosis with extracellular and hepatobiliary contrast agents. With extracellular contrast agents, fibrosis is noted as linear delayed enhancement often seen best on 5- to 10-minute delays (*B*), whereas on arterial phase imaging there is no evidence of abnormal enhancement (*A*). On T2-weighted imaging, fibrous tissue is hyperintense (*C*). Typically on hepatobiliary phase imaging (*D*), fibrosis is hypointense relative to the hepatic parenchyma, but in this case an extracellular contrast agent was administered prior to gadoxetate disodium and, therefore, the fibrous tissue is isointense to the hepatic parenchyma, whereas the HCC is hypointense (*D*).

Since the 1995 International Working Party categorized hepatocellular nodules, the terms, *regenerative nodule* and *dysplastic nodule*, have become common in radiology.[19]

- Regenerative or cirrhotic nodules typically measure less than 2 cm, are homogeneous, and are isointense to the background parenchyma on contrast-enhanced imaging and can be hyperintense on hepatobiliary phase imaging (**Fig. 7**). On gross pathology, cirrhotic nodules are those that are indistinguishable from background nodules, and, because in cirrhotic livers they are not truly regenerative, the term regenerative nodule is being replaced with *cirrhotic nodule*.[20]
- Siderotic nodules are characteristically T1 hyperintense and T2 hypointense due to their increased iron content and are benign, although there is debate as to whether these should be termed regenerative/cirrhotic nodules or dysplastic nodules.[21] If all the nodules within a liver are similarly iron laden, they should be termed, cirrhotic nodules, with the term, *siderotic nodule*, reserved for a nodule that is uniquely iron laden compared with the background liver.
- Dysplastic nodules, unlike cirrhotic nodules, are distinct from background nodules on gross

pathology. On imaging, dysplastic nodules may be larger (ie, measuring more than 2 cm), be mildly hypointense on hepatobiliary phases, or have heterogeneous internal signal or an enhancement pattern on postcontrast imaging that differentiates them from the background cirrhotic nodules.[22] Distinguishing high-grade dysplastic nodules from early or well-differentiated hepatocellular carcinoma (HCC) can be difficult, because even on pathology the diagnosis is frequently in question.

It is believed that nodules in the cirrhotic liver progress sequentially from regenerative/cirrhotic nodules to dysplastic nodules and then to HCCs, although this has not been demonstrated.[21] The diagnosis of HCC is discussed elsewhere in this issue by Roth and colleagues.

## METABOLIC/STORAGE DISEASES
### Hepatosteatosis

Nonalcoholic fatty liver disease (NAFLD) describes the hepatic manifestation of the metabolic syndrome and is associated with obesity, diabetes, and dydslipidemia. The main conundrum for clinicians is separating out those patients who have reversible hepatosteatosis, termed *dormant disease*, and those who have a progressive

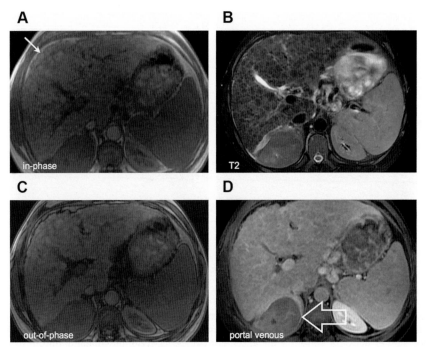

**Fig. 7.** Cirrhotic nodules and HCC. Innumerable benign cirrhotic nodules are noted throughout the liver measuring less than 2 cm. These nodules all demonstrate the characteristic T1 hyperintensity (*A, arrow*) and T2 hypointensity (*B*) and do not contain fat (*C*). These should not be termed siderotic nodules because they are not distinct nodules. In contrast, the HCC is hyperintense on T2-weighted imaging and T1 hypointense. Additionally on postcontrast images (*D*), the nodules enhanced identically to the background hepatic parenchyma whereas the HCC washes out on the portal venous phase (*arrow*).

inflammatory form, termed *nonalcoholic steatohe-patitis (NASH)*. Hepatosteatosis also occurs in the setting of alcoholic liver disease as well as numerous other settings, including steroid use and chemotherapy administration. Patients who develop fibrosis can go on to develop cirrhosis and its complications, including portal hypertension and HCC. A recent study showed, using MR elastography, that NAFLD patients with NASH but no fibrosis had higher hepatic stiffness measurements than patients with simple steatosis.[23] Hepatosteatosis can present with diffuse or geographic involvement, which is often best seen on IP and out-of-phase GRE imaging. Both forms can have associated nodular sparing or focal fat that can be misinterpreted as a focal liver lesion if not careful during interpretation (**Fig. 8**).[24] Focal fat is frequently seen along the falciform ligament and gallbladder fossa, which is thought related to differences in portal venous drainage. MR imaging quantification of hepatic fat is discussed previously.

### Iron Overload

Hepatic iron deposition is broken down into primary and secondary causes (**Table 1**). Primary hemochromatosis is a hereditary disease caused by

increased intestinal absorption of iron. Additionally, in primary hemochromatosis, there is a defect in the RES such that the excess iron does not accumulate within the RES. This results in iron being deposited in the liver, heart, pancreas, and skin (eg bronze diabetes) (**Fig. 9**). Secondary causes of hepatic iron deposition are termed, *hemosiderosis*, and are most commonly due to multiple blood transfusions. Because of the intact RES in hemosiderosis, iron is deposited within the Kupffer cells in the liver, whereas in primary hemochromatosis, iron is deposited within hepatocytes. Additionally, in hemosiderosis, iron deposition spares the pancreas and involves the spleen and bone marrow. Hepatic iron content is often measured using MR imaging in both diseases to follow the efficacy of treatment. Methods of detecting and quantifying hepatic iron deposition are described previously. There is a wide range in normal T2*/R2* values in patients,[25] making it difficult to use MR imaging for detection in patients with mild iron overload.

### Wilson Disease

Wilson disease is an autosomal recessive disease where there is increased intestinal uptake of copper that is deposited in various tissues throughout

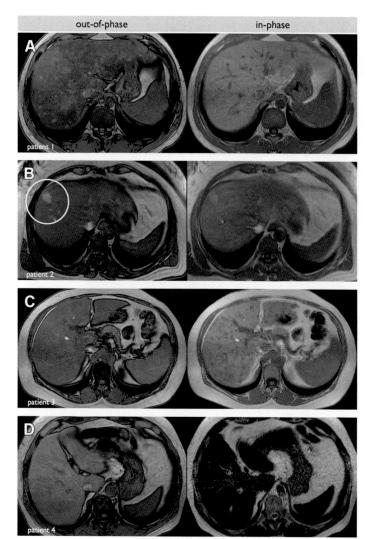

Fig. 8. Effect of fat on signal intensity on IP and out-of-phase imaging. Patient 1 (A) demonstrates diffuse patchy fatty infiltration with heterogeneous loss of signal throughout the liver on out-of-phase imaging relative to IP images. Patient 2 (circle, B) demonstrates focal fatty sparing in segment 8 with loss of signal in the adjacent hepatic parenchyma on OP images causing increased contrast with the unaffected region. Patient 3 (C) demonstrates diffuse nodular focal fatty sparing where the loss of signal in the adjacent parenchyma on out-of-phase imaging masks the spared regions. Patient 4 (D) demonstrates the opposite effect on IP and out-of-phase images whereby there is increased signal on the out-of-phase images relative to in phase images due to iron deposition.

the body, including the liver, cornea, and basal ganglia. In the liver, deposited copper results in an inflammatory response often with the development of hepatosteatosis, which then progresses to macronodular cirrhosis. Patients with Wilson disease develop T1 hyperintense and T2 hypointense nodules that resolve with chelation therapy, which are reportedly due to deposition of copper and its

| Table 1 | |
|---|---|
| **Comparison of primary and secondary hemochromatosis** | |
| **Primary Hemochromatosis** | **Secondary Hemochromatosis** |
| Genetically inherited defect (HFE gene) results in increased intestinal uptake | Often iatrogenic, due to multiple transfusions or iron replacement therapy |
| RES abnormal | Intact RES |
| Iron deposited in the liver, heart, pancreas, and skin | Iron deposited in the liver, spleen, and bone marrow |
| Hepatic iron in the hepatocytes | Hepatic iron in Kupffer cells (the RES) |
| Treated with phlebotomy | Treated with iron chelation |

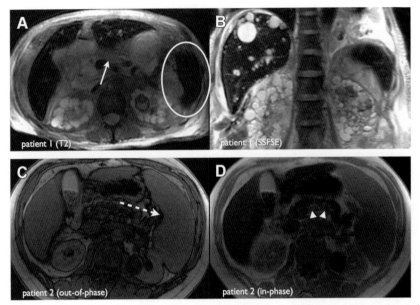

**Fig. 9.** Primary versus secondary hemochromatosis (hemosiderosis). In secondary hemochromatosis (hemosiderosis), the excess iron is deposited within the RES and, therefore, there is low signal on T2 and T2*-weighted images in the liver and spleen (*circle, A; B*), whereas the pancreas is not affected (*arrow, A*). In primary hemochromatosis (*bottom row*), the RES is injured and subsequently iron does not accumulate within the RES. This results in an altered biodistribution whereby iron is deposited in the liver, pancreas, cornea, and skin. There is low signal on the IP images in the pancreas (*arrowheads, D*) and liver whereas the signal intensity in the spleen remains (*dashed arrow, C; D*). Because the IP echo is acquired after the out-of-phase echo, there is lower signal in voxels that contain iron due to T2* effects.

paramagnetic effect (**Fig. 10**).[26,27] But given that these nodules appear identical to regenerative nodules, it is not a useful sign in differentiating Wilson from other causes of cirrhosis nor is it clear that these are copper-laden nodules rather than cirrhosis-associated nodules.

### Glycogen and Lipid Storage Diseases

Storage diseases are a heterogeneous group of inherited disorders that result in the accumulation of various metabolites used in either glycogen or lipid synthesis (see **Table 1**). Glycogen storage diseases are broken up into 12 subtypes, and a majority share hepatomegaly as a presenting symptom. Type 1, or von Gierke disease, is the most common form accounting for more than 90% of cases. The role of imaging in glycogen storage disease is not to differentiate the subtypes or severity of disease, which is typically done biochemically or genetically, but rather to evaluate for the development of HCCs, adenomas, and cirrhosis (**Fig. 11**).[28] Adenomas in glycogen storage disease are typically β-catenin associated and have an increased risk of malignant degeneration.[29] Nonetheless, there has been limited work using MR spectroscopy to quantify glycogen content within the liver.[30,31] Lipid storage diseases

also present typically with hepatomegaly but are not at risk of developing adenomas or HCC and, therefore, the most common finding in this heterogeneous group is hepatosteatosis, although some cases can progress to cirrhosis.

### INFECTIOUS AND INFLAMMATORY/GRANULOMATOUS
### Amyloidosis

Amyloidosis is used to describe a family of disease that all result in the deposition of misfolded proteins in soft tissues throughout the body.[32] The most common type of systemic amyloidosis is the immunoglobulin light chain form (primary amyloidosis) in which plasma cells produce excess monoclonal light chains; 10% to 15% of patients with multiple myeloma develop this disease. Less common forms of systemic amyloidosis can be related to infections or hereditary disease and often are caused by proteins synthesized in the liver. Hepatic amyloidosis is a common finding in patients with systemic amyloidosis, although rarely do patients develop clinically significant liver disease. MR imaging findings are nonspecific and often only show hepatomegaly and, as result, MR often is not helpful to assess in diagnosing hepatic involvement.

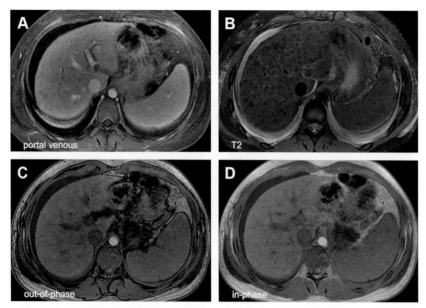

**Fig. 10.** Wilson disease. A 19-year-old patient with Wilson disease and evidence of cirrhosis. On portal venous imaging (A) the nodules are hypointense. There are numerous cirrhotic nodules that are T2 hypointense (B), but there is no evidence of signal loss on IP imaging (D) compared with out-of-phase imaging (C), because copper does not have the same paramagnetic effects as iron.

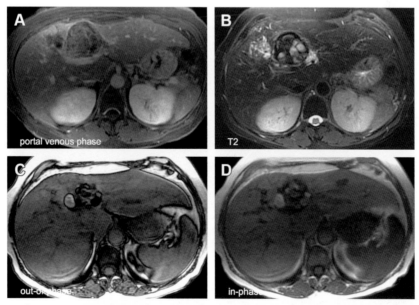

**Fig. 11.** Type 1 glycogen storage disease (von Gierke) with adenomas. Patients with glycogen storage disease develop hepatomegally due to glycogen deposition, although otherwise the hepatic parenchyma appears unremarkable. They are at risk for developing adenomas and HCCs. In this patient, a large adenoma can be seen in segment 4A with macroscopic fat (A, B). There is evidence of signal loss to suggest fat deposition on IP and OP, including both microscopic fat with loss of signal and macroscopic fat with India ink artifact on the OP images (C, D).

## Sarcoidosis

Sarcoidosis is characterized by the development of noncaseating granulomas most commonly involving mediastinal lymph nodes and the pulmonary parenchyma (90% of cases). Although sarcoid granulomas are noted histologically in the liver in up to 80% of patients, as few as 5% of patients have imaging findings of hepatic sarcoidosis.[33] Typically, hepatic involvement is subclinical, although in chronic cases, patients can develop cholestasis and uncommonly cirrhosis. The hepatic granulomas are often not apparent on MR, although on contrast-enhanced studies, multiple small ill-defined nodules can be appreciated (**Fig. 12**). Lesions are more easily appreciated in the spleen due to the relatively high intrinsic T1 and T2 hyperintensity of the splenic tissue, allowing for better contrast ratio to the hypointense and hypoenhancing nodules from splenic noncaseating granulomas. A majority of patients with hepatic and splenic involvement have thoracic involvement aiding in the diagnosis.

## VASCULAR
### Budd-Chiari Syndrome

Budd-Chiari syndrome is caused by obstruction of hepatic venous outflow from the liver. It can occur at multiple levels: type 1 occurs at the inferior vena cava (IVC); type 2 involves occlusion in the major hepatic veins; and type 3 occurs in the small hepatic veins.[34] The end result is venous stasis and increased portal pressure. In primary Budd-Chiari syndrome, there is occlusion in the main hepatic veins due to endoluminal lesions, such as webs or diaphragms. Hepatic venous thromboses are also included in the primary form, often seen in the setting of hypercoagulable patients. In the secondary form, the obstruction is due to compression from outside of the hepatic veins, often due to mass effect from tumors. Imaging plays an important role in the diagnosis because the disease can be heterogeneously distributed throughout the liver, meaning that a biopsy may provide a false-negative result.

In an acute setting, hepatomegaly and marked ascites develop, and if there is not enough time to develop collateral drainage, centrilobular necrosis occurs. Typically, there is decreased peripheral enhancement due to the venous stasis with relatively preserved central enhancement (**Fig. 13**).[35] Chronically, collateral drainage pathways develop, resulting in nodular regeneration within an affected liver and atrophy and fibrosis in the hepatic segments affected by chronic venous obstruction (**Fig. 14**). Unlike the acute setting, ascites is less commonly seen due to improved venous collaterals. T2-weighted images often demonstrate increased signal in affected regions of the liver due to increased parenchymal edema.

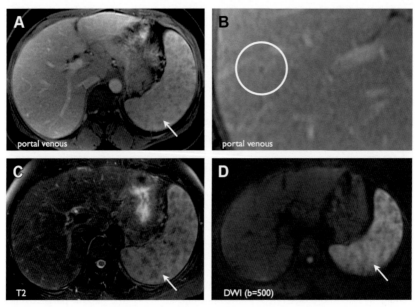

**Fig. 12.** Hepatic sarcoidosis. Innumerable small hepatic lesions can be appreciated on postcontrast T1-weighted images (*A; circle, B*), although lesions are much better appreciated in the spleen due to the intrinsic high T2 and restricted diffusion within the spleen, allowing for better contrast between spleen and the small granulomas (*arrows, A, B,* and *C*).

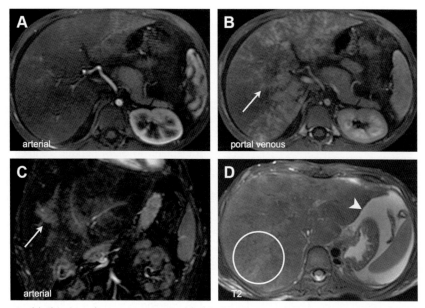

**Fig. 13.** Acute Budd-Chiari syndrome. In acute Budd-Chiari syndrome, there is relative preservation of the central flow with decreased perfusion to the peripheral liver due to venous stasis (*A, B, C, arrows*). On T2-weighted imaging, there is patchy increased T2 signal due to periportal edema secondary to increased sinusoidal pressures (*circle, D*). Also note the significant amount of ascites more commonly seen in the acute setting (*arrowhead, D*).

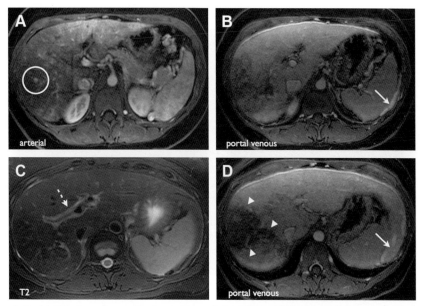

**Fig. 14.** Chronic Budd-Chiari syndrome. In the setting of chronic Budd-Chiari syndrome, collateral pathways for hepatic venous flow form, in this case primarily draining the left lobe of the liver (*arrow, B; C*), whereas the regions of the liver with persistent venous drainage obstruction (*arrowheads, D*) demonstrate abnormal perfusion due to the increase venous congestion. The increased pressure within the sinusoids results in periportal edema that can be seen on T2-weighted images (*dashed arrow, C*). As affected parenchyma regains venous drainage, regenerative nodules form that are seen as hyperenhancing lesions on the arterial phase (*circle, A*). Also note the absence of ascites on the T2-weighted image (*C*).

The key observation in the initial imaging study is to differentiate Budd-Chiari syndrome from congestive hepatopathy. In Budd-Chiari syndrome, the hepatic veins are obliterated or slitlike, whereas in congestive hepatopathy, they are enlarged and dilated. Additionally, the hepatic veins do not enhance in Budd-Chiari syndrome. Once a diagnosis has been made, the focus becomes on differentiating regenerating nodules from HCC. Unlike in cirrhotic livers, Budd-Chiari syndrome–associated regenerative nodules are truly regenerative and should not be termed cirrhotic nodules. The caudate lobe often has a separate venous drainage into the IVC and, therefore, can hypertrophy and mimic a mass and may show early and persistent enhancement.

## Passive Hepatic Congestion

Passive hepatic congestion is typically secondary to severe right-sided heart failure. The hepatic findings on MR imaging are nonspecific and include heterogeneous enhancement and periportal edema on T2-weighted images. What differentiates these findings from Budd-Chiari syndrome or other disease is that the hepatic veins and IVC are enlarged and there may be associated cardiac enlargement and signs of right-sided heart failure. If the process is longstanding, then fibrosis and cirrhosis can develop, typically in a micronodular pattern.

## Sinusoidal Obstruction Syndrome

Although SOS is often lumped together with Budd-Chiari syndrome, it should be considered a distinct entity. Previously termed hepatic veno-occlusive disease, SOS can be a complication of chemotherapy administration most commonly in patients with colorectal cancer treated with oxaloplatin but can also occur in conjunction with numerous other chemotherapy agents and after bone marrow transplant. In SOS, hepatic venules become obstructed from sloughed sinusoidal endothelial cells,[36] resulting in heterogeneous hepatic enhancement. The hepatic veins are attenuated but patent. On gadoxetate-enhanced studies, there can be diffuse or heterogeneous hypointensity on the hepatobiliary phase (**Fig. 15**).[37]

## DISCUSSION

MR imaging provides a unique tool for evaluating diffuse liver disease. In particular, multiecho sequences are becoming the gold standard in evaluation and quantification of hepatic fat and iron. MR elastography promises to play a larger role in the early detection of hepatic fibrosis. Unfortunately, a majority of the diffuse liver diseases lack specific features on MR imaging, yet a solid understanding of the different pathologic processes allows radiologists to provide a more informed interpretation.

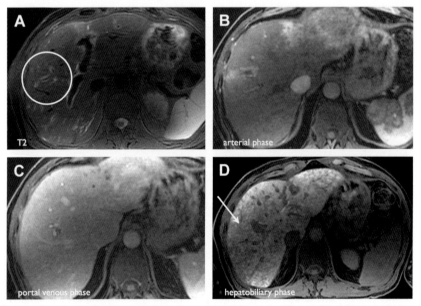

**Fig. 15.** SOS in a patient treated with oxaliplatin for colorectal cancer. T2-weighted images demonstrate hyperintensity in the region of severely affected sinusoids (*circle A*), whereas dynamic contrast enhancement shows early enhancement on arterial phases (*B*), which becomes isointense on the portal venous phase (*C*). Hepatobiliary phase images 20 minutes after the administration of gadoxetate demonstrate heterogeneous reticular hypointensity throughout the hepatic parenchyma (*arrow, D*).

## REFERENCES

1. Sirlin CB, Reeder SB. Magnetic resonance imaging quantification of liver iron. Magn Reson Imaging Clin N Am 2010;18(3):359–81, ix.
2. Gandon Y, Olivié D, Guyader D, et al. Non-invasive assessment of hepatic iron stores by MRI. Lancet 2004;363(9406):357–62.
3. St Pierre TG, Clark PR, Chua-anusorn W, et al. Noninvasive measurement and imaging of liver iron concentrations using proton magnetic resonance. Blood 2005;105(2):855–61.
4. Wood JC, Enriquez C, Ghugre N, et al. MRI R2 and R2* mapping accurately estimates hepatic iron concentration in transfusion-dependent thalassemia and sickle cell disease patients. Blood 2005; 106(4):1460–5.
5. Reeder SB, Cruite I, Hamilton G, et al. Quantitative assessment of liver fat with magnetic resonance imaging and spectroscopy. J Magn Reson Imaging 2011;34(4):729–49.
6. Qayyum A, Goh JS, Kakar S, et al. Accuracy of liver fat quantification at MR imaging: comparison of out-of-phase gradient-echo and fat-saturated fast spin-echo techniques–initial experience. Radiology 2005;237(2):507–11.
7. Dixon WT. Simple proton spectroscopic imaging. Radiology 1984;153(1):189–94.
8. Fishbein MH, Gardner KG, Potter CJ, et al. Introduction of fast MR imaging in the assessment of hepatic steatosis. Magn Reson Imaging 1997;15(3):287–93.
9. Reeder SB, Hu HH, Sirlin CB. Proton density fat-fraction: a standardized mr-based biomarker of tissue fat concentration. J Magn Reson Imaging 2012;36(5):1011–4.
10. Hernando D, Kramer JH, Reeder SB. Multipeak fat-corrected complex R2* relaxometry: theory, optimization, and clinical validation. Magn Reson Med 2013;70(5):1319–31.
11. Kühn JP, Hernando D, Munoz Del Rio A, et al. Effect of multipeak spectral modeling of fat for liver iron and fat quantification: correlation of biopsy with MR imaging results. Radiology 2012;265(1): 133–42.
12. Bydder M, Yokoo T, Hamilton G, et al. Relaxation effects in the quantification of fat using gradient echo imaging. Magn Reson Imaging 2008;26(3):347–59.
13. Yu H, Shimakawa A, McKenzie CA, et al. Multiecho water-fat separation and simultaneous R2* estimation with multifrequency fat spectrum modeling. Magn Reson Med 2008;60(5):1122–34.
14. Venkatesh SK, Yin M, Ehman RL. Magnetic resonance elastography of liver: technique, analysis, and clinical applications. J Magn Reson Imaging 2013;37(3):544–55.
15. Girometti R, Furlan A, Bazzocchi M, et al. Diffusion-weighted MRI in evaluating liver fibrosis: a feasibility study in cirrhotic patients. Radiol Med 2007;112(3): 394–408.
16. Yin M, Talwalkar JA, Glaser KJ, et al. Assessment of hepatic fibrosis with magnetic resonance elastography. Clin Gastroenterol Hepatol 2007;5(10): 1207–13.e2.
17. Wang Y, Ganger DR, Levitsky J, et al. Assessment of chronic hepatitis and fibrosis: comparison of MR elastography and diffusion-weighted imaging. Am J Roentgenol 2011;196(3):553–61.
18. Rustogi R, Horowitz J, Harmath C, et al. Accuracy of MR elastography and anatomic MR imaging features in the diagnosis of severe hepatic fibrosis and cirrhosis. J Magn Reson Imaging 2012;35(6): 1356–64.
19. International Working Party. Terminology of nodular hepatocellular lesions. Hepatology 1995;22(3): 983–93.
20. International Consensus Group for Hepatocellular NeoplasiaThe International Consensus Group for Hepatocellular Neoplasia. Pathologic diagnosis of early hepatocellular carcinoma: a report of the international consensus group for hepatocellular neoplasia. Hepatology 2009;49(2):658–64.
21. Jeong YY, Yim NY, Kang HK. Hepatocellular carcinoma in the cirrhotic liver with helical CT and MRI: imaging spectrum and pitfalls of cirrhosis-related nodules. Am J Roentgenol 2005;185(4):1024–32.
22. Kogita S, Imai Y, Okada M, et al. Gd-EOB-DTPA-enhanced magnetic resonance images of hepatocellular carcinoma: correlation with histological grading and portal blood flow. Eur Radiol 2010; 20(10):2405–13.
23. Chen J, Talwalkar JA, Yin M, et al. Early detection of nonalcoholic steatohepatitis in patients with nonalcoholic fatty liver disease by using MR elastography. Radiology 2011;259(3):749–56.
24. Hamer OW, Aguirre DA, Casola G, et al. Fatty liver: imaging patterns and pitfalls. Radiographics 2006; 26(6):1637–53.
25. Schwenzer NF, Machann J, Haap MM, et al. T2* relaxometry in liver, pancreas, and spleen in a healthy cohort of one hundred twenty-nine subjects-correlation with age, gender, and serum ferritin. Invest Radiol 2008;43(12):854–60.
26. Kozic D, Svetel M, Petrovic I, et al. Regression of nodular liver lesions in Wilson's disease. Acta Radiol 2006;47(7):624–7.
27. Ko S, Lee T, Ng S, et al. Unusual liver MR findings of Wilson's disease in an asymptomatic 2-year-old girl. Abdom Imaging 1998;23(1):56–9.
28. Manzia TM, Angelico R, Toti L, et al. Glycogen storage disease type Ia and VI associated with hepatocellular carcinoma: two case reports. Transplant Proc 2011;43(4):1181–3.
29. Shanbhogue A, Shah S, Zaheer A, et al. Hepatocellular adenomas: current update on genetics,

taxonomy, and management. J Comput Assist To-mogr 2011;35(2):159–66.

30. Roser W, Beckmann N, Wiesmann U, et al. Absolute quantification of the hepatic glycogen content in a patient with glycogen storage disease by 13C magnetic resonance spectroscopy. Magn Reson Imaging 1996;14(10):1217–20.

31. Ouwerkerk R, Pettigrew RI, Gharib AM. Liver metabolite concentrations measured with 1H MR spectroscopy. Radiology 2012;265(2):565–75.

32. Merlini G, Seldin DC, Gertz MA. Amyloidosis: pathogenesis and new therapeutic options. J Clin Oncol 2011;29(14):1924–33.

33. Ferreira A, Ramalho M, de Campos RO, et al. Hepatic sarcoidosis: MR appearances in patients with chronic liver disease. Magn Reson Imaging 2013; 31(3):432–8.

34. Janssen HL, Garcia-Pagan JC, Elias E, et al. Budd-Chiari syndrome: a review by an expert panel. J Hepatol 2003;38(3):364–71.

35. Brancatelli G, Vilgrain V, Federle MP, et al. Budd-Chiari syndrome: spectrum of imaging findings. Am J Roentgenol 2007;188(2):W168–76.

36. Rubbia-Brandt L. Sinusoidal obstruction syndrome. Clin Liver Dis 2010;14(4):651–68.

37. Shin NY, Kim MJ, Lim JS, et al. Accuracy of gadoxetic acid-enhanced magnetic resonance imaging for the diagnosis of sinusoidal obstruction syndrome in patients with chemotherapy-treated colorectal liver metastases. Eur Radiol 2012;22(4):864–71.

# MR Imaging of the Biliary System

Benjamin L. Yam, MD, Evan S. Siegelman, MD*

## KEYWORDS

- Biliary • Gallbladder • Bile ducts • Magnetic resonance imaging
- Magnetic resonance cholangiopancreatography • MR imaging • MRCP

## KEY POINTS

- Variant biliary ductal drainage should be identified on preoperative imaging in patients undergoing partial hepatectomy, whether for liver donation or disease resection.
- Low or medial insertion of the cystic duct into the extrahepatic duct should be identified on preoperative imaging in patients undergoing cholecystectomy to minimize accidental ligation of the common duct.
- Impaired concentration of cholesterol within bile in ill patients can be determined with chemical shift imaging.
- Hyperintense signal within the biliary system on T1-weighted sequences is related to high bilirubin content and is present within cholestasis, pigment stones, and biliary casts.
- Cholangiocarcinoma and gallbladder carcinoma typically demonstrate arterial phase enhancement with persistent enhancement into the portal venous phase, related to the fibrotic nature of these neoplasms.

## INTRODUCTION

Although ultrasound, computed tomography (CT), and cholescintigraphy play essential roles in the evaluation of suspected biliary abnormalities, magnetic resonance (MR) imaging and magnetic resonance cholangiopancreatography (MRCP) can be used to evaluate inconclusive findings and provide a comprehensive noninvasive assessment of the biliary tract and gallbladder. MRCP has become widely used for evaluating the biliary tree and can be performed instead of diagnostic endoscopic retrograde cholangiopancreatography (ERCP) and percutaneous transhepatic cholangiography for many patients. Conventional MR sequences allow for additional evaluation of the biliary system and adjacent structures. This article reviews standard MR and MRCP techniques,

clinical applications, and pitfalls. Normal biliary anatomy and variants are discussed, particularly as they pertain to preoperative planning. A spectrum of benign and malignant biliary processes is reviewed, emphasizing MR findings that aid in characterization.

## MR TECHNIQUE

For the evaluation of suspected biliary disease, the authors suggest a standard abdominal MR protocol consisting of unenhanced T1-weighted, T2-weighted, diffusion-weighted pulse sequences, and dynamic postcontrast images, supplemented by MRCP. Patients can fast 3 to 6 hours before the study to decrease the amount of residual fluid within the stomach and bowel, decrease duodenal peristalsis, and promote gallbladder filling.

Disclosures: None.
Department of Radiology, Hospital of the University of Pennsylvania, Perelman School of Medicine at the University of Pennsylvania, 34th and Spruce Streets, Philadelphia, PA 19104-4283, USA
* Corresponding author.
*E-mail address:* Evan.Siegelman@uphs.upenn.edu

Radiol Clin N Am 52 (2014) 725–755
http://dx.doi.org/10.1016/j.rcl.2014.02.011

MRCP is a technique that provides noninvasive evaluation of the biliary tree and exploits the high water content of bile while reducing background signal from adjacent soft tissues by using heavily T2-weighted sequences (echo times >180 ms). This technique is particularly useful in cases with low pretest probability requiring biliary intervention, whereby a negative result precludes the need for an invasive ERCP.[1] MRCP is also advantageous in cases of suspected high-grade obstruction and surgically altered biliary anatomy that might make ERCP difficult or impossible to perform. Several different pulse sequences may be used to generate an MRCP, and the particular technique may be tailored to the individual. MRCP sequences commonly include a combination of thin multislice acquisitions and thick multislab techniques.[2–4] Both methods derive from variants of single-shot fast spin-echo techniques with long echo times that allow for short acquisition times.[2,5]

MRCP may be acquired using 2D or 3D techniques, with 3D isotropic MRCP providing higher spatial resolution because of the thinner sections without intersection gaps. Isotropic 3D thin-section MRCP may be performed in the coronal oblique plane as 1.5-mm sections. These source thin images can be postprocessed in multiple planes to generate maximum intensity projections (MIPs). If the patient is unable to breathe regularly, an alternative to the respiratory-triggered thin slices are 2D heavily T2-weighted single-shot single-slab coronal projection images that vary from 3 to 8 cm in width that can be acquired in less than 3 seconds. Source thin sections should be reviewed in conjunction with thick slabs and MIPs to distinguish real lesions from artifacts related to volume averaging.

Conventional multiplanar abdominal MR sequences are obtained for the evaluation of the duct walls and periductal soft tissues. T1-weighted gradient-echo and single-shot T2-weighted fast spin-echo sequences may be obtained as a breath-hold to minimize motion artifact. Respiratory-triggered T2-weighted fast spin-echo sequences generate images with high spatial resolution. Dynamic postcontrast imaging is commonly acquired using 3D isotropic volumetric fat-saturated T1-weighted sequences during the arterial, portal venous, equilibrium, and delayed phases.

## HEPATOBILIARY-SPECIFIC CONTRAST AGENTS

Dual pharmacokinetic gadolinium-based contrast agents demonstrate both renal and hepatic excretion, producing positive-contrast T1-weighted functional MRCPs, because the contrast agent is excreted by the biliary system. Both gadobenate dimeglumine (Gd-BOPTA; Multihance) and gadoxetate disodium (Gd-EOB-DPTA; Eovist) accumulate within hepatocytes with subsequent excretion into the biliary system and can provide a complementary functional way to depict the biliary tree.[6,7] Approximately 4% of the injected dose of gadobenate dimeglumine is eliminated via the hepatobiliary system, with hepatobiliary phase imaging performed 1 to 2 hours after injection.[8] Fifty percent of the injected dose of gadoxetate disodium is eliminated in bile with hepatobiliary phase imaging performed 20 minutes following injection.[8]

## PITFALLS AND ARTIFACTS

Susceptibility artifacts associated with surgical clips, metallic stents, pneumobilia, or adjacent bowel gas, particularly on gradient-echo sequences, may obscure pathology or result in pseudolesions leading to false-positive results (**Fig. 1**). When an artifact is suspected, review of the fast spin-echo sequences may aid in clarification.

Respiratory motion artifacts may be produced due to irregular diaphragmatic excursion and resultant suboptimal triggering during breathing-averaged acquisitions, possibly resulting in misregistration of the bile ducts, which can appear discontinuous, stenotic, or duplicated, particularly on MRCP MIP reconstructions. In addition, partial voluming on MIP images may result in a failure to detect small intraductal filling defects. Source thin sections should be reviewed in conjunction with thick slabs and MIPs to distinguish real lesions from artifacts related to volume averaging.

Pulsation artifact arising from vessels adjacent to the extrahepatic duct, typically the right hepatic artery as it crosses the posterior aspect of the common bile duct (CBD), may mimic an intraductal filling defect or short segment stricture on MRCP and appear more pronounced on the MIP image (**Fig. 2**).[9] The absence of upstream ductal dilation should suggest the absence of a stricture or a mass.

The use of Gd-EOB-DPTA can introduce another potential artifact by shortening T2 relaxation times of gadolinium in excreted bile and thus reducing the bile T2 signal intensity of delayed sequences, possibly producing spurious intraductal filling defects on T2-weighted images. Thus, one should consider performing T2-weighted MRCP pulse sequences before injection of Gd-EOB DPTA.[10]

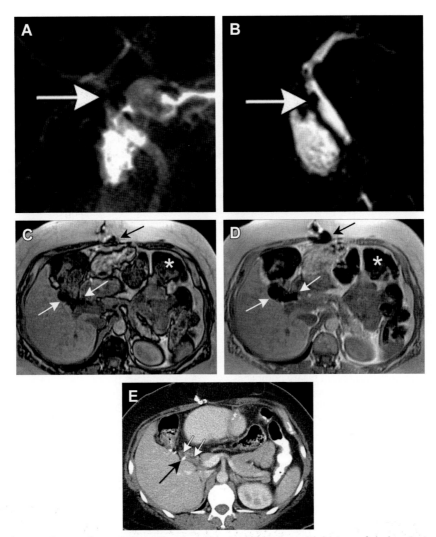

**Fig. 1.** Pseudostenosis secondary to clip artifact in a 48-year-old woman with history of cholecystectomy presenting with right upper quadrant pain. (*A*) Coronal thick-slab MRCP image shows an apparent stenotic lesion within the common hepatic duct (*arrow*). No intrahepatic biliary ductal dilation is present. (*B*) Coronal image from a thin-section 3D MRCP shows a polypoid lesion within the common hepatic duct (*arrow*) with asymmetric luminal narrowing. T1-weighted out-of-phase (*C*) and in-phase (*D*) images show susceptibility artifact within the cholecystectomy bed due to metallic surgical clips, which blooms on the in-phase image (*white arrows*). Note the presence of blooming within the clips in the anterior abdominal wall (*black arrows*) and within gas-containing bowel segments (*asterisks*). (*E*) Corresponding CT demonstrates metallic cholecystectomy clips (*black arrow*) adjacent to a normal caliber common hepatic duct (*white arrows*).

## NORMAL AND VARIANT BILIARY ANATOMY

Classic biliary anatomy is present in 60% of the population (**Fig. 3**). Several biliary ductal variants should be identified on MR and MRCP before partial hepatectomy for resection of disease or living donor transplantation (**Table 1**). One common biliary variant is known as a crossover variant and is characterized by drainage of the right posterior hepatic duct into the main left hepatic duct (**Fig. 4**). This variant occurs in 13% to 19% of the population.[11–13] In the "triple confluence" pattern, present in 11% to 19% of individuals, the right posterior hepatic duct drains into the confluence of the main right and left hepatic ducts.[11,12] Both the crossover and the triple confluence variants are important to identify before left hepatectomy, as inadvertent injury to one of the variant right hepatic ductal branches may result in biliary leakage, stricture, or ligation, causing atrophy and fibrosis of the associated right hepatic segments.[12] Biliary ductal variants should be identified on

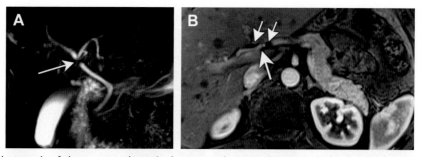

Fig. 2. Pseudostenosis of the common hepatic duct secondary to adjacent right hepatic artery in a 51-year-old man presenting with right upper quadrant pain. (*A*) Coronal MRCP MIP image demonstrates signal void at the level of the proximal common hepatic duct in the region of the hepatic hilum (*arrow*). No upstream biliary ductal dilatation is identified. (*B*) Axial postcontrast fat-suppressed T1 image depicts a right hepatic artery (*large arrow*) crossing the common hepatic duct (*small arrows*) in the region of the pseudostenosis seen on MRCP.

preoperative imaging in right hepatic lobe donors, because the presence of variant anatomy may warrant more than one ductal anastomosis in the transplant recipient.[14]

An aberrant or accessory anterior or posterior right hepatic duct empties directly into the common hepatic duct (CHD) or cystic duct in 7.4% of the population (see **Fig. 4C**). This anatomic variant is important to recognize to prevent biliary complications in patients undergoing right hepatic transplant donation or cholecystectomy.[11,12,15] Ligation of an aberrant or accessory right duct can lead to exclusion of the biliary segments drained by the duct, with resultant segmental right hepatic atrophy.

Laparoscopic cholecystectomy is currently the most commonly performed surgical procedure in the United States. Lack of recognition of variant cystic duct anatomy can contribute to postprocedural morbidity. A low insertion of the cystic duct into the distal third of the CBD (9%), or an aberrant insertion of the cystic duct into the medial CBD (10%–17%), increases the risk of injury to the adjoining CBD (**Fig. 5**).[12,16] In patients with low or medial cystic duct insertion, the surgeon may prefer to avoid dissection of the cystic duct to its distal insertion and instead leave a longer cystic duct remnant.[13]

An anomalous pancreaticobiliary junction exists when the common channel formed by the confluence of the CBD and main pancreatic duct is greater than 15 mm. This variant may result in reflux of pancreatic exocrine sections into the CBD, which predisposes patients to develop choledochal cysts, calculi, cholangitis, pancreatitis, and neoplasms (**Fig. 6**).[17]

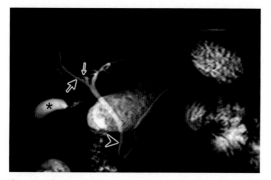

Fig. 3. Classic biliary anatomy. Coronal thick-slab MRCP shows the anterior branch of the right hepatic duct (*large arrow*) joining the posterior branch of the right hepatic duct (*small arrow*) to form the main right hepatic duct, which then joins with the left hepatic duct to form the common hepatic duct. The gallbladder (*asterisk*) communicates with the extrahepatic duct via the cystic duct, distal to which it is termed the common bile duct (*arrowhead*).

**Table 1**
**Biliary tree variants of surgical interest**

| Variant | Prevalence (%) |
| --- | --- |
| Posterior branch of the right hepatic duct draining into the left hepatic duct | 13–19 |
| Triple confluence of the intrahepatic ducts | 11–19 |
| Anterior or posterior branch of the right hepatic duct draining into the common hepatic or cystic duct | 7.4 |
| Low insertion of the cystic duct into the common bile duct | 9 |
| Medial insertion of the cystic duct into the common bile duct | 10–17 |
| Long parallel course of the cystic duct | 2–25 |

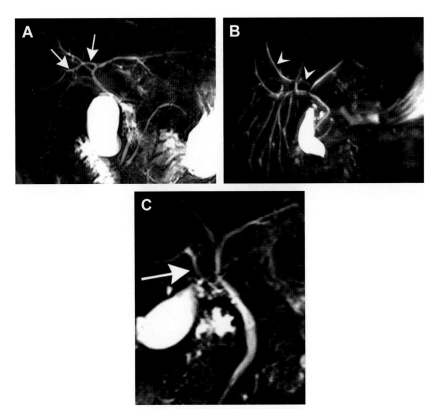

**Fig. 4.** Variant biliary ductal anatomy. (*A*) Coronal oblique thick-slab MRCP image shows drainage of the right posterior branch (*arrows*) into the left hepatic duct. (*B*) Coronal MRCP MIP image shows the right anterior branch (*arrowheads*) draining into the left hepatic duct. (*C*) Coronal thick-slab MRCP image demonstrates drainage of the right posterior branch directly into the cystic duct (*arrow*).

## CONGENITAL BILIARY LESIONS

The ductal plate is the embryologic precursor of the intrahepatic bile ducts, forming a cylindrical sleeve that surrounds the intrahepatic portal branches.[18] If bile duct remodeling undergoes arrest or derangement, congenital ductal plate malformations develop.[18] Biliary hamartomas, also known as Von Meyenburg complexes, are ductal plate malformations caused by failure of the small intrahepatic interlobular bile ducts to involute and are more common in women.[19] On conventional T2-weighted and MRCP sequences, biliary hamartomas appear as multiple intrahepatic hyperintense cystic lesions measuring less than 1.5 cm that do not communicate with the biliary tree (**Fig. 7**). Although these hamartomas do not usually enhance, variable patterns of enhancement have been described, including rim and homogeneous enhancement. Rim enhancement may represent compressed normal hepatic parenchyma.[18] To minimize unnecessary anxiety for patients and referring clinicians, the authors often report these lesions as benign cysts as opposed to biliary hamartomas.

Cystic hepatic lesions are noted in 13% to 74% of individuals with autosomal-dominant polycystic kidney disease and may represent either biliary hamartomas or peribiliary cysts.[20] Peribiliary cysts represent ductal plate malformations of the medium-sized intrahepatic ducts, appearing on MR imaging as nonenhancing T1 hypointense, T2 hyperintense, round to ovoid intrahepatic cysts of various sizes that do not communicate with the biliary tree (**Fig. 8**).[18,21]

Choledochal cysts reflect congenital dilatation of all or part of the extrahepatic or intrahepatic bile ducts. Although most choledochal cysts are diagnosed during childhood, up to 20% present in adults, more commonly in women.[22–24] Choledochal cysts are categorized into 5 types according their morphologic pattern of cystic dilatation using the Todani classification (**Table 2**).[22] Aside from type V (Caroli disease, see later discussion), choledochal cysts are not considered ductal plate abnormalities. An underlying anomalous pancreaticobiliary junction is present in up to half of patients and is thought to predispose choledochal cyst development by allowing reflux of pancreatic

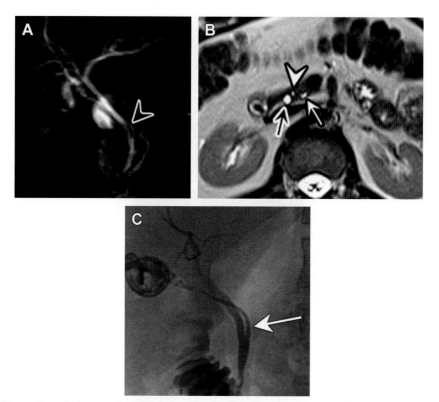

Fig. 5. MR illustration of a low medial insertion of the cystic duct. (A) Coronal thick-slab MRCP image shows low medial insertion of the cystic duct into the common bile duct (*arrowhead*), a normal anatomic variant. (B) Corresponding axial T2-weighted image shows the cystic duct (*arrowhead*) located medial to the common bile duct (*black arrow*). The main pancreatic duct is partially visualized (*white arrow*). (C) Fluoroscopic image obtained during percutaneous cholecystostomy tube placement in a different patient depicts the cystic duct (*arrow*) inserting medially into the common bile duct.

enzymes into the bile ducts during sphincter of Oddi contraction and causing upstream ductal wall weakening with subsequent dilatation.[24] Distal obstruction has been postulated as another causative factor.[24]

Type I choledochal cysts are confined to the extrahepatic duct and are subdivided into type Ia (diffuse) cysts, involving the entire extrahepatic bile duct, type Ib (focal) cysts, involving a focal segment of the extrahepatic bile duct, and type Ic (fusiform) cysts, which involve only the CBD (see Fig. 6). Type IV choledochal cysts demonstrate multifocal dilatations and are subdivided into type IVa, which involves both the intrahepatic and the extrahepatic bile ducts, and type IVb, which manifests as multiple saccular dilatations

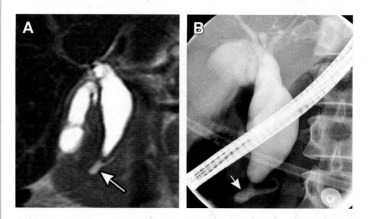

Fig. 6. Anomalous pancreaticobiliary junction with type 1a choledochal cyst in a 59-year-old man. (A) Coronal T2-weighted image shows a common pancreaticobiliary channel (*arrow*) and diffuse fusiform dilatation of the extrahepatic bile duct, representing a type Ia choledochal cyst. (B) Corresponding ERCP showing an elongated pancreaticobiliary junction (*arrow*).

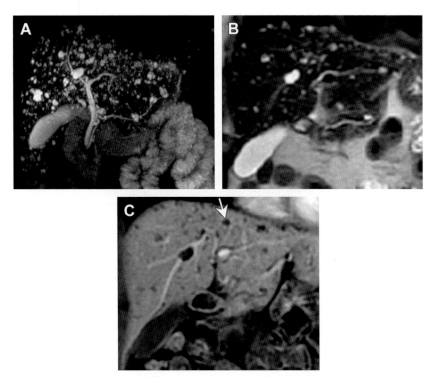

**Fig. 7.** MR depiction of multiple benign biliary hamartomas in a 72-year-old woman. Coronal MRCP MIP (*A*) and coronal T2-weighted (*B*) images show multiple (less than 15 mm) hyperintense cysts that do not communicate with the biliary tree, consistent with biliary hamartomas. (*C*) Gadolinium-enhanced fat-suppressed T1-weighted image demonstrates rimlike peripheral enhancement of a hamartoma (*arrow*).

of the extrahepatic duct (**Fig. 9**). The type V chole-dochal cyst, also known as Caroli disease, is an autosomal-recessive disease associated with ductal plate malformations, leading to varying degrees of inflammation and segmental fusiform or saccular dilatation of the larger intrahepatic bile ducts. On enhanced MR or CT, an associated central dot sign further supports this diagnosis, visualized as a focus of contrast enhancement within a central portal venous branch that is cir-cumferentially surrounded by a dilated intrahe-patic bile duct (**Fig. 10**).[25,26] Intraductal calculi may also be present within the dilated ducts. Car-oli disease is associated with congenital hepatic fibrosis, as well as fibrocystic renal anomalies such as autosomal-recessive polycystic kidney

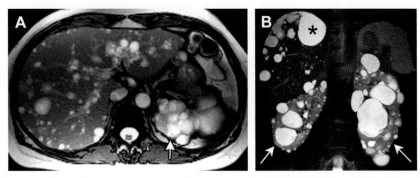

**Fig. 8.** Peribiliary cysts in a 43-year-old woman with history of autosomal-dominant polycystic kidney disease. Axial balanced steady-state free precession (*A*) and fat-suppressed coronal T2-weighted HASTE (*B*) images show the typical appearance of peribiliary cysts as well-marginated homogeneously hyperintense cysts of varying sizes (*asterisk*) scattered throughout the liver without wall or internal enhancement. Note that the cysts do not communicate with the biliary tree. No wall or internal enhancement was present on postcontrast imaging (not shown). Coexistent enlarged polycystic kidneys are present (*arrows* in *A* and *B*).

Table 2
Todani classification of choledochal cysts

| Type | Morphologic Pattern of Cystic Dilatation | Frequency |
|------|------------------------------------------|-----------|
| Ia | Diffuse dilatation of the extrahepatic duct | 80–90 |
| Ib | Focal dilatation of the extrahepatic duct | |
| Ic | Fusiform dilatation of the CBD | |
| II | True diverticula arising from the extrahepatic duct | 2 |
| III | Focal ectasia of the intramural segment of the distal CBD (choledochocele) | 4–5 |
| IVa | Fusiform dilatation of the intrahepatic and extrahepatic bile ducts | 10 |
| IVb | Multifocal saccular dilatation of the extrahepatic | |
| V | Multifocal dilatation of the intrahepatic bile ducts (Caroli disease) | Rare |

disease, medullary sponge kidney, and medullary cystic disease.[27] Congenital hepatic fibrosis manifests as dilatation of only the very small intrahepatic bile ducts. When congenital hepatic fibrosis is seen in combination with Caroli disease, the entity is known as Caroli syndrome. Intraductal stones, cirrhosis, portal hypertension, cholangiocarcinoma, pancreatitis, and intrahepatic abscesses are complications that can be evaluated by imaging.

## BILE

Bile exhibits variable signal intensity depending on its proportions of water, cholesterol, and conjugated salts. In the nonfasting state, recently excreted dilute bile demonstrates low T1 and high T2 signal, similar to free water. During fasting, water molecules become bound to macromolecules within concentrated bile, resulting in restricted motion and shortening of the T1 and T2 relaxation times. As the lipid-rich bile-containing bound water layers due to gravity, high T1-dependent and low T2-dependent signal may be present within the gallbladder.[28] On T1-weighted in-phase and out-of-phase imaging, loss of signal intensity results from the lipid component of concentrated bile (Fig. 11).

In ill fasting patients, decreased signal loss on out-of-phase imaging reflects the inability of the gallbladder to concentrate bile, sometimes indicating an underlying gallbladder inflammatory process (Fig. 12).[28] When hyperintense bile is noted on opposed-phase images, one should search for imaging findings of cholecystitis.

Occasionally, cholestatic regions within the liver manifest as segmental areas of high T1 signal that may be associated with ductal dilatation but without a correlate mass lesion. Such regions correspond histologically to biliary ductal proliferation and bile deposition within hepatocytes.[29]

## CHOLELITHIASIS

Cholelithiasis is present in approximately 10% of the population, often incidentally detected.

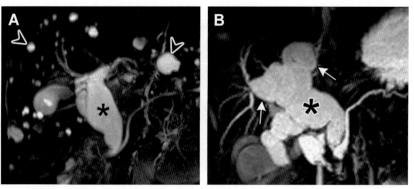

Fig. 9. Two different MR illustrations of type IVa choledochal cysts. (A) Coronal MRCP MIP image in a 72-year-old man shows diffuse dilatation of the extrahepatic and left central intrahepatic ducts, representing a type IVa choledochal cyst (asterisk). Scattered biliary hamartomas are also seen (arrowheads). (B) Coronal MRCP MIP image in a 3-year-old girl shows dilation of the entire extrahepatic (asterisk) and portions of the central intrahepatic biliary ducts (arrows), consistent with a type IVa choledochal cyst. Note that the peripheral intrahepatic bile ducts remain normal in caliber.

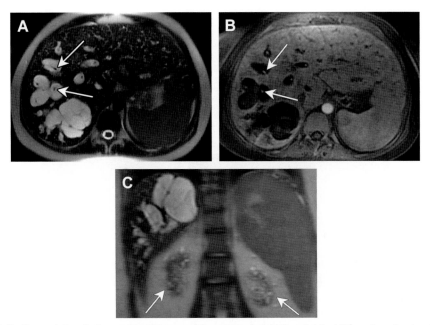

**Fig. 10.** MR findings of Caroli disease in a 19-year-old woman. Axial T2-weighted (*A*) and contrast enhanced fat-suppressed T1-weighted (*B*) images show predominantly right-sided intrahepatic biliary ductal dilation extending to the periphery with enhancing portal venules (*arrows*) located centrally within dilated intrahepatic ducts (*central dot sign*). No complicating cholangiocarcinoma is present. (*C*) Coronal T2-weighted image shows small cysts throughout both kidneys (*arrows*), reflecting autosomal-recessive polycystic kidney disease. Splenomegaly is also present, secondary to portal hypertension.

Gallstones are more prevalent in middle-aged and older women.[30] Although often asymptomatic, gallstones may produce acute or chronic abdominal pain, with or without associated inflammation.

Gallstones may intermittently become obstructed within the gallbladder neck, producing symptoms of biliary colic. Gallstones are classified as cholesterol or pigment stones. Cholesterol stones are

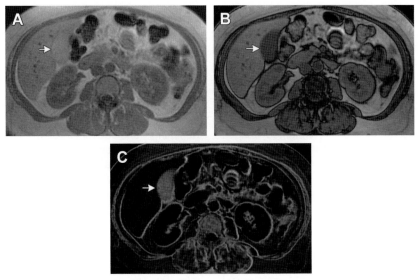

**Fig. 11.** MR illustration of normal lipid content of gallbladder bile in a 53-year-old woman with no symptoms related to the biliary system. Axial T1-weighted in-phase (*A*) and out-of-phase (*B*) images demonstrate signal dropout of bile (*arrows*), reflecting lipid-rich concentrated bile within a normally functioning gallbladder. (*C*) Corresponding subtraction image (opposed-phase image subtracted from the in-phase image) confirms the presence of normal lipid-rich bile within the gallbladder (*arrow*).

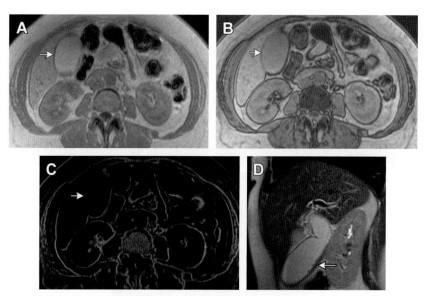

**Fig. 12.** Follow-up MR of the same patient in **Fig. 11** four years later, who now presents with right upper quadrant pain and abnormal liver function tests. Axial T1-weighted in-phase (*A*) and out-of-phase (*B*) images now show relatively less bile signal dropout of bile (*arrows*), reflecting impaired gallbladder concentrating ability. (*C*) Corresponding subtraction image demonstrates a relative decrease in bile lipid content (*arrow*) when compared with earlier study seen in **Fig. 11**C. (*D*) Sagittal T2-weighted image shows a dilated gallbladder containing dependent layering gallstones and sludge (*arrow*). There is no gallbladder mural thickening or pericholecystic fluid. Cholecystectomy specimen revealed chronic cholecystitis.

composed of at least 50% cholesterol and account for approximately 80% of gallstones in the United States.[30] Cholesterol stones typically have low signal intensity on both T1-weighted and T2-weighted imaging.[31]

Pigment stones have a smaller cholesterol component and a larger percentage of other constituents, including calcium bilirubinate and protein macromolecules. Although pigment stones also demonstrate low signal surrounded by hyperintense bile on T2-weighted sequences, these stones demonstrate a more variable range of signal intensities on T1-weighted sequences, in part related to the degree of hydration, with most appearing hyperintense on T1-weighted images (**Table 3**). In vitro studies suggest that the presence of metal ions within pigment stones cause T1 shortening of adjacent protons, thus appearing hyperintense (**Fig. 13**).[32] Although pigment stones

are easily fragmented by endoscopic lithotripsy, cholesterol stones tend to be harder in consistency and more resistant to fragmentation.[33]

Biliary sludge, or microlithiasis, is a common gallbladder finding distinct from concentrated bile and consists of a suspension of T2 hypointense particulate matter less than 2 mm.[34,35] Although biliary sludge often resolves or persists over time without clinical consequence, it may evolve into discrete stones or cause cholecystitis, cholangitis, or acute pancreatitis.[36]

Bile duct stones occur in 10% to 15% of patients with cholelithiasis. MRCP has very high sensitivity (91%–98%) and specificity (88%) for depicting choledocholithiasis, comparable to ERCP and endoscopic sonography, even for stones smaller than 5 mm.[37,38] MRCP may detect calculi as small as 2 mm, with higher sensitivities when viewed with thin-slice acquisitions of 3 mm or less (**Fig. 14**).

Bile is a dynamic fluid and may produce flow voids simulating a stone, particularly where the cystic duct joins the CHD on axial T2-weighted MRCP and single-shot fast spin-echo sequences (**Fig. 15**). The nondependent nature of this intraductal void should raise suspicion of a flow artifact. Review of the coronal sequences or axial images acquired with steady-state free precession sequences can differentiate between a stone

| Table 3 | | |
| --- | --- | --- |
| **Gallstone signal characteristics** | | |
| **Gallstone Type** | **T1 Signal Intensity** | **T2 Signal Intensity** |
| Cholesterol | ↓ | ↓ |
| Pigment | ↑ | ↓ |

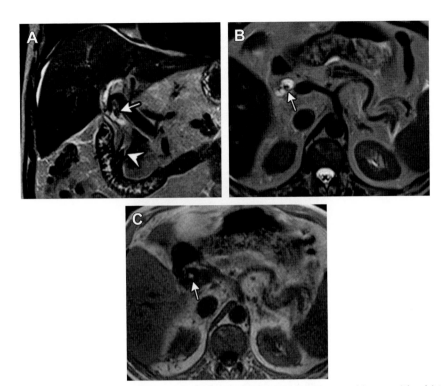

**Fig. 13.** MR detection and characterization of pigment cholelithiasis in a 61-year-old-man with a history of hepatitis C cirrhosis status post-orthotopic liver transplantation, presenting with epigastric abdominal pain, jaundice, and clay-colored stools. (*A*) Coronal T2-weighted MR image reveals a hypointense stone within the extrahepatic bile duct at the level of the cystic duct stump insertion (*arrow*) and an additional stone within the distal common bile duct (*arrowhead*), with extrahepatic ductal dilation. Axial T2-weighted (*B*) and T1-weighted (*C*) images at the level of the cystic duct stump insertion show a dependent T2 hypointense and T1 hyperintense stone within the dilated extrahepatic duct (*arrows*), consistent with a pigment stone.

and artifact. Additional mimics of biliary stones include pneumobilia, debris, mucin, hemorrhage, and tumor within the biliary tree. Pneumobilia is characterized by its nondependent signal voids and use of T1 in-phase and out-of-phase sequences, which demonstrate blooming of gas on the in-phase sequences with longer echo times (**Fig. 16**).

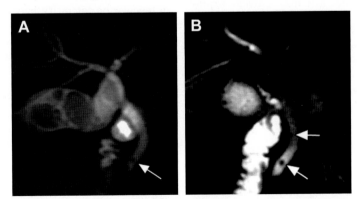

**Fig. 14.** Comparison of thick-slab and think-slice MRCP in the detection of common bile duct stones in a 38-year-old man with a history of cholelithiasis and abnormal liver function tests. (*A*) Coronal thick-slab MRCP shows a 3-mm stone within the distal common bile duct (*arrow*). Several gallstones are present within the gallbladder. (*B*) Single thin-slice image from a coronal 3D MRCP shows the distal common bile duct stone to greater advantage, as well as an additional 2-mm stone within the mid common bile duct not previously seen on the thick-slab image (*arrows*). Decreased volume-averaging with surrounding bile improves conspicuity of choledocholithiasis on thin sections.

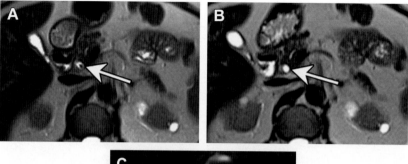

**Fig. 15.** False-positive choledocholithiasis secondary to flowing bile. (*A*) Axial T2-weighted fast spin-echo image shows a nondependent signal void within the extrahepatic bile duct (*arrow*) encircled by hyperintense bile. (*B*) The signal void is no longer seen on a separate axial T2-weighted fast spin-echo sequence obtained during the same study, confirming a pseudo-filling defect related to flow artifact (*arrow*). (*C*) Coronal single thick-slab MRCP image demonstrates no filling defects within the extrahepatic biliary tree. No potential stone was present on any other pulse sequence and this patient had no signs of symptoms to suggest choledocholithiasis.

## CHOLECYSTITIS

Acute cholecystitis typically occurs because of gallstone impaction within the cystic duct or gallbladder neck. Although ultrasound and CT are frequently the first imaging modalities used in the setting of suspected cholecystitis, they may miss an obstructing stone. MR may provide higher sensitivity for detection of an impacted gallbladder neck stone in acute cholecystitis.[39,40] An impacted stone may be detected on axial T2-weighted sequences and MRCP as a rounded or polygonal hypointense filling defect larger than the diameter of the cystic duct. When hepatobiliary contrast agents are used, the lack of gallbladder filling on hepatobiliary phases implies cystic duct obstruction.[41]

The diagnosis of acute cholecystitis on MR is based on the presence of gallstones, often impacted in the cystic duct or gallbladder neck, gallbladder wall thickening greater than 3 mm, gallbladder wall edema, gallbladder distension (diameter >40 mm), pericholecystic fluid, and perihepatic fluid between the liver and the right hemidiaphragm or abdominal wall (**Fig. 17**).[39,40,42] The presence of one or more of these, in the

appropriate clinical setting, confers a diagnostic sensitivity of 88% and specificity of 89%.[43] A thickened gallbladder wall that demonstrates diffuse or patchy T2 hyperintensity on fat-saturated images suggests an active inflammatory process (**Fig. 18A–D**).[41] Extension of inflammation to involve the pericholecystic fat appears as areas of reticular or patchy T2 hyperintense signal. On postcontrast fat-saturated T1-weighted images, enhancement of the gallbladder wall, pericholecystic fat, and intrahepatic periportal tissues may be seen, supporting the diagnosis of acute cholecystitis.

Isolated gallbladder wall thickening is not sufficient for diagnosing acute cholecystitis, because wall thickening is nonspecific and may be present in other conditions, including chronic cholecystitis, adenomyomatosis, gallbladder carcinoma, and edema secondary to extracholecystic or systemic disease, including hepatic dysfunction, hepatitis, and kidney failure. The cause of gallbladder wall edema in the setting of cirrhosis is incompletely understood but is likely multifactorial and related to factors such as elevated portal and cholecystic venous pressures and hypoproteinemia.[44] In cases of acute hepatitis, hepatic parenchymal

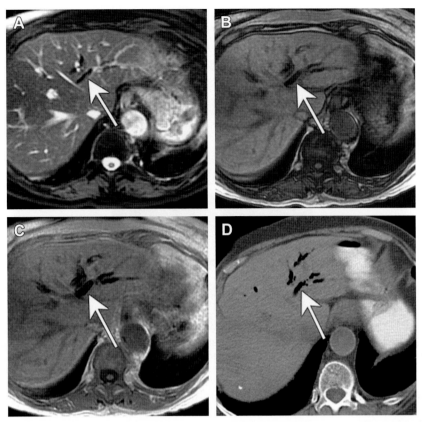

**Fig. 16.** Pneumobilia in an 82-year-old woman with abdominal pain following sphincterotomy. (*A*) Axial fat-suppressed T2-weighted image shows curvilinear low signal intensity in the distribution of the left-sided bile ducts (*arrow*). Axial T1-weighted in-phase (*B*) and out-of-phase images (*C*) demonstrate blooming of the pneumobilia on in-phase imaging due to the susceptibility effects of gas (*arrows*). (*D*) Corresponding unenhanced axial CT image confirming pneumobilia (*arrow*).

necrosis and inflammation may lead to layered gallbladder edema and thickening, reflecting inflammation and hyperemia within the serosal and muscular layers adjacent to the liver.[45]

Acalculous cholecystitis represents 5% to 10% of cases of acute cholecystitis and typically occurs in critically ill patients as a result of bile stasis and increased lithogenicity. Total parenteral nutrition, ischemia, and vasoactive mediators contribute to the development of the disease.[46]

Hemorrhagic cholecystitis may be seen as a complication of acute cholecystitis. On MR imaging, hemorrhage within the gallbladder wall, lumen, or pericholecystic tissues typically demonstrates high signal on T1-weighted sequences related to methemoglobin within subacute blood products.[47] On T2-weighted sequences and MRCP, hemorrhage or clot within the gallbladder and biliary tract demonstrate low signal intensity, which may result in nonvisualization of the gallbladder. Hemorrhagic bile tends to layer, producing a fluid-fluid level, with the T2-dependent

hypointense deoxyhemoglobin and methemoglobin within the hemorrhagic bile. In cases of gallbladder perforation, hemorrhagic bile may be present within the peritoneal cavity or adjacent hepatic parenchyma.

## ADENOMYOMATOSIS

Adenomyomatosis is a benign noninflammatory condition seen in up to 87% of cholecystectomy specimens, characterized by proliferation of the mucosal epithelium with deep and branching invaginations (Rokitansky-Aschoff sinuses) into a thickened tunica muscularis.[48] Associated gallstones are present in most patients.[30] On T2-weighted sequences, bile-filled Rokitansky-Aschoff sinuses appear as hyperintense intramural cysts within the thickened wall, producing the "string-of-pearls" sign that carries a 92% specificity for adenomyomatosis; this sign has a lower sensitivity of 62%, as sinuses less than 3 mm and sinuses containing inspissated proteinaceous

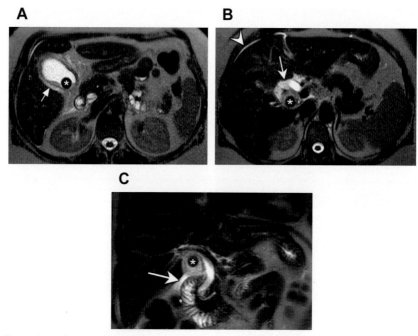

**Fig. 17.** MR illustration of acute cholecystitis in a 52-year-old woman presenting with abdominal pain. (*A*) Axial T2-weighted image shows findings typical of acute cholecystitis, including a dilated gallbladder containing a gall-stone (*asterisk*), dependent hypointense biliary sludge, and diffuse hyperintense gallbladder wall thickening (*arrow*), indicating an acute inflammatory process. Axial (*B*) and coronal (*C*) T2-weighted images at the level of the gallbladder neck show an impacted gallstone (*asterisk*), pericholecystic fluid (*arrows*), and perihepatic fluid (*arrowhead*).

bile or small calculi result in reduced or absent T2 signal and may be occult on MR imaging (**Fig. 19**).[49,50] Localized, segmental, and diffuse adenomyomatosis of the gallbladder may be present. Localized adenomyomatosis is usually present within the gallbladder fundus as focal semilunar or crescentic thickening.[48] In the segmental form, focal circumferential thickening in the midportion gives the gallbladder an "hour-glass" configuration.[51]

## GALLBLADDER CARCINOMA

Gallbladder carcinoma is the most common carcinoma of the biliary tree, with an incidence of 2 to 3 new cases per 100,000 individuals per year.[52] This entity is more common in women and the elderly and typically presents with advanced-stage disease with invasion of the adjacent liver and local nodal metastases. The advanced stage at diagnosis accounts for its poor prognosis, with a 5-year survival rate of only 5%.[53] Associated gall-stones that are present in 70% to 90% of patients cause long-standing gallbladder wall irritation, which increases the risk of developing carcinoma.[54] Chronic irritation may lead to "porcelain" gallbladder, characterized by calcific encrustation

of the gallbladder wall. Although early studies suggested up to a 60% chance of carcinoma development in patients with porcelain gallbladder, more recent studies suggest an incidence of less than 10%.[55–57] Greater than 90% of gallbladder carcinomas are adenocarcinomas, with small cell and squamous cell carcinomas rarely seen.[58] Serum carcinoembryonic antigen levels greater than 4 ng/mL, in the appropriate setting, carry a 93% specificity and a sensitivity of 50%.[53]

On imaging, gallbladder carcinoma manifests as focal or diffuse infiltrative mural thickening, an intraluminal polypoid mass, or a soft tissue mass replacing the gallbladder (**Fig. 20**). Focal or diffuse mural thickening of greater than 1 cm and asymmetric thickening are suggestive of carcinoma. On T1-weighted images, the tumor often demonstrates intermediate or low signal. On T2-weighted sequences, the tumor usually appears heterogeneously hyperintense to the liver. Restriction on diffusion-weighted imaging may improve sensitivity and increase confidence in distinguishing gallbladder carcinoma from benign causes of gallbladder wall thickening.[59]

The intraluminal polypoid form of gallbladder carcinoma comprises approximately 25% of cases. These masses demonstrate broad-based

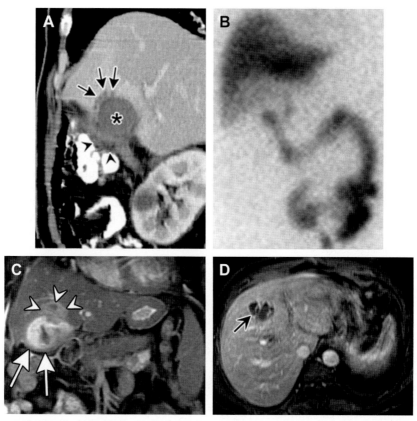

**Fig. 18.** Perforated acute cholecystitis with pericholecystic abscess in a 58-year-old man who presented with fever, postprandial pain, and abnormal liver function tests. (*A*) Initial enhanced sagittal reformatted CT image shows a dilated gallbladder (*asterisk*) and inflammatory pericholecystic stranding (*arrowheads*), representing acute cholecystitis. Several hypoattenuating pericholecystic abscesses are seen at the gallbladder-liver interface (*arrows*). (*B*) A 60-minute image from a nuclear hepatobiliary scan performed 1 day later shows tracer uptake within the liver and small bowel without radiotracer within the gallbladder fossa, consistent with acute cholecystitis. Additional imaging following morphine injection did not show tracer within the gallbladder. The patient was managed with percutaneous cholecystostomy. On follow-up MR imaging performed 5 days following the initial CT for persistent symptoms despite ongoing treatment, coronal fat-suppressed T2-weighted image (*C*) shows marked irregular gallbladder wall thickening with heterogeneous high signal (*arrows*) and extension of the pericholecystic abscesses into the hepatic parenchyma (*arrowheads*). (*D*) Axial postcontrast fat-suppressed T1-weighted image depicts the hepatic abscess as a rim-enhancing multilocular mass (*arrow*).

mural attachments with signal characteristics similar to those of the infiltrative form. Intraluminal polypoid carcinomas enhance moderately and homogeneously in the early postcontrast phases and rarely demonstrate necrosis or calcification.[31,60] Although there may be overlap in the appearances of intraluminal polypoid carcinomas and benign polyps, findings that favor malignancy include size greater than 1 cm along with early and prolonged enhancement. Benign polyps tend to enhance early, with subsequent washout.[61] Gallbladder metastases may demonstrate imaging features similar to gallbladder carcinoma and should be considered in the context of a known primary malignancy (**Fig. 21**).

Approximately 68% of gallbladder carcinomas manifest as diffusely infiltrative mass lesions involving the gallbladder fossa, with extension into the hepatic parenchyma in up to 65% of cases.[58] Nonvisualization of the gallbladder lumen, soft tissue replacement of the gallbladder fossa, engulfed stones, and liver invasion suggest the diagnosis. On MR, intermediate T1 signal and heterogeneous hyperintense T2 signal may be observed, and early and prolonged enhancement into the delayed phases is usually seen on dynamic postcontrast imaging.[30,61,62]

The most commonly used staging system for gallbladder cancer is that developed by the American Joint Committee on Cancer (AJCC)/International

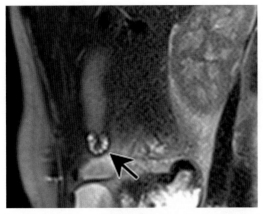

Fig. 19. MR illustration of asymptomatic focal fundal adenomyomatosis in a 42-year-old woman. Sagittal T2-weighted MR image shows focal fundal gallbladder wall thickening with hyperintense intramural cystic foci in a string of pearls configuration (*arrow*), representing the dilated Rokitansky-Aschoff sinuses of adenomyomatosis.

Union Against Cancer (UICC) (**Table 4**).[63] Agreement on criteria for resectability with curative intent for higher stages of gallbladder carcinoma is not universal.[64] In general, stage I carcinoma confined to the gallbladder wall is completely resectable and treated patients have 5-year survival rates of nearly 100%.[65] Unfortunately most tumors present at an advanced stage, extending beyond the gallbladder wall. With the exception of resectable focally invasive stage IIA disease, stage II–IV disease tends to be unresectable for curative intent. Tumor that invades the main portal vein, hepatic artery, or at least 2 extrahepatic organs or structures typically connotes unresectability.

MR has greater than 95% sensitivity for hepatic invasion and 92% sensitivity for the detection of metastatic lymphadenopathy.[30,62] Postgadolinium imaging is particularly useful in evaluating tumor extent, invasion of adjacent soft tissue structures, metastases, and involvement of the adjacent portal veins and hepatic arteries.[31,62,66] When tumor abuts the bile duct, microscopic invasion should be suspected even in the absence of biliary duct dilatation.[31,66]

## INFECTIOUS CHOLANGITIS

Acute bacterial cholangitis is a potentially life-threatening infection, usually arising in the setting of bile duct obstruction, with ensuing bacterial contamination, stagnant bile, and increased biliary pressures.[67,68] Choledocholithiasis accounts for up to 80% of cases of acute cholangitis. Patients typically present with right upper quadrant pain,

fever, and jaundice. Complications include sepsis, hepatic abscesses, portal vein thrombosis, and bile peritonitis. Imaging is helpful for detecting portal vein thrombosis and hepatic abscesses that may be unsuspected clinically.[67] On MR, the CBD shows diffuse, concentric wall thickening with associated periductal edema and mural enhancement, with or without pneumobilia. Within the liver, focal or diffuse intrahepatic ductal dilation, usually in combination with smooth, symmetric wall thickening, has been described.[69] Enhancement of intrahepatic duct walls is present in up to 92% of cases and is best identified on delayed postcontrast sequences (**Fig. 22**).[69] T2-weighted images may reveal peribiliary or wedge-shaped areas of high signal that enhance.[69] Marked inhomogeneous parenchymal enhancement in the arterial is more often present in patients with acute suppurative cholangitis.[70] An avidly enhancing and enlarged papilla measuring greater than 10 mm has 60% sensitivity and 86% specificity for suppurative cholangitis.[70] Endoscopic or percutaneous biliary decompression is necessary in such cases, because treatment with antibiotics alone is associated with mortality rates of 87% to 100%, owing to the limited excretion of antibiotics into the biliary tree.[71]

Recurrent pyogenic cholangitis (RPC), also known as Oriental cholangiohepatitis, is characterized by recurrent episodes of infectious cholangitis. RPC is associated with malnutrition and biliary parasitosis, such as ascariasis and clonorchiasis. Chronic biliary colonization by parasites induces persistent inflammation and eventual ductal fibrosis, which leads to stricture formation, bile stasis, and stone formation, predisposing patients to recurrent bacterial infections.[72,73] RPC is most prevalent in Southeast Asia and is associated with people of low socioeconomic status who live in rural regions. However, cases are presenting in Western countries because of increased immigration.[74] Patients typically present with recurrent episodes of right upper quadrant pain, fever, jaundice, and leukocytosis. MR and MRCP findings consist of varying degrees of intrahepatic and extrahepatic ductal structuring and dilatation.[75] Intraductal calculi are present in 80% of patients, most of which are T1 hyperintense secondary to the presence of bile pigment.[76] Strictures of the peripheral intrahepatic ducts result in decreased branching and abrupt tapering, giving an "arrowhead" appearance, with disproportionate dilation of the central and extrahepatic bile ducts. Pneumobilia is common due to reflux during stone passage through the ampulla. Thickened periportal spaces may also be present,

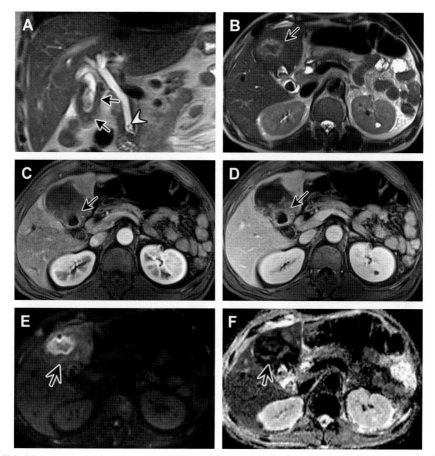

**Fig. 20.** Gallbladder carcinoma in a 64-year-old man who presented with right upper quadrant pain. (*A*) Coronal T2-weighted image shows infiltrative nodular wall thickening of the gallbladder body and fundus (*arrows*), intraluminal gallstones, choledocholithiasis (*arrowhead*), and extrahepatic bile duct dilation. (*B*) Axial T2-weighted image shows gallbladder wall thickening and intraluminal gallstones. Immediately anterior to the gallbladder within the medial left hepatic lobe, there is a poorly marginated mass demonstrating a thick hyperintense rim and an isointense central necrotic cavity (*arrow*), representing tumor extension into the liver. Note that differentiating between perforated gallbladder carcinoma and adjacent tumor extension into liver may be challenging. In this patient, a tumor extension was found at surgery. Axial fat-suppressed postcontrast T1-weighted images in the arterial (*C*) and delayed (*D*) phases demonstrate an ill-defined liver interface and progressive enhancement of the gallbladder wall and contiguous pericholecystic mass (*arrows*), consistent with gallbladder carcinoma with tumor infiltration of the adjacent liver. (*E*) Axial diffusion-weighted image with a b-value of 800 s/mm$^2$ (*E*) and corresponding apparent diffusion coefficient (ADC) map (*F*) depict restricted diffusion within the necrotic tumor (*arrows*).

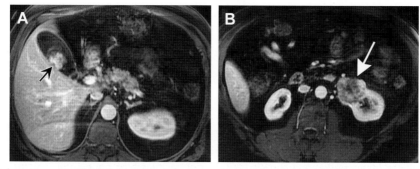

**Fig. 21.** MR depiction of gallbladder metastasis from renal cell carcinoma in a 59-year-old woman. (*A*) Axial postcontrast fat-suppressed T1-weighted image shows a lobulated enhancing polypoid intraluminal mass arising from the lateral wall of the gallbladder (*arrow*), representing biopsy-proven metastatic renal cell carcinoma. (*B*) Axial postcontrast fat-suppressed T1-weighted image at the level of the kidneys demonstrates a heterogeneously enhancing exophytic left renal mass, representing the patient's primary renal cell carcinoma (*arrow*).

**Table 4**
**AJCC staging system for gallbladder cancer**

**Primary Tumor (T)**

| | |
|---|---|
| TX | Primary tumor cannot be assessed |
| T0 | No evidence of primary tumor |
| Tis | Carcinoma in situ |
| T1 | Tumor invades lamina propria or muscular layer |
| T1a | Tumor invades lamina propria |
| T1b | Tumor invades muscular layer |
| T2 | Tumor invades perimuscular connective tissue; no extension beyond serosa or into liver |
| T3 | Tumor perforates the serosa (visceral peritoneum) and/or directly invades the liver and/or one other adjacent organ or structure, such as the stomach, duodenum, colon, pancreas, omentum, or extrahepatic bile ducts |
| T4 | Tumor invades main portal vein or hepatic artery or invades at least 2 extrahepatic organs or structures |

**Regional Lymph Nodes (N)**

| | |
|---|---|
| NX | Regional lymph nodes cannot be assessed |
| N0 | No regional lymph node metastasis |
| N1 | Metastases to nodes along the cystic duct, common bile duct, hepatic artery, and/or portal vein |
| N2 | Metastases to periaortic, pericaval, superior mesenteric artery, and/or celiac artery lymph nodes |

**Distant Metastasis (M)**

| | |
|---|---|
| M0 | No distant metastasis |
| M1 | Distant metastasis |

**Anatomic Stage/Prognostic Groups**

| Stage | T | N | M |
|---|---|---|---|
| 0 | Tis | N0 | M0 |
| I | T1 | N0 | M0 |
| II | T2 | N0 | M0 |
| IIIA | T3 | N0 | M0 |
| IIIB | T1–3 | N1 | M0 |
| IVA | T4 | N0–1 | M0 |
| IVB | Any T | N2 | M0 |
| | Any T | Any N | M1 |

*From* Edge SB, American Joint Committee on Cancer, American Cancer Society. AJCC cancer staging manual. 7th edition. New York, London: Springer; 2010; with permission.

owing to periductal inflammation and fibrosis.[73,76] Chronic intrahepatic duct obstruction or portal vein thrombosis may lead to lobar or segmental atrophy. Atrophy most often affects the left lateral

segment of the left lobe and posterior segments of the right hepatic lobe. RPC is associated with an increased risk of cholangiocarcinoma that develops in up to 15% of patients (**Fig. 23**).[74] Treatment of RPC involves removal of intraductal stones to maintain patency of the common duct and treatment of any underlying infection.

Although bacterial infection is the most common cause of infectious cholangitis in Western countries, parasites play an important role in other parts of the world, either as causative agents or as a predisposing factor to bacterial superinfection. *Ascaris lumbricoides* affects 25% of the world's population and is the third most common helminthic infection in the United States, after hookworm and trichuriasis.[77] Larvae mature in the small bowel and then migrate to the bile ducts.[78,79] Biliary ascariasis is more common in patients following biliary surgeries, such as cholecystectomy, and is presumed to be related to CBD ectasia.[78,79] On MR, the ascaris worm appears as an elongated T2 hypointense intraductal structure, coiled within or parallel to the bile duct (**Fig. 24**). Occasionally, the fluid-filled gastrointestinal tract of the worm may demonstrate T2 hyperintensity. Diagnosis may be made by fecal examination and removal of the worms may be accomplished by ERCP.

## STRICTURE

When biliary duct dilation is identified on MR, a search for distal obstruction is warranted. In the absence of an obstructing calculus, a stricture should be excluded. MRCP can depict an area of narrowing caused by a malignant lesion and upstream ductal dilatation with a sensitivity of 95%.[80] However, differentiation between benign and malignant causes can be challenging in some patients, because the morphologies of benign and malignant strictures have overlapping features.[80] The specificity of MRCP for differentiating between benign and malignant strictures varies widely, from 30% to 98%.[81] In general, benign strictures tend to have smooth borders with tapered margins, whereas malignant strictures are suggested by irregular, asymmetric stenosis with shouldered margins. Cross-sectional T1-weighted and T2-weighted sequences add specificity, and the presence of an associated mass lesion is suggestive of a malignant cause.[80] Strictures of the distal extrahepatic duct may be benign, such as in cases related to prior choledocholithiasis or pancreatitis, or malignant, secondary to pancreatic adenocarcinoma, distal cholangiocarcinoma, ampullary carcinoma, or duodenal carcinoma. Intrahepatic strictures are

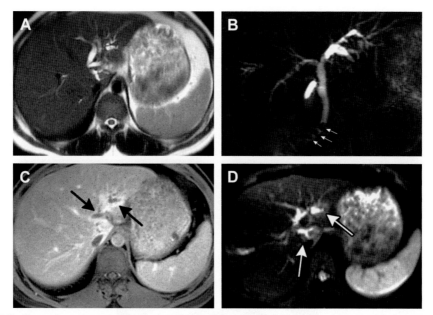

**Fig. 22.** MR findings of acute ascending cholangitis and choledocholithiasis in a 35-year-old man presenting with right upper quadrant pain and fever. (*A*) Axial T2-weighted image shows left-sided intrahepatic biliary ductal dilatation. (*B*) Coronal thick-slab MRCP shows 3 common bile duct stones (*arrows*) with upstream extrahepatic and left intrahepatic ductal dilatation. (*C*) Axial delayed postcontrast fat-suppressed T1-weighted image demonstrates periductal enhancement surrounding dilated left intrahepatic ducts (*arrows*), consistent with cholangitis. (*D*) Axial diffusion-weighted image with b-value of 50 s/mm² shows patchy hyperintensity within the left hepatic lobe in a periductal distribution (*arrows*), indicating active inflammation.

more likely related to an inflammatory process or invasion by gallbladder carcinoma. Malignant strictures secondary to metastatic disease can occur anywhere along the biliary tract and are typically due to extrinsic compression by metastases involving the periductal soft tissues and lymph nodes. Intraductal metastases are rarely seen and are typically from colorectal cancer, which has a propensity to grow along epithelial surfaces.[82]

There is a wide spectrum of nonneoplastic causes of biliary stricture, with iatrogenic injury accounting for up to 80% of cases, especially following cholecystectomy.[83,84] Benign strictures can occur in 0.2% to 0.7% of cholecystectomy patients, predominantly involving the common hepatic duct or CBD.[84,85] In patients who have undergone orthotopic liver transplantation, biliary stricture is the most common biliary complication, seen in 8% to 30% of patients.[86] These strictures may be anastomotic or nonanastomotic. Anastomotic strictures usually occur secondary to fibrosis, while nonanastomotic strictures result from biliary ischemia induced by hepatic artery thrombosis or stenosis.[87] Nonanastomotic strictures most commonly originate at the hilum and may progress to involve the intrahepatic ducts.[88] Balloon dilatation may be used to treat benign biliary strictures.

Diffuse intrahepatic and extrahepatic strictures are more likely secondary to postsurgical complications, intra-arterial chemotherapy, radiation exposure, or autoimmune diseases.

## PRIMARY SCLEROSING CHOLANGITIS

Primary sclerosing cholangitis (PSC) is an idiopathic, chronic inflammatory process involving the intrahepatic and extrahepatic bile ducts, seen predominantly in men in the third to fourth decade. The diagnosis of PSC is made from clinical, laboratory, and imaging findings. Initial clinical presentation may be nonspecific constitutional or cholestatic symptoms. PSC is associated with inflammatory bowel disease in 55% to 75% of patients, most commonly ulcerative colitis. MR imaging and MRCP are useful for both establishing the diagnosis of PSC and monitoring progression of disease by allowing assessment of the intrahepatic and extrahepatic biliary tree as well as the hepatic parenchyma and to screen for the development of malignancy. MRCP is comparable to ERCP for the detection of PSC, with a sensitivity of 80% to 88% and specificity of 87% to 99%.[89] MRCP characteristically shows a pattern of multifocal intrahepatic and extrahepatic stenoses alternating between segments of dilated and normal

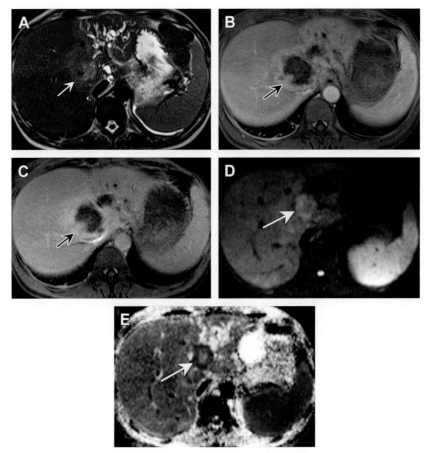

**Fig. 23.** Intrahepatic cholangiocarcinoma in a 43-year-old woman with a history of recurrent pyogenic cholangitis. (*A*) Axial T2-weighted image shows an ill-defined heterogeneously hyperintense mass within the central liver (*arrow*), left-sided intrahepatic biliary ductal dilatation, and mild atrophy of the left lateral hepatic lobe. Axial fat-suppressed postcontrast T1-weighted images in the arterial (*B*) and delayed (*C*) phases show a necrotic mass with a thick irregular soft tissue rim demonstrating progressive enhancement (*arrows*), consistent with cholangiocarcinoma. Viable tumor exhibits restricted diffusion on axial diffusion-weighted image with a b-value of 800 s/mm$^2$ (*D*) and corresponding reduced signal on the ADC map (*E*) (*arrows* in *D* and *E*). Note that signal characteristics of the tumor are similar to those of spleen on T2-weighted and diffusion-weighted sequences.

caliber ducts, giving a beaded appearance (**Fig. 25**). Isolated intrahepatic ductal involvement is seen in 25% of patients, whereas isolated extrahepatic duct involvement is rare.[90] Limitations of MRCP include lower detection in the early stages of stenosis and overestimation of the extent of focal strictures.[6] PSC remains difficult to treat because of progressive bile duct destruction. Medical management involves ursodiol, antibiotics, and immunomodulators including methotrexate and steroids.[91] Dominant symptomatic strictures may be treated with balloon dilatation, with or without stenting.

Progressive PSC eventually leads to biliary cirrhosis, characterized by diffuse peripheral hepatic atrophy with prominent central regenerative nodules.[92,93] A hypertrophied caudate lobe is identified in 68% to 98% of patients.[93] Atrophy of the left lobe helps distinguish PSC from other causes of cirrhosis, which typically demonstrate left lobe hypertrophy (**Fig. 26**). Enlarged reactive perihepatic portal lymph nodes may also be identified. Most patients with PSC eventually advance to biliary cirrhosis and subsequent failure, necessitating liver transplantation, with a 5-year survival rate of 85%.[90]

Postgadolinium images in the late arterial phase may demonstrate peripheral areas of hyperenhancement within the liver. These areas of hyperenhancement are likely secondary to transient hepatic intensity differences, whereby increased arterial flow compensates for decreased portal venous flow in areas of bile duct obstruction.[93,94] Periportal T2 hyperintensity and delayed

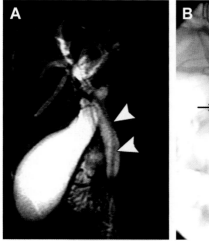
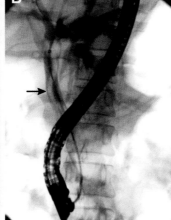
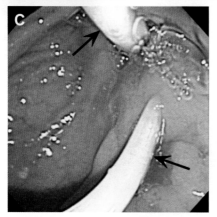

Fig. 24. MR and endoscopic depiction of an ascariasis worm in a 40-year-old woman with abdominal pain. (*A*) MIP image generated from a coronal MRCP demonstrates a linear filling defect within the extrahepatic duct (*arrowheads*), representing the ascariasis worm. (*B*) Corresponding ERCP image shows the ascariasis worm within the extrahepatic duct (*arrow*). A balloon is inflated proximally to facilitate worm removal. (*C*) Photograph obtained during ERCP and sphincterotomy shows the worm exiting the duodenal papilla (*arrows*).

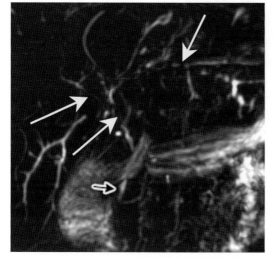

Fig. 25. MRCP depiction of PSC in a 41-year-old woman. Coronal MRCP MIP shows multifocal alternating segments of stricturing (*long arrows*) and normal duct caliber throughout the intrahepatic and extrahepatic biliary tree. The distal common bile duct is indicated by a small arrow for reference.

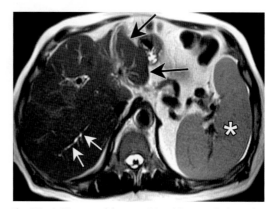

Fig. 26. A 72-year-old man with a history of ulcerative colitis, PSC, and cirrhosis. Axial T2-weighted image shows preferential left hepatic lobe atrophy (*black arrows*), typically seen in patients with PSC as opposed to other causes of cirrhosis. Splenomegaly (*asterisk*) and segmental irregular duct dilation within segment 6 (*white arrows*) are also present.

enhancement may surround segments of the portal tracts due to fibrotic replacement, sometimes in a hepatic segmental or lobar distribution (**Fig. 27**).[95]

## PRIMARY BILIARY CIRRHOSIS

Primary biliary cirrhosis (PBC) is an autoimmune disease characterized by acute and chronic inflammation of the small to medium bile ducts, primarily affecting middle-aged women. Patients present with clinical features of cholestasis and most have elevated antimitochondrial antibodies. PBC is sometimes associated with other autoimmune processes such as Sjogren syndrome, CREST syndrome, Raynaud phenomenon, inflammatory bowel disease, and autoimmune hepatitis. On MR, a periportal halo sign, observed in about 43% of PBC patients, is thought to represent a portal triad surrounded by an area of parenchymal loss and rimmed by regenerative nodules.[96]

T2-weighted sequences and postgadolinium T1-weighted images in the portal or equilibrium phases demonstrate the periportal halo as a 5- to 10-mm hypointense rim surrounding a hyperintense central area (**Fig. 28**).[96] Cholestatic symptoms are initially medically managed with ursodiol, with the subsequent addition of colchicine and methotrexate if treatment response is inadequate.[97]

## CHOLANGIOCARCINOMA

Cholangiocarcinoma is an adenocarcinoma arising from the bile ducts, either intrahepatic or extrahepatic. Intrahepatic cholangiocarcinoma is the second most common primary liver malignancy after hepatocellular carcinoma and is more common in men. Clinical symptoms include upper abdominal pain, ascites, weight loss, jaundice, weakness, nausea, and vomiting.[98]

Imaging features of intrahepatic cholangiocarcinomas differ according to pattern of growth, which

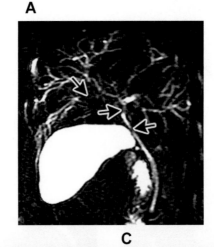

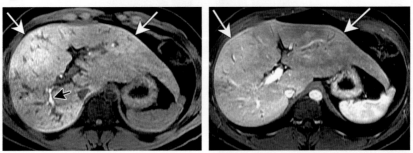

**Fig. 27.** Active PSC in a 21-year-old man with a history of inflammatory bowel disease and abnormal liver function tests. (*A*) Coronal thick-slab MRCP image shows multifocal intrahepatic and extrahepatic biliary stenoses (*arrows*) alternating with segments of mild biliary ductal dilation. (*B*) Axial fat-suppressed T1-weighted image depicts high intraluminal signal within dilated intrahepatic bile ducts (*black arrow*), as well as peripheral wedge-shaped areas of high signal intensity without an associated mass lesions, indicating cholestasis (*white arrows*). (*C*) Axial postcontrast fat-suppressed T1-weighted image in the portal venous phase shows persistent peripheral wedge-shaped areas of enhancement (*arrows*) corresponding to areas of cholestasis in (*B*), reflecting parenchymal fibrosis.

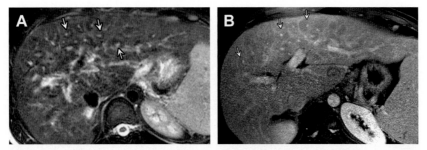

Fig. 28. MR illustration of the periportal halo sign in a 30-year-old man with PBC. Axial T2-weighted (*A*) and Gd-EOB-DPTA-enhanced fat-suppressed T1-weighted (*B*) images depict the periportal halo sign of PBC as central hyperintense portal triads encircled by low-signal intensity rims (*arrows*) measuring less than 10 mm in diameter. The caudate and left lateral hepatic lobes are hypertrophied, indicating cirrhosis. Note ghosting artifact within the liver due to aortic pulsation along the phase-encoding direction in (*B*). The spleen is enlarged.

include mass-forming, periductal infiltrating, and intraductal variants.[99] Mass-forming intrahepatic cholangiocarcinomas are irregularly marginated and demonstrate low T1 and high T2 signal intensity. In some cases of intrahepatic cholangiocarcinoma, central hypointense areas can be demonstrated on T2-weighted images, reflecting fibrotic components.[100]

Following contrast administration, the mass usually demonstrates irregular peripheral enhancement with gradual centripetal filling, which persists in the delayed phase and is related to the fibrotic component.[99] Associated findings include ductal dilation peripheral to the mass, transient hepatic intensity differences, capsular retraction, and encasement of the hepatic vessels, usually without thrombosis.[99] The intraductal variant is rare and typically appears on MR as an intraductal filling defect on T2 sequences that enhances on post-contrast imaging. When this form occurs within the smaller intrahepatic ducts, it may manifest as ductal dilation, with or without a visible intraductal polypoid mass. Intraductal enhancement may be seen.

Extrahepatic cholangiocarcinomas comprise 20% to 30% of cases and most commonly present as sclerosing strictures but may also present as nodular tumors or, rarely, as papillary lesions.[101] Extrahepatic cholangiocarcinomas are categorized by location as hilar cholangiocarcinomas, also called Klatskin tumors, and distal cholangiocarcinomas. Hilar cholangiocarcinomas account for 60% to 70% of extrahepatic cholangiocarcinomas and carry a poor prognosis, with a 5-year survival rate of less than 5%.[101] Klatskin tumors originate from the CHD and main hepatic ducts and spread in an infiltrating pattern in greater than 70%, with exophytic or polypoid forms seen less commonly.[102] On MR, these tumors most often appear as ill-defined hilar lesions demonstrating hypointense or isointense signal on T1-weighted sequences and hyperintense or isointense signal on T2-weighted sequences.[103,104] Bile duct wall thickening greater than 5 mm and upstream biliary ductal dilatation support the diagnosis. Enhancement patterns of Klatskin tumors are variable, but these lesions typically demonstrate early arterial phase enhancement of bile ducts with persistence of enhancement into the portal venous phase.[103] Lesions with a larger fibrotic component tend to demonstrate heterogeneous and delayed enhancement.

MR and MRCP are helpful for determining the level of obstruction and assessing peripheral extent of bile duct involvement (**Fig. 29**). Duct involvement may extend from the level of the CHD to the second-order intrahepatic ducts. MRCP accurately depicts the extent of involvement in most cases, with rates of detection and characterization similar to ERCP.[80,103] At MRCP, a signal void between the right and left hepatic ducts is typical of infiltrative cholangiocarcinoma, and associated ductal wall thickening may be observed on axial sequences. Malignant strictures caused by cholangiocarcinomas are usually abrupt, with asymmetric luminal narrowing and irregularity. Chronic tumor obstruction of a single hepatic lobe and invasion of the supplying portal vein causes proximal intrahepatic ductal dilation and parenchymal atrophy, known as the atrophy-hypertrophy complex.

The infiltrative growth pattern and proximity to the portal vein and hepatic artery result in lower resectability rates of 20% to 40%.[105] Several different staging systems exist for classifying Klatskin tumors, including the modified Bismuth-Corlette, AJCC/UICC, and Memorial Sloan-Kettering Cancer Center (MSKCC) staging systems.[63,106] The MSKCC system was developed to determine tumor resectability by imaging. Under this system,

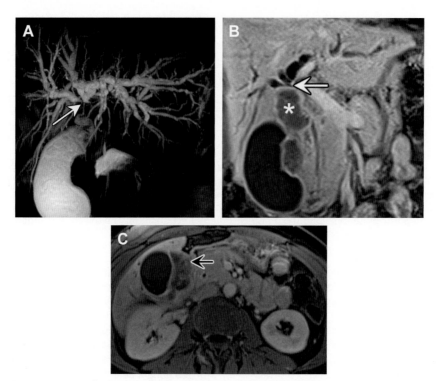

**Fig. 29.** MR imaging–MRCP illustration of hilar cholangiocarcinoma in a 53-year-old woman presenting with abdominal pain and jaundice. (*A*) Coronal MRCP MIP image shows diffuse intrahepatic biliary ductal dilation with abrupt termination at the confluence of the right and left hepatic ducts (*arrow*). The common bile duct is normal in caliber distal to the site of obstruction. A polypoid signal void is seen along the medial gallbladder, related to tumor invasion. (*B*) Coronal postcontrast fat-suppressed T1-weighted image in the delayed phase shows the site of ductal obstruction (*arrow*) due to a hypoenhancing hilar mass (*asterisk*) with contiguous extension inferiorly to involve the medial aspect of the gallbladder. (*C*) Axial postcontrast fat-suppressed T1-weighted image in the delayed phase shows enhancement of the tumor invading the medial gallbladder (*arrow*), typical of cholangiocarcinoma. Multiple intraluminal gallstones are faintly seen.

resectability is determined by the presence of hepatic cirrhosis, extent of biliary tree involvement, vascular encasement, hepatic lobar atrophy, and local and distant metastases (**Box 1**).

MR/MRCP determines the extent of bile duct tumors with 71% to 96% accuracy.[107] Dynamic gadolinium-enhanced imaging and diffusion-weighted sequences are helpful for determining the extent of parenchymal invasion, and periductal enhancement on delayed postcontrast MR imaging corresponds to periductal tumor spread with 93% accuracy.[108,109]

Thirty percent to 95% of Klatskin tumors at or above the hepatic duct bifurcation exhibit caudate lobe infiltration, and several studies demonstrate improved 5-year survival in patients who have undergone caudate lobe resection when compared with bile duct resection alone.[110,111]

Distal cholangiocarcinoma comprises a minority of extrahepatic cholangiocarcinomas and is usually of the periductal infiltrative variety. Although differentiating distal cholangiocarcinoma from other malignant strictures may be challenging, a long segment of extrahepatic duct involvement is more suggestive of cholangiocarcinoma (**Fig. 30**). When the intrapancreatic portion of the CBD is affected, the absence of main and accessory pancreatic ductal involvement favors cholangiocarcinoma over pancreatic adenocarcinoma.[112]

## BILIARY CYSTADENOMA AND CYSTADENOCARCINOMA

Biliary cystadenomas and cystadenocarcinomas are rare, multilocular cystic tumors of biliary origin, most commonly intrahepatic and communicating with a duct.[25,113] More than 85% of these tumors occur in middle-aged women and have histologic components that are similar to ovarian stroma.[114,115] Clinical symptoms are often related to mass effect by the lesion, manifesting as intermittent pain or biliary obstruction.[113] Biliary cystadenomas are considered premalignant, with a tendency to recur.[116,117] The tumors are lined by mucin-secreting cells and contain internal fluid that may be proteinaceous or mucinous and occasionally contain gelatinous, purulent, or hemorrhagic components.[118]

MR imaging features reflect pathologic features; biliary cystadenomas typically appear as cystic masses with a well-marginated capsule, internal septa, and mural nodules, with rare capsular calcification (**Fig. 31**).[118] Although imaging features of cystadenomas and cystadenocarcinomas overlap, malignant cystadenocarcinomas tend to have a thicker wall and thicker internal septa and more often contain intratumoral papillary and polypoid projections.[119] Malignancy is suggested by the presence of lymphadenopathy and metastases. In both cystadenomas and cystadenocarcinomas, the internal fluid contents typically demonstrate homogeneous T1 hypointense and T2 hyperintense signal, but may vary depending on the presence of protein or hemorrhage. Because biliary cystadenomas and cystadenocarcinomas are often indistinguishable by imaging, both are treated with surgical resection.

## POSTSURGICAL EVALUATION

Biliary-enteric anastomoses (most commonly either a Roux-en-Y choledochojejunostomy or a hepaticojejunostomy) are often created during surgical treatment of both benign and malignant conditions. MRCP is preferred over ERCP for the evaluation of these cases, as the altered anatomy makes ERCP challenging. MR and MRCP are useful for postoperative evaluation of anastomotic

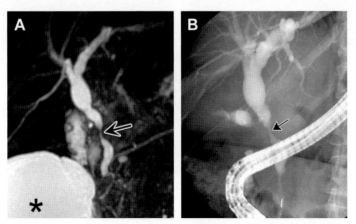

Fig. 30. MRCP-ERCP depiction of a distal cholangiocarcinoma in a 72-year-old woman who presented with abdominal pain and abnormal liver function tests. (*A*) Coronal MRCP MIP image shows focal asymmetric narrowing of the suprapancreatic portion of the common bile duct (*arrow*) with upstream ductal dilation in this patient with biopsy-proven distal cholangiocarcinoma. Note that the main pancreatic duct is normal in caliber. A renal cyst is partially visualized (*asterisk*). (*B*) Corresponding ERCP image shows focal stricturing and luminal irregularity of the common bile duct (*arrow*) with upstream ductal dilatation.

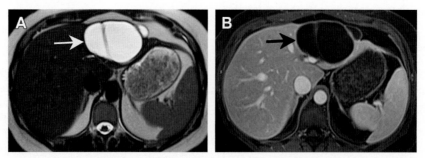

**Fig. 31.** MR findings of a nonaggressive biliary cystadenoma in a 45-year-old woman. (*A*) Axial T2-weighted image shows a hyperintense multilocular septated cystic mass within the left lateral lobe of the liver (*arrow*). (*B*) Axial postcontrast fat-suppressed T1-weighted image shows enhancement of the outer capsule and thin septa (*arrow*). The lack of thick septa, intracystic hemorrhage, solid components, and solid enhancement argue against this lesion being a biliary cystadenocarcinoma. The lesion was excised at the time of surgery for a pancreatic neuroendocrine tumor (not shown).

patency and potential early and late complications, such as biliary leak, obstruction, cholangitis, and calculi.[120,121] Following biliary-enteric anastomosis, isolated bile duct dilatation is not sufficient to diagnose a stricture, because residual preexisting ductal dilatation is often present despite a patent anastomosis. However, when ductal dilatation is associated with narrowing at the anastomotic site, functional stenosis should be considered. This information aids treatment planning for symptomatic patients who may benefit from techniques such as ductal cannulation and drainage or balloon dilatation. One limitation of MRCP is the inability to assess bile flow and definitively document patency. Hepatobiliary contrast agents have the potential to help differentiate strictures from patent anastomoses on postcontrast hepatobiliary phase imaging and can detect the

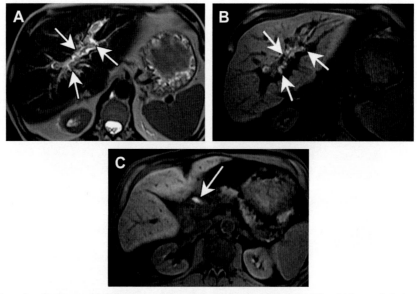

**Fig. 32.** MR imaging findings of biliary cast syndrome in a 68-year-old man with a history of cirrhosis and hepatocellular carcinoma status post-liver transplantation 4 years earlier. (*A*) Axial T2-weighted image demonstrates dilated intrahepatic bile ducts containing a branching intraluminal filling defect with a "staghorn" configuration (*arrows*), representing a biliary cast, with surrounding hyperintense bile. (*B*) Axial fat-suppressed T1-weighted image shows dilated intrahepatic bile ducts and hyperintense signal within the biliary cast (*arrows*), reflecting its relatively high bilirubin content. (*C*) Axial fat-suppressed T1-weighted image inferiorly shows a tubular hyperintensity (*arrow*) within the transplant hepatic artery consistent with subacute thrombus, contributing to biliary ischemia and subsequent cast formation in this patient.

presence of bile leak by depicting the presence of excreted gadolinium into the peritoneal cavity.[120,122]

Biliary cast syndrome (BCS) has been observed in up to 18% of liver transplant recipients.[123,124] BCS refers to an aggregate of hardened intraluminal material conforming to the shape of the biliary ducts, sometimes demonstrating a "staghorn calculus" configuration.[125] Biliary casts are composed of bilirubin as well as components of bile acids, cholangiocyte fragments, and bacteria. Proposed causes of BCS include biliary ischemia, acute cellular rejection, biliary infection, and biliary obstruction.[123,124] On T2-weighted MR sequences and MRCP, biliary casts appear as filling defects within the biliary tree, usually adherent to the duct walls.[126] On T1-weighted sequences, biliary casts appear as hyperintense linear or branching material within the biliary tree due to the relatively higher bilirubin composition (**Fig. 32**).[127]

## SUMMARY

MR and MRCP provide comprehensive noninvasive evaluation of the biliary system and are effective for localizing and characterizing a spectrum of benign and malignant processes involving the biliary tree and gallbladder. Familiarity with the MR and MRCP imaging features associated with each process allows for the accurate diagnosis and classification of disease, thus enabling optimal clinical and surgical management.

## REFERENCES

1. Barish MA, Yucel EK, Ferrucci JT. Magnetic resonance cholangiopancreatography. N Engl J Med 1999;341(4):258–64.
2. Sodickson A, Mortele KJ, Barish MA, et al. Three-dimensional fast-recovery fast spin-echo MRCP: comparison with two-dimensional single-shot fast spin-echo techniques. Radiology 2006;238(2): 549–59.
3. Soto JA, Barish MA, Alvarez O, et al. Detection of choledocholithiasis with MR cholangiography: comparison of three-dimensional fast spin-echo and single- and multisection half-Fourier rapid acquisition with relaxation enhancement sequences. Radiology 2000;215(3):737–45.
4. Zhang J, Israel GM, Hecht EM, et al. Isotropic 3D T2-weighted MR cholangiopancreatography with parallel imaging: feasibility study. AJR Am J Roentgenol 2006;187(6):1564–70.
5. Miyazaki T, Yamashita Y, Tsuchigame T, et al. MR cholangiopancreatography using HASTE (half-Fourier acquisition single-shot turbo spin-echo)

6. sequences. AJR Am J Roentgenol 1996;166(6): 1297–303.
6. Heller SL, Lee VS. MR imaging of the gallbladder and biliary system. Magn Reson Imaging Clin N Am 2005;13(2):295–311.
7. Reiner CS, Merkle EM, Bashir MR, et al. MRI assessment of biliary ductal obstruction: is there added value of T1-weighted gadolinium-ethoxybenzyl-diethylenetriamine pentaacetic acid-enhanced MR cholangiography? AJR Am J Roentgenol 2013; 201(1):W49–56.
8. Seale MK, Catalano OA, Saini S, et al. Hepatobiliary-specific MR contrast agents: role in imaging the liver and biliary tree. Radiographics 2009; 29(6):1725–48.
9. Watanabe Y, Dohke M, Ishimori T, et al. Diagnostic pitfalls of MR cholangiopancreatography in the evaluation of the biliary tract and gallbladder. Radiographics 1999;19(2):415–29.
10. Ringe KI, Gupta RT, Brady CM, et al. Respiratory-triggered three-dimensional T2-weighted MR cholangiography after injection of gadoxetate disodium: is it still reliable? Radiology 2010; 255(2):451–8.
11. Yu J, Turner MA, Fulcher AS, et al. Congenital anomalies and normal variants of the pancreaticobiliary tract and the pancreas in adults: part 1, Biliary tract. AJR Am J Roentgenol 2006;187(6): 1536–43.
12. Mortele KJ, Rocha TC, Streeter JL, et al. Multimodality imaging of pancreatic and biliary congenital anomalies. Radiographics 2006;26(3):715–31.
13. Mortele KJ, Ros PR. Anatomic variants of the biliary tree: MR cholangiographic findings and clinical applications. AJR Am J Roentgenol 2001; 177(2):389–94.
14. Marcos A, Ham JM, Fisher RA, et al. Surgical management of anatomical variations of the right lobe in living donor liver transplantation. Ann Surg 2000;231(6):824–31.
15. Suhocki PV, Meyers WC. Injury to aberrant bile ducts during cholecystectomy: a common cause of diagnostic error and treatment delay. AJR Am J Roentgenol 1999;172(4):955–9.
16. MacFadyen BV Jr, Vecchio R, Ricardo AE, et al. Bile duct injury after laparoscopic cholecystectomy. The United States experience. Surg Endosc 1998;12(4):315–21.
17. Sugiyama M, Baba M, Atomi Y, et al. Diagnosis of anomalous pancreaticobiliary junction: value of magnetic resonance cholangiopancreatography. Surgery 1998;123(4):391–7.
18. Brancatelli G, Federle MP, Vilgrain V, et al. Fibropolycystic liver disease: CT and MR imaging findings. Radiographics 2005;25(3):659–70.
19. Tohme-Noun C, Cazals D, Noun R, et al. Multiple biliary hamartomas: magnetic resonance features

with histopathologic correlation. Eur Radiol 2008; 18(3):493–9.

20. Levine E, Cook LT, Grantham JJ. Liver cysts in autosomal-dominant polycystic kidney disease: clinical and computed tomographic study. AJR Am J Roentgenol 1985;145(2):229–33.

21. Terada T, Nakanuma Y. Congenital biliary dilatation in autosomal dominant adult polycystic disease of the liver and kidneys. Arch Pathol Lab Med 1988; 112(11):1113–6.

22. Todani T, Watanabe Y, Fujii T, et al. Congenital choledochal cyst with intrahepatic involvement. Arch Surg 1984;119(9):1038–43.

23. Todani T, Watanabe Y, Narusue M, et al. Congenital bile duct cysts: classification, operative procedures, and review of thirty-seven cases including cancer arising from choledochal cyst. Am J Surg 1977;134(2):263–9.

24. Wiseman K, Buczkowski AK, Chung SW, et al. Epidemiology, presentation, diagnosis, and outcomes of choledochal cysts in adults in an urban environment. Am J Surg 2005;189(5):527–31 [discussion: 531].

25. Mortele KJ, Ros PR. Cystic focal liver lesions in the adult: differential CT and MR imaging features. Radiographics 2001;21(4):895–910.

26. Choi BI, Yeon KM, Kim SH, et al. Caroli disease: central dot sign in CT. Radiology 1990;174(1): 161–3.

27. Griffin N, Yu D, Alexander Grant L. Magnetic resonance cholangiopancreatography: pearls, pitfalls, and pathology. Semin Ultrasound CT MR 2013; 34(1):32–43.

28. Hricak H, Filly RA, Margulis AR, et al. Work in progress: nuclear magnetic resonance imaging of the gallbladder. Radiology 1983;147(2):481–4.

29. Hashimoto M, Akabane Y, Heianna J, et al. Segmental high intensity on T1-weighted hepatic MR images. Abdom Imaging 2005;30(1):60–4.

30. Catalano OA, Sahani DV, Kalva SP, et al. MR imaging of the gallbladder: a pictorial essay. Radiographics 2008;28(1):135–55 [quiz: 324].

31. Gore RM, Yaghmai V, Newmark GM, et al. Imaging benign and malignant disease of the gallbladder. Radiol Clin North Am 2002;40(6):1307–23, vi.

32. Ukaji M, Ebara M, Tsuchiya Y, et al. Diagnosis of gallstone composition in magnetic resonance imaging: in vitro analysis. Eur J Radiol 2002;41(1):49–56.

33. Tsai HM, Lin XZ, Chen CY, et al. MRI of gallstones with different compositions. AJR Am J Roentgenol 2004;182(6):1513–9.

34. Ko CW, Sekijima JH, Lee SP. Biliary sludge. Ann Intern Med 1999;130(4 Pt 1):301–11.

35. Lee NK, Kim S, Lee JW, et al. MR appearance of normal and abnormal bile: correlation with imaging and endoscopic finding. Eur J Radiol 2010;76(2): 211–21.

36. Lee SP, Nicholls JF, Park HZ. Biliary sludge as a cause of acute pancreatitis. N Engl J Med 1992; 326(9):589–93.

37. Romagnuolo J, Bardou M, Rahme E, et al. Magnetic resonance cholangiopancreatography: a meta-analysis of test performance in suspected biliary disease. Ann Intern Med 2003;139(7):547–57.

38. Aube C, Delorme B, Yzet T, et al. MR cholangiopancreatography versus endoscopic sonography in suspected common bile duct lithiasis: a prospective, comparative study. AJR Am J Roentgenol 2005;184(1):55–62.

39. Park MS, Yu JS, Kim YH, et al. Acute cholecystitis: comparison of MR cholangiography and US. Radiology 1998;209(3):781–5.

40. Loud PA, Semelka RC, Kettritz U, et al. MRI of acute cholecystitis: comparison with the normal gallbladder and other entities. Magn Reson Imaging 1996;14(4):349–55.

41. Kim KW, Park MS, Yu JS, et al. Acute cholecystitis at T2-weighted and manganese-enhanced T1-weighted MR cholangiography: preliminary study. Radiology 2003;227(2):580–4.

42. Altun E, Semelka RC, Elias J Jr, et al. Acute cholecystitis: MR findings and differentiation from chronic cholecystitis. Radiology 2007;244(1):174–83.

43. Hakansson K, Leander P, Ekberg O, et al. MR imaging in clinically suspected acute cholecystitis. A comparison with ultrasonography. Acta Radiol 2000;41(4):322–8.

44. Son JY, Kim YJ, Park HS, et al. Diffuse gallbladder wall thickening on computed tomography in patients with liver cirrhosis: correlation with clinical and laboratory variables. J Comput Assist Tomogr 2011;35(5):535–8.

45. Jung SE, Lee JM, Lee K, et al. Gallbladder wall thickening: MR imaging and pathologic correlation with emphasis on layered pattern. Eur Radiol 2005; 15(4):694–701.

46. Barie PS, Eachempati SR. Acute acalculous cholecystitis. Gastroenterol Clin North Am 2010;39(2): 343–57, x.

47. Bradley WG Jr. MR appearance of hemorrhage in the brain. Radiology 1993;189(1):15–26.

48. Levy AD, Murakata LA, Abbott RM, et al. From the archives of the AFIP. Benign tumors and tumorlike lesions of the gallbladder and extrahepatic bile ducts: radiologic-pathologic correlation. Armed Forces Institute of Pathology. Radiographics 2002;22(2):387–413.

49. Kim MJ, Oh YT, Park YN, et al. Gallbladder adenomyomatosis: findings on MRI. Abdom Imaging 1999;24(4):410–3.

50. Haradome H, Ichikawa T, Sou H, et al. The pearl necklace sign: an imaging sign of adenomyomatosis of the gallbladder at MR cholangiopancreatography. Radiology 2003;227(1):80–8.

51. Hwang JI, Chou YH, Tsay SH, et al. Radiologic and pathologic correlation of adenomyomatosis of the gallbladder. Abdom Imaging 1998;23(1):73–7.

52. Carriaga MT, Henson DE. Liver, gallbladder, extra-hepatic bile ducts, and pancreas. Cancer 1995;75(Suppl 1):171–90.

53. Bartlett DL. Gallbladder cancer. Semin Surg Oncol 2000;19(2):145–55.

54. Hsing AW, Gao YT, Han TQ, et al. Gallstones and the risk of biliary tract cancer: a population-based study in China. Br J Cancer 2007;97(11):1577–82.

55. Pandey M, Shukla VK. Lifestyle, parity, menstrual and reproductive factors and risk of gallbladder cancer. Eur J Cancer Prev 2003;12(4):269–72.

56. Towfigh S, McFadden DW, Cortina GR, et al. Porcelain gallbladder is not associated with gallbladder carcinoma. Am Surg 2001;67(1):7–10.

57. Stephen AE, Berger DL. Carcinoma in the porcelain gallbladder: a relationship revisited. Surgery 2001;129(6):699–703.

58. Levy AD, Murakata LA, Rohrmann CA Jr. Gallbladder carcinoma: radiologic-pathologic correlation. Radiographics 2001;21(2):295–314 [questionnaire: 549–55].

59. Kim SJ, Lee JM, Kim H, et al. Role of diffusion-weighted magnetic resonance imaging in the diagnosis of gallbladder cancer. J Magn Reson Imaging 2013;38(1):127–37.

60. Yoshimitsu K, Honda H, Jimi M, et al. MR diagnosis of adenomyomatosis of the gallbladder and differentiation from gallbladder carcinoma: importance of showing Rokitansky-Aschoff sinuses. AJR Am J Roentgenol 1999;172(6):1535–40.

61. Tseng JH, Wan YL, Hung CF, et al. Diagnosis and staging of gallbladder carcinoma. Evaluation with dynamic MR imaging. Clin Imaging 2002;26(3):177–82.

62. Kim JH, Kim TK, Eun HW, et al. Preoperative evaluation of gallbladder carcinoma: efficacy of combined use of MR imaging, MR cholangiography, and contrast-enhanced dual-phase three-dimensional MR angiography. J Magn Reson Imaging 2002;16(6):676–84.

63. Edge SB, American Joint Committee on Cancer, American Cancer Society. AJCC cancer staging manual. 7th edition. New York, London: Springer; 2010.

64. Murakami Y, Uemura K, Sudo T, et al. Prognostic factors of patients with advanced gallbladder carcinoma following aggressive surgical resection. J Gastrointest Surg 2011;15(6):1007–16.

65. Shirai Y, Yoshida K, Tsukada K, et al. Inapparent carcinoma of the gallbladder. An appraisal of a radical second operation after simple cholecystectomy. Ann Surg 1992;215(4):326–31.

66. Schwartz LH, Black J, Fong Y, et al. Gallbladder carcinoma: findings at MR imaging with MR cholangiopancreatography. J Comput Assist Tomogr 2002;26(3):405–10.

67. Hanau LH, Steigbigel NH. Acute (ascending) cholangitis. Infect Dis Clin North Am 2000;14(3):521–46.

68. Kimura Y, Takada T, Kawarada Y, et al. Definitions, pathophysiology, and epidemiology of acute cholangitis and cholecystitis: Tokyo guidelines. J Hepatobiliary Pancreat Surg 2007;14(1):15–26.

69. Bader TR, Braga L, Beavers KL, et al. MR imaging findings of infectious cholangitis. Magn Reson Imaging 2001;19(6):781–8.

70. Lee NK, Kim S, Lee JW, et al. Discrimination of suppurative cholangitis from nonsuppurative cholangitis with computed tomography (CT). Eur J Radiol 2009;69(3):528–35.

71. Nagino M, Takada T, Kawarada Y, et al. Methods and timing of biliary drainage for acute cholangitis: Tokyo guidelines. J Hepatobiliary Pancreat Surg 2007;14(1):68–77.

72. Catalano OA, Sahani DV, Forcione DG, et al. Biliary infections: spectrum of imaging findings and management. Radiographics 2009;29(7):2059–80.

73. Heffernan EJ, Geoghegan T, Munk PL, et al. Recurrent pyogenic cholangitis: from imaging to intervention. AJR Am J Roentgenol 2009;192(1):W28–35.

74. Al-Sukhni W, Gallinger S, Pratzer A, et al. Recurrent pyogenic cholangitis with hepatolithiasis–the role of surgical therapy in North America. J Gastrointest Surg 2008;12(3):496–503.

75. Jain M, Agarwal A. MRCP findings in recurrent pyogenic cholangitis. Eur J Radiol 2008;66(1):79–83.

76. Kim MJ, Cha SW, Mitchell DG, et al. MR imaging findings in recurrent pyogenic cholangitis. AJR Am J Roentgenol 1999;173(6):1545–9.

77. Shah OJ, Zargar SA, Robbani I. Biliary ascariasis: a review. World J Surg 2006;30(8):1500–6.

78. Bethony J, Brooker S, Albonico M, et al. Soil-transmitted helminth infections: ascariasis, trichuriasis, and hookworm. Lancet 2006;367(9521):1521–32.

79. Astudillo JA, Sporn E, Serrano B, et al. Ascariasis in the hepatobiliary system: laparoscopic management. J Am Coll Surg 2008;207(4):527–32.

80. Park MS, Kim TK, Kim KW, et al. Differentiation of extrahepatic bile duct cholangiocarcinoma from benign stricture: findings at MRCP versus ERCP. Radiology 2004;233(1):234–40.

81. Kim MJ, Mitchell DG, Ito K, et al. Biliary dilatation: differentiation of benign from malignant causes–value of adding conventional MR imaging to MR cholangiopancreatography. Radiology 2000;214(1):173–81.

82. Riopel MA, Klimstra DS, Godellas CV, et al. Intrabiliary growth of metastatic colonic adenocarcinoma: a pattern of intrahepatic spread easily confused with primary neoplasia of the biliary tract. Am J Surg Pathol 1997;21(9):1030–6.

83. Judah JR, Draganov PV. Endoscopic therapy of benign biliary strictures. World J Gastroenterol 2007;13(26):3531–9.

84. Martin RF, Rossi RL. Bile duct injuries. Spectrum, mechanisms of injury, and their prevention. Surg Clin North Am 1994;74(4):781–803 [discussion: 805–7].

85. Pitt HA, Kaufman SL, Coleman J, et al. Benign postoperative biliary strictures. Operate or dilate? Ann Surg 1989;210(4):417–25 [discussion: 426–7].

86. Barriga J, Thompson R, Shokouh-Amiri H, et al. Biliary strictures after liver transplantation. Predictive factors for response to endoscopic management and long-term outcome. Am J Med Sci 2008;335(6):439–43.

87. Lerut J, Gordon RD, Iwatsuki S, et al. Biliary tract complications in human orthotopic liver transplantation. Transplantation 1987;43(1):47–51.

88. Ito K, Siegelman ES, Stolpen AH, et al. MR imaging of complications after liver transplantation. AJR Am J Roentgenol 2000;175(4):1145–9.

89. Berstad AE, Aabakken L, Smith HJ, et al. Diagnostic accuracy of magnetic resonance and endoscopic retrograde cholangiography in primary sclerosing cholangitis. Clin Gastroenterol Hepatol 2006;4(4):514–20.

90. Karlsen TH, Schrumpf E, Boberg KM. Update on primary sclerosing cholangitis. Dig Liver Dis 2010;42(6):390–400.

91. Lee YM, Kaplan MM. Primary sclerosing cholangitis. N Engl J Med 1995;332(14):924–33.

92. Bader TR, Beavers KL, Semelka RC. MR imaging features of primary sclerosing cholangitis: patterns of cirrhosis in relationship to clinical severity of disease. Radiology 2003;226(3):675–85.

93. Ito K, Mitchell DG, Outwater EK, et al. Primary sclerosing cholangitis: MR imaging features. AJR Am J Roentgenol 1999;172(6):1527–33.

94. Elsayes KM, Oliveira EP, Narra VR, et al. MR and MRCP in the evaluation of primary sclerosing cholangitis: current applications and imaging findings. J Comput Assist Tomogr 2006;30(3):398–404.

95. Dusunceli E, Erden A, Erden I, et al. Primary sclerosing cholangitis: MR cholangiopancreatography and T2-weighted MR imaging findings. Diagn Interv Radiol 2005;11(4):213–8.

96. Wenzel JS, Donohoe A, Ford KL 3rd, et al. Primary biliary cirrhosis: MR imaging findings and description of MR imaging periportal halo sign. AJR Am J Roentgenol 2001;176(4):885–9.

97. Kaplan MM, Gershwin ME. Primary biliary cirrhosis. N Engl J Med 2005;353(12):1261–73.

98. Lewis RB, Lattin GE Jr, Makhlouf HR, et al. Tumors of the liver and intrahepatic bile ducts: radiologic-pathologic correlation. Magn Reson Imaging Clin N Am 2010;18(3):587–609, xii.

99. Chung YE, Kim MJ, Park YN, et al. Varying appearances of cholangiocarcinoma: radiologic-pathologic correlation. Radiographics 2009;29(3):683–700.

100. Maetani Y, Itoh K, Watanabe C, et al. MR imaging of intrahepatic cholangiocarcinoma with pathologic correlation. AJR Am J Roentgenol 2001;176(6):1499–507.

101. Aljiffry M, Walsh MJ, Molinari M. Advances in diagnosis, treatment and palliation of cholangiocarcinoma: 1990-2009. World J Gastroenterol 2009;15(34):4240–62.

102. Choi BI, Lee JM, Han JK. Imaging of intrahepatic and hilar cholangiocarcinoma. Abdom Imaging 2004;29(5):548–57.

103. Vogl TJ, Schwarz WO, Heller M, et al. Staging of Klatskin tumours (hilar cholangiocarcinomas): comparison of MR cholangiography, MR imaging, and endoscopic retrograde cholangiography. Eur Radiol 2006;16(10):2317–25.

104. Masselli G, Gualdi G. Hilar cholangiocarcinoma: MRI/MRCP in staging and treatment planning. Abdom Imaging 2008;33(4):444–51.

105. Gores GJ. Cholangiocarcinoma: current concepts and insights. Hepatology 2003;37(5):961–9.

106. Jarnagin WR, Fong Y, DeMatteo RP, et al. Staging, resectability, and outcome in 225 patients with hilar cholangiocarcinoma. Ann Surg 2001;234(4):507–17 [discussion: 517–9].

107. Choi JY, Kim MJ, Lee JM, et al. Hilar cholangiocarcinoma: role of preoperative imaging with sonography, MDCT, MRI, and direct cholangiography. AJR Am J Roentgenol 2008;191(5):1448–57.

108. Park HS, Lee JM, Choi JY, et al. Preoperative evaluation of bile duct cancer: MRI combined with MR cholangiopancreatography versus MDCT with direct cholangiography. AJR Am J Roentgenol 2008;190(2):396–405.

109. Masselli G, Manfredi R, Vecchioli A, et al. MR imaging and MR cholangiopancreatography in the preoperative evaluation of hilar cholangiocarcinoma: correlation with surgical and pathologic findings. Eur Radiol 2008;18(10):2213–21.

110. Tabata M, Kawarada Y, Yokoi H, et al. Surgical treatment for hilar cholangiocarcinoma. J Hepatobiliary Pancreat Surg 2000;7(2):148–54.

111. Nimura Y, Kamiya J, Kondo S, et al. Aggressive preoperative management and extended surgery for hilar cholangiocarcinoma: Nagoya experience. J Hepatobiliary Pancreat Surg 2000;7(2):155–62.

112. Matos C, Serrao E, Bali MA. Magnetic resonance imaging of biliary tumors. Magn Reson Imaging Clin N Am 2010;18(3):477–96, x.

113. Singh Y, Winick AB, Tabbara SO. Multiloculated cystic liver lesions: radiologic-pathologic differential diagnosis. Radiographics 1997;17(1):219–24.

114. Devaney K, Goodman ZD, Ishak KG. Hepatobiliary cystadenoma and cystadenocarcinoma. A light microscopic and immunohistochemical study of 70 patients. Am J Surg Pathol 1994;18(11):1078–91.

115. Colombari R, Tsui WM. Biliary tumors of the liver. Semin Liver Dis 1995;15(4):402–13.

116. Woods GL. Biliary cystadenocarcinoma: case report of hepatic malignancy originating in benign cystadenoma. Cancer 1981;47(12):2936–40.

117. Ishak KG, Willis GW, Cummins SD, et al. Biliary cystadenoma and cystadenocarcinoma: report of 14 cases and review of the literature. Cancer 1977;39(1):322–38.

118. Buetow PC, Midkiff RB. MR imaging of the liver. Primary malignant neoplasms in the adult. Magn Reson Imaging Clin N Am 1997;5(2):289–318.

119. Powers C, Ros PR, Stoupis C, et al. Primary liver neoplasms: MR imaging with pathologic correlation. Radiographics 1994;14(3):459–82.

120. Kandasamy D, Sharma R, Seith Bhalla A, et al. MR evaluation of biliary-enteric anastomotic stricture: does contrast-enhanced T1W MRC provide additional information? Clin Res Hepatol Gastroenterol 2011;35(8–9):563–71.

121. Ragozzino A, De Ritis R, Mosca A, et al. Value of MR cholangiography in patients with iatrogenic bile duct injury after cholecystectomy. AJR Am J Roentgenol 2004;183(6):1567–72.

122. Boraschi P, Donati F. Biliary-enteric anastomoses: spectrum of findings on Gd-EOB-DTPA-enhanced MR cholangiography. Abdom Imaging 2013;38(6):1351–9.

123. Gor NV, Levy RM, Ahn J, et al. Biliary cast syndrome following liver transplantation: predictive factors and clinical outcomes. Liver Transpl 2008;14(10):1466–72.

124. Srinivasaiah N, Reddy MS, Balupuri S, et al. Biliary cast syndrome: literature review and a single centre experience in liver transplant recipients. Hepatobiliary Pancreat Dis Int 2008;7(3):300–3.

125. Tung BY, Kimmey MB. Biliary complications of orthotopic liver transplantation. Dig Dis 1999;17(3):133–44.

126. Sandblom P, Essinger A. Stones or clots in the biliary tract. A diagnostic dilemma. Acta Chir Scand 1981;147(8):673–83.

127. Kinner S, Umutlu L, Dechene A, et al. Biliary complications after liver transplantation: addition of T1-weighted images to MR cholangiopancreatography facilitates detection of cast in biliary cast syndrome. Radiology 2012;263(2):429–36.

# MR Imaging of the Pancreas

Erin O'Neill, MD, Nancy Hammond, MD, Frank H. Miller, MD*

## KEYWORDS

- Pancreas • Pancreas magnetic resonance • Magnetic resonance imaging
- Magnetic resonance cholangiopancreatography (MRCP) • Pancreatic cancer • Acute pancreatitis
- Chronic pancreatitis • Cystic pancreatic masses

## KEY POINTS

- Magnetic resonance (MR) imaging of the pancreas is useful as both a problem-solving tool based on computed tomography or sonography as well as an initial imaging examination of choice.
- MR is particularly useful in the evaluation of both acute and chronic pancreatitis as well as their complications.
- MR cholangiopancreatographyis useful in the detection and evaluation of pancreatic ductal anomalies, including pancreas divisum and annular pancreas.
- MR can help evaluate different forms of pancreatitis, including autoimmune and groove pancreatitis.
- MR can also be used to help delineate and better define both cystic and solid neoplasms of the pancreas.

## INTRODUCTION

Magnetic resonance (MR) imaging of the pancreas is useful as both a problem-solving tool based on computed tomography (CT) or sonographic findings and is increasingly being used as the initial imaging examination of choice. With newer imaging sequences such as diffusion-weighted imaging, MR offers improved ability to detect and characterize lesions, as well as identify and stage tumors and inflammation. In addition, MR cholangiopancreatography (MRCP) can be used to visualize the biliary and pancreatic ductal system. In this article, the use of MR to evaluate the pancreas, including recent advances, is reviewed, and the normal appearance of the pancreas on different imaging sequences, as well as inflammatory diseases, congenital abnormalities, and neoplasms of the pancreas, are discussed.

## TECHNIQUE

At our institution, we routinely perform MRCP with our standard pancreatic MR imaging protocol. Our standard protocol is outlined in **Table 1**.

### Normal MR Appearance of the Pancreas

The unenhanced and dynamic gadolinium-enhanced T1-weighted sequences with fat suppression best evaluate the pancreatic parenchyma. On the T1-weighted fat-suppressed sequences, the pancreas shows high signal intensity, because of the presence of aqueous protein. The pancreatic signal should be homogenous and at least equal to or greater than the liver in signal intensity.[1–3] On T2-weighted images, the signal intensity of the pancreas is variable; however, these sequences are useful for evaluating the pancreatic duct and biliary system, pancreatic and peripancreatic

Department of Radiology, Feinberg School of Medicine, Northwestern Memorial Hospital, Northwestern University, 676 North Saint Clair Street, Suite 800, Chicago, IL 60611, USA
* Corresponding author.
E-mail address: fmiller@northwestern.edu

Radiol Clin N Am 52 (2014) 757–777
http://dx.doi.org/10.1016/j.rcl.2014.02.006
0033-8389/14/$ – see front matter © 2014 Elsevier Inc. All rights reserved.

| Table 1 |
|---|
| **Example of comprehensive pancreas MR imaging protocol** |

| Protocol Step | Sequence |
|---|---|
| Precontrast images | T2-weighted single-shot fast spin-echo |
| | T1-weighted in-phase and opposed-phase gradient-echo |
| | Diffusion-weighted imaging |
| | T2-weighted fat-suppressed fast spin-echo |
| | Three-dimensional T1-weighted fat-suppressed spoiled gradient-echo |
| | T2-weighted MRCP (navigator triggered three-dimensional or rapid acquisition with relaxation enhancement) |
| Postcontrast images | Dynamic three-dimensional T1-weighted fat-suppressed spoiled gradient-echo (in pancreatic, portal venous, and equilibrium phases) |

edema, fluid collections, cystic neoplasms, and endocrine tumors.[1,2]

On gadolinium-enhanced fat-suppressed sequences, the normal pancreas maintains its high T1 signal intensity and shows homogenous enhancement, because of its rich vascular network. The pancreas is hyperintense relative to the other abdominal organs on the early gadolinium-enhanced images and becomes isointense to the liver on delayed gadolinium-enhanced images. Focal pancreatic masses are best identified and evaluated using a combination of unenhanced and early gadolinium-enhanced T1-weighted sequences. The venous and delayed phases of gadolinium-enhanced sequences are best for detecting peripancreatic and periportal lymphadenopathy as well as peritoneal metastases.[1]

MRCP uses heavily T2-weighted sequences to evaluate the pancreatic duct and biliary tract. These sequences are essential in identifying ductal stones or strictures and aid in evaluating for the presence of ductal communication with cystic lesions of the pancreas.[1,4] There is good correlation between MRCP and endoscopic retrograde cholangiopancreatography (ERCP) in evaluation of the pancreatic duct.[5] An advantage of ERCP over MRCP is that it is both diagnostic and therapeutic, allowing the endoscopist to perform sphincterotomy and remove

common duct stones.[6] However, unlike ERCP, MRCP is noninvasive and provides a useful road map for the endoscopist when ERCP is planned. Unlike ERCP, it can evaluate areas proximal to an obstruction and detect pseudocysts that do not communicate with the main pancreatic duct.[1]

Secretin-enhanced MRCP may be considered when evaluating for chronic pancreatitis or ductal anomalies. Secretin temporarily distends the pancreatic ducts by inducing pancreatic secretions and increasing the tone of the sphincter of Oddi, with maximal effect occurring at 7 to 10 minutes after administration. Secretin-enhanced MRCP can detect subtle side branch dilatation in mild chronic pancreatitis, complex ductal anomalies, and stenosis of the pancreatic duct.[7,8] Secretin can also be used to assess the exocrine response of the pancreas, either quantitatively or semiquantitatively. With quantitative assessment, exocrine response of the pancreas is obtained by measuring pancreatic flow output and total excreted volume of pancreatic fluid released into the duodenum after secretin injection.[7–12] With semiquantitative assessment, evaluation of the exocrine response of the pancreas is based on the amount of duodenal and small bowel filling with pancreatic fluid after secretin injection. Normal quantitative exocrine function consists of complete filling of the duodenum with pancreatic fluid output. Suboptimal quantitative exocrine function consists of filling only a portion of the duodenum.[7,8] Another use for secretin-enhanced MRCP is to show pancreatic duct injury, which can occur as a sequela from trauma, surgery, or severe pancreatitis.[7]

Diffusion-weighted imaging serves as an excellent adjunct to routine abdominal MR imaging. Diffusion-weighted imaging detects random water motion within cellular tissues and produces a representative apparent diffusion coefficient (ADC) value.[13–15] Because of the increased motion of water molecules in simple pancreatic cysts, these lesions show high signal intensity on low b value images, lower signal intensity on high b value images, and high signal intensity on ADC images. In contrast, solid neoplasms show increased signal on low b value images, relatively high signal on high b value images, and low ADC values because of restricted water motion.[13] This low ADC value in solid neoplasms is believed to be caused by the decreased extracellular space from dense cellularity and extracellular fibrosis, which accounts for the restricted water diffusion.[13,16]

Diffusion-weighted imaging may allow earlier detection of pancreatic neoplasms, as well as detection of liver and lymph node metastases, which are not always so apparent on other sequences. In addition, the presence of restricted diffusion in a liver lesion can sometimes characterize small lesions as suspicious for metastases. However, diffusion-weighted imaging can have limitations in distinguishing malignant from benign pancreatic lesions or lymph nodes, because both can show restricted diffusion.[13]

## PANCREATITIS
### Acute Pancreatitis

According to the revised Atlanta classification for acute pancreatitis,[17] the diagnosis of acute pancreatitis is usually based on clinical and laboratory values, particularly within the first week of symptoms, when only clinical parameters are considered important for treatment planning. However, after the first week, morphologic criteria, determined by imaging studies, are used in conjunction with clinical findings to help guide clinicians in their treatment plan.

Although CT is most commonly used in the evaluation of acute pancreatitis, MR imaging has been shown to be more sensitive than CT in the detection of acute pancreatitis, particularly mild cases.[1,3,18] MR imaging may show the development of morphologic changes of the pancreas in both acute and chronic pancreatitis at an earlier stage than CT.[19] MR imaging with MRCP can identify underlying causes of pancreatitis, such as choledocholithiasis, abnormalities of the pancreatic duct, or pancreatic neoplasm.[1,3,18]

Using the Atlanta classification, pancreatitis is divided into 2 forms: acute interstitial pancreatitis and necrotizing pancreatitis.[17] On unenhanced T1-weighted fat-suppressed and dynamic contrast-enhanced images, imaging features of acute interstitial pancreatitis include diffuse or focal enlargement of the pancreas, loss of the normal T1-weighted signal intensity, and decreased and delayed enhancement (**Fig. 1**). However, with mild acute pancreatitis, T1-weighted sequences

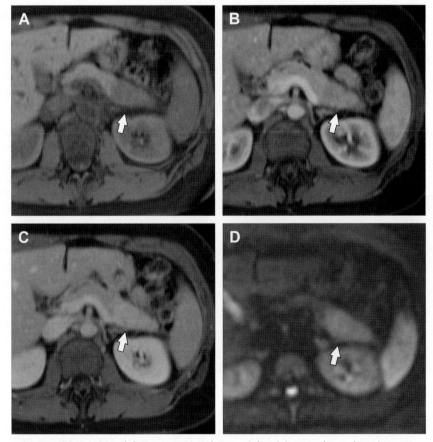

Fig. 1. Acute pancreatitis on MR. (*A*) Fat-suppressed T1-weighted image shows hypointense pancreatic tail (*arrow*). (*B*) Early contrast-enhanced T1-weighted image shows decreased enhancement of the pancreatic tail with minimal adjacent fat stranding consistent with acute pancreatitis (*arrow*). (*C*) Venous phase image shows delayed enhancement of the pancreatic tail (*arrow*). (*D*) Diffusion-weighted image (b 500 s/mm$^2$) shows increased signal in the pancreatic tail (*arrow*).

with fat suppression may appear normal.[1,3,19] T2-weighted fat-suppressed sequences can show peripancreatic edema and fluid collections. MRCP may be normal or show relative compression of the pancreatic duct by the surrounding edematous pancreas and may help in identifying the underlying cause of pancreatitis.[1] Diffusion-weighted imaging may show restricted diffusion in pancreatitis; however, it may not be specific, because both acute and chronic pancreatitis can show restricted diffusion.[20]

With necrotizing pancreatitis, there often is high signal intensity on T1-weighted images secondary to hemorrhage and lack of pancreatic enhancement from necrosis (**Fig. 2**).[1] These areas can be focal, segmental, or diffuse and are usually poorly defined.[2,21,22] T2-weighted sequences can show low signal intensity in areas of pancreatic necrosis and high signal intensity in areas of liquefaction.[2]

MR imaging effectively shows complications resulting from pancreatitis, including pancreatic duct disruption, hemorrhage, venous thrombosis, arterial pseudoaneurysms, and peripancreatic fluid collections. Hemorrhage can result from either necrotizing pancreatitis or rupture of a pseudoaneurysm. A pseudoaneurysm appears as a round structure that follows blood pool on contrast-enhanced sequences and typically arises from the splenic, gastroduodenal, or pancreaticoduodenal arteries (**Fig. 3**). Acute venous thrombi appear as intravascular filling defects on contrast-enhanced images, usually within the splenic, portal, or superior mesenteric veins.

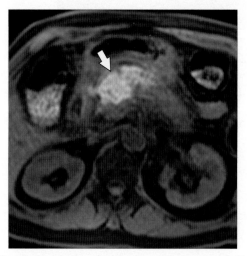

Fig. 2. Necrotizing pancreatitis. Fat-suppressed T1-weighted image shows high signal intensity within the pancreatic head and body (*arrow*), compatible with hemorrhage in this patient with necrotizing pancreatitis.

With chronic thrombosis, the normal vein may not be identified, but collateral vessels are present.[2,3]

Another complication of acute pancreatitis is the development of pancreatic and peripancreatic fluid collections. Peripancreatic fluid collections are divided into 4 types based on the morphologic type of acute pancreatitis (interstitial edematous pancreatitis or necrotizing pancreatitis), presence of a capsule, contents of the collection, age of the collection (either <4 weeks or >4 weeks), and presence or absence of infection. With interstitial edematous pancreatitis, the collections comprise fluid and are either acute peripancreatic fluid collections or pseudocysts, depending on the age of the collection and the presence or absence of a capsule. With acute necrotizing pancreatitis, collections comprise necrotic debris and fluid and are either acute necrotic collections or areas of walled-off necrosis, depending on the age of the collection and the presence or absence of a capsule. All of these collections can be either sterile or infected.[17,23]

Fluid collections are usually best evaluated on T2-weighted sequences and contrast-enhanced T1-weighted fat-suppressed sequences. Acute peripancreatic fluid collections are homogenous nonencapsulated fluid collections adjacent to the pancreas.[23] These collections usually develop within 48 hours and resolve spontaneously within 2 to 4 weeks.[18] A pseudocyst, in contrast, usually appears as a homogenous encapsulated unilocular or multilocular fluid collection that may or may not communicate with the pancreatic duct. Although ERCP can often better show the site of communication between the pseudocyst and the pancreatic duct, MRCP is more sensitive in detecting pseudocysts, because only about half of pseudocysts are seen to fill with contrast on ERCP. In addition, unlike ERCP, MR imaging can characterize the composition of the pseudocyst better, including the presence of hemorrhagic, proteinaceous, or necrotic components.[1,22,23]

Acute necrotic collections, as the name implies, are composed of tissue from pancreatic or peripancreatic fat necrosis secondary to the release of pancreatic enzymes. These collections are nonencapsulated homogeneous or heterogeneous collections found in the pancreatic or peripancreatic regions. This entity is in contrast to areas of walled-off necrosis, which show a capsule. It has been shown that the solid elements of both of these collections are better depicted with MR imaging than with CT.[18,24,25] It is important to distinguish these 2 entities, because the treatment of walled-off pancreatic necrosis is surgical resection or drainage, whereas acute

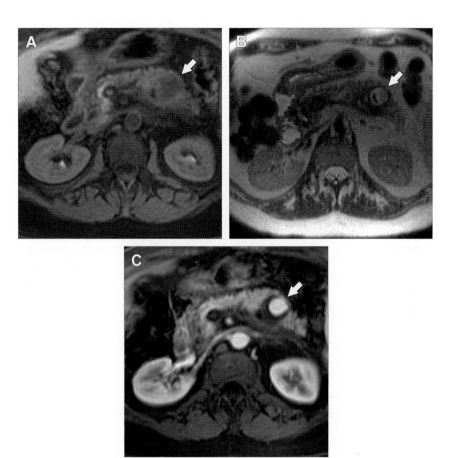

**Fig. 3.** Cystic-appearing mass, emphasizing the importance of intravenous contrast. (*A*) Fat-suppressed T1-weighted image shows a hypointense lesion in the pancreatic tail (*arrow*) in a patient with a history of pancreatitis. (*B*) T2-weighted image shows the lesion (*arrow*) is high signal, suggestive of a cystic lesion. In a patient with a history of pancreatitis, the lesion may suggest a pseudocyst, but it is important to consider other causes. (*C*) Gadolinium-enhanced T1-weighted image shows enhancement following blood pool of the cystic mass consistent with a pseudoaneurysm (*arrow*) and emphasizes the importance of contrast to exclude a vascular lesion before biopsy.

necrotic collections require only surgery in the setting of superimposed infection.[17,26]

In patients without a known history of pancreatitis, it can be difficult to differentiate a pancreatic fluid collection from a cystic pancreatic neoplasm. However, the presence of dependent debris layering within a cystic pancreatic lesion is highly specific for the diagnosis of a pancreatic fluid collection and generally is not seen in cystic neoplasms.[27]

## Chronic Pancreatitis

Chronic pancreatitis is a chronic inflammatory process causing pancreatic fibrosis, atrophy, and calcifications and results in irreversible pancreatic exocrine and endocrine dysfunction. Although MR imaging is less sensitive than CT for the detection of calcifications, MR imaging is more sensitive for the early findings of chronic pancreatitis, before the development of the calcifications, because the attenuation of the pancreas remains normal on CT in chronic pancreatitis, even with advanced disease (**Fig. 4**).[1] The MR imaging diagnosis is based on multiple characteristics, including the signal intensity and enhancement pattern of the pancreas, as well as the morphologic characteristics of the pancreatic parenchyma and the pancreatic duct. One of the early findings of chronic pancreatitis is loss of the normal high T1 signal of the pancreas on T1 fat-suppressed images. This finding is secondary to a decreased amount of proteinaceous fluid within the pancreas from chronic inflammation and fibrosis. There can also be decreased enhancement on the early contrast-enhanced sequences, with more pronounced delayed enhancement of the pancreas secondary to chronic fibrosis, atrophy, and loss of the

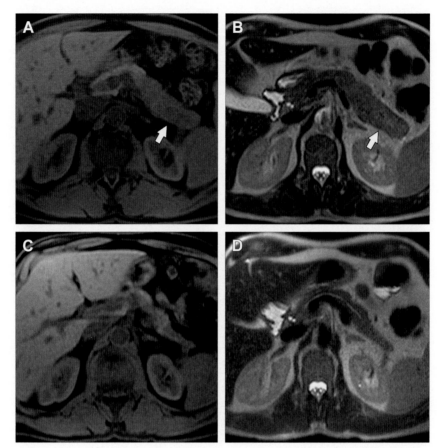

**Fig. 4.** Acute pancreatitis developing into chronic pancreatitis. (*A*) T1-weighted image shows mild enlargement and loss of the normal signal of the pancreatic tail (*arrow*). (*B*) T2-weighted image shows enlargement of the pancreatic tail (*arrow*), with mild peripancreatic fat stranding. (*C*) Subsequent follow-up MR imaging after the acute presentation had resolved shows findings compatible with chronic pancreatitis. T1-weighted image shows progressive pancreatic atrophy with heterogeneous loss of the normal T1 signal of the pancreatic tail. (*D*) T2-weighted image from follow-up MR shows interval atrophy of the pancreatic tail, with mild prominence of the pancreatic duct.

pancreatic vascular supply.[28,29] In older patients, there may be normal age-related fibrosis and relative decreased signal intensity of the pancreas.

The use of secretin-enhanced MRCP can help identify early findings of chronic pancreatitis before the development of morphologic changes seen on conventional MR imaging. First, there can be decreased or complete lack of pancreatic duct distension after secretin administration. Normal duct distension is considered when there is 1 mm or greater increase in duct diameter more than that of baseline. Less than 1 mm of duct distension after secretin administration suggests the possibility of impaired pancreatic ductal compliance, which can be seen in chronic pancreatitis. Second, dilated side branches can be shown after secretin administration in chronic pancreatitis, a finding that is not seen in normal patients. Secretin increases flow of pancreatic

secretions into side branches as well as the main pancreatic duct, enabling earlier detection of dilated side branches. With chronic pancreatitis, areas of fibrosis at the junction of the side branches and main pancreatic duct may interrupt the pancreatic secretion flow and lead to dilatation of the side branches. Third, there can be decreased filling of the duodenum with pancreatic secretions in patients with chronic pancreatitis, which can be used to assess pancreatic exocrine function. Normal pancreatic exocrine function is considered when pancreatic fluid goes into at least the third portion of the duodenum; impaired exocrine function occurs when pancreatic fluid fills only the proximal duodenum (**Figs. 5** and **6**).[8]

Late findings of chronic pancreatitis include pancreatic atrophy, pseudocyst formation, and pancreatic duct abnormalities. Duct abnormalities are best evaluated on thin-section T2-weighted

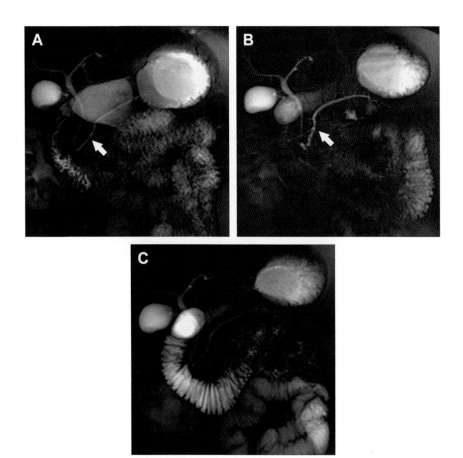

**Fig. 5.** Normal secretin study. (*A*) Before and (*B*) after the administration of secretin, there is mild increase in duct distension (*arrows*), a normal finding. (*C*) After the administration of secretin, there is complete filling of the duodenum.

HASTE (half Fourier single-shot turbo spin-echo) and MRCP images. In a normal pancreas, the diameter of the main pancreatic duct is about 2 mm, and the side branches are not usually visualized. However, with chronic pancreatitis, there can be pancreatic duct dilatation, pancreatic ductal strictures and irregularities, and visualization of dilated side branches, leading to the chain of lakes appearance. Although CT is helpful to show calcifications associated with chronic pancreatitis, MR has advantages in showing the location of the stones within the pancreatic duct on T2-weighted images.[1,3]

Although MR is highly sensitive and specific in distinguishing between pancreatic carcinoma and chronic pancreatitis,[28] at times, differentiating between the two can be difficult on MR, because decreased T1-weighted fat-suppressed signal intensity, decreased and delayed enhancement, peripancreatic fat infiltration, pancreatic duct dilatation and obstruction, and restricted diffusion can be seen in both processes. An inflammatory mass within the head of the pancreas can mimic a pancreatic neoplasm.[29] Findings that favor chronic pancreatitis include an irregular appearance of the duct, presence of calcifications, diffuse pancreatic involvement, and the duct-penetrating sign, in which the normal or smoothly stenotic pancreatic duct penetrates the inflammatory mass. Findings that favor carcinoma include a smoothly dilated pancreatic duct with abrupt cutoff, a mass located at the site of obstruction with distal pancreatic atrophy, obliteration of the perivascular fat, and the double-duct sign, with dilatation of both the pancreatic and common bile duct.[28,29] However, two things must be kept in mind when trying to distinguish between chronic pancreatitis and adenocarcinoma: adenocarcinoma can be superimposed on patients with chronic pancreatitis, and a pancreatic mass can cause upstream pancreatitis.[29]

## Groove Pancreatitis

Groove pancreatitis is a focal chronic pancreatitis that occurs in the pancreaticoduodenal groove,

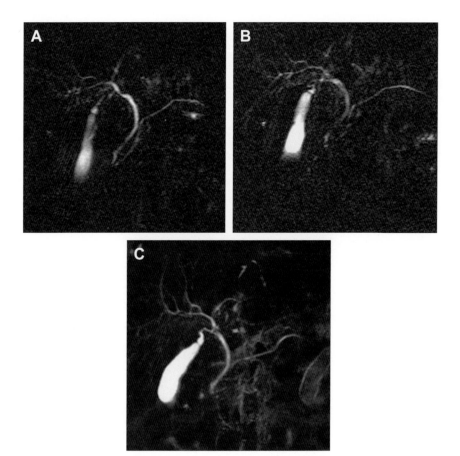

**Fig. 6.** Abnormal secretin from chronic pancreatitis. MRCP (*A*) before and (*B*) after the administration of secretin shows lack of pancreatic duct distension, a finding suggesting impaired ductal compliance (*C*) Delayed image obtained after secretin shows lack of duodenal filling.

located between the head of the pancreas, duodenum, and the common bile duct. The pancreatic parenchyma is typically spared or only slightly involved.[30] Several causes of this inflammatory process have been implicated, including previous biliary disease, peptic ulcers, gastric resections, pancreatic head or duodenal wall cysts, and heterotopic pancreatic tissue within the duodenum.[30] There are 2 forms of groove pancreatitis: pure and segmental. The pure form affects the groove only, whereas the segmental form extends to the pancreatic head.[29] Nevertheless, both types can lead to stenosis of the pancreatic duct, which can in turn lead to diffuse chronic pancreatitis.[30]

Imaging findings of groove pancreatitis relate to the fibrotic nature of the process and include a T1 hypointense mass located between the head of the pancreas and the duodenum (**Fig. 7**), with delayed enhancement secondary to the presence of fibrotic scar tissue.[29] On T2-weighted sequences, the signal of the mass can be variable, depending on the stage of the disease. A subacute process shows increased T2 signal secondary to edema,

whereas a chronic process shows decreased T2 signal secondary to fibrosis. There can be associated chronic inflammatory changes of the pancreatic head, leading to decreased T1 signal of the pancreatic head, diffuse pancreatic atrophy, and pancreatic duct dilatation. Chronic inflammatory changes involving the duodenum with wall thickening, stenosis, and delayed wall enhancement may be present.[30] On MRCP, groove pancreatitis usually shows smooth tapering of the distal common bile duct secondary to the adjacent edema and fibrosis,[29] which can in turn lead to mild proximal biliary dilatation.[30] MRCP can show cystic lesions within the groove or the duodenal wall and can depict their relationship with the ductal system.[30]

## Autoimmune Pancreatitis

Autoimmune pancreatitis is a type of chronic pancreatitis characterized by lymphocytic infiltration and pancreatic fibrosis, leading to pancreatic dysfunction.[31] Patients typically present with

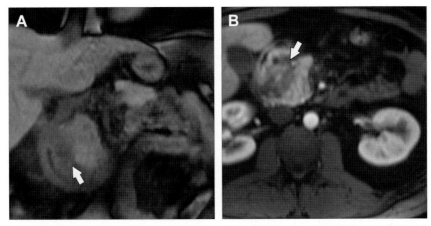

**Fig. 7.** Groove pancreatitis. (*A*) Coronal T1 fat-suppressed image shows low signal abnormality in the pancreatic groove between the pancreas and duodenum (*arrow*). (*B*) Axial contrast-enhanced T1-weighted image shows decreased enhancement (*arrow*) of the abnormality.

painless jaundice secondary to pancreatic duct narrowing with absence of the typical history of previous episodes of acute pancreatitis or alcohol abuse.[29] Autoimmune pancreatitis is important to distinguish clinically from other forms of pancreatitis, because the process is reversible; pancreatic function can return to normal, and treatment is with steroids.[32] Autoimmune pancreatitis can also affect other organ systems, including the biliary system, lungs, kidneys, retroperitoneum, and salivary glands. Increase of IgG4 level is the best serologic marker for this disease and can help in diagnosis.[33]

The typical appearance of autoimmune pancreatitis on MR imaging (**Fig. 8**) is diffuse pancreatic enlargement with featureless borders, decreased T1 fat-suppressed signal intensity, increased T2 signal intensity, and delayed enhancement. A rim-like capsule of decreased T1 fat-suppressed signal intensity and increased T2 signal intensity with associated delayed enhancement is suggestive of fibrosis. MRCP can show diffuse or segmental irregular narrowing of the main pancreatic duct as well as the intrahepatic and common bile duct[31–33]; however, these findings are more reliably visualized on ERCP.[34] The involvement of the main pancreatic duct is characteristic of this entity and usually resolves after appropriate management with steroids.[32]

Sometimes, autoimmune pancreatitis may mimic a mass and present as a focal lesion within the pancreas with or without associated duct dilatation and distal pancreatic atrophy, making it difficult to distinguish from pancreatic adenocarcinoma. Hur and colleagues[31] found that certain findings favor mass-forming autoimmune pancreatitis over adenocarcinoma, including multiplicity, geographic shape, delayed enhancement, capsulelike rim

enhancement, low ADC value, and segmental strictures of the common bile duct or main pancreatic duct. Imaging findings, serology features, and other organ involvement may allow assessment of steroid response for the diagnosis of autoimmune pancreatitis. However, biopsy may be required for the diagnosis and distinction from cancer.

## ANATOMIC VARIANTS
### Pancreas Divisum

Pancreas divisum is the most common congenital variant of the pancreatic duct and occurs when the dorsal and ventral ducts fail to fuse with each other during gestation. The pancreatic head and uncinate process are drained by the ventral pancreatic duct, which opens through the major papilla. The pancreatic body and tail are drained by the dorsal pancreatic duct, which opens via the minor papilla.[3,35]

MRCP depicts the absence of communication between the ventral and dorsal duct systems (**Fig. 9**). The long and narrow dorsal duct drains via the minor papilla. The short ventral duct joins the distal bile duct and drains via the major papilla. It is postulated that impaired drainage of the major duct through the minor papilla results in increased endoluminal pressure, which may increase the risk of pancreatitis.[3,36–39] Although patients with pancreas divisum may have acute pancreatitis, most patients with this anatomic variant are asymptomatic.

### Annular Pancreas

Annular pancreas is an uncommon congenital anomaly in which pancreatic tissue completely or incompletely encircles the second portion of the duodenum. Patients can be asymptomatic or can

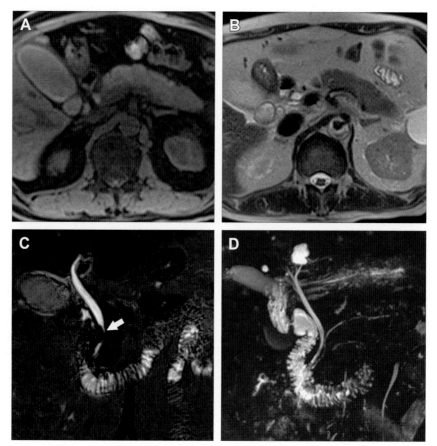

**Fig. 8.** Autoimmune pancreatitis. (*A*) T1-weighted image shows fusiform enlargement of the pancreatic body and tail, with loss of the normal T1 signal. (*B*) T2-weighted image shows fusiform enlargement and peripancreatic fat stranding. Incidental note is made of an exophytic left renal cyst. (*C*) Coronal MRCP image shows focal narrowing involving the distal common bile duct (*arrow*), accounting for the patient's presentation with painless jaundice. (*D*) MRCP image shows resolution of the focal area of narrowing of the common bile duct after the patient was treated with steroids.

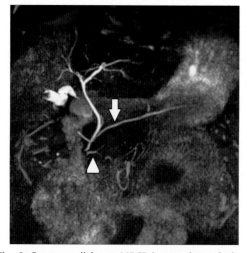

**Fig. 9.** Pancreas divisum. MRCP image shows lack of communication between the ventral (*arrowhead*) and dorsal (*white arrow*) pancreatic ducts, consistent with pancreas divisum.

present in infancy to adulthood with duodenal obstruction or stenosis, chronic pancreatitis, or biliary obstruction. MR shows hyperintense pancreatic tissue encircling the relatively hypointense duodenum on T1-weighted fat-suppressed sequences (**Fig. 10**).[3,35] MRCP can also be used to show the pancreatic duct encircling the duodenum.[3]

## PANCREATIC NEOPLASMS
### Adenocarcinoma

Pancreatic adenocarcinoma is the most common pancreatic neoplasm; however, by the time patients usually present, only about 10% to 15% are considered potentially operable candidates.[3] Pancreatic adenocarcinomas located within the pancreatic head usually present earlier than pancreatic body and tail lesions secondary to involvement of the common bile duct, leading to jaundice and other symptoms. Because of

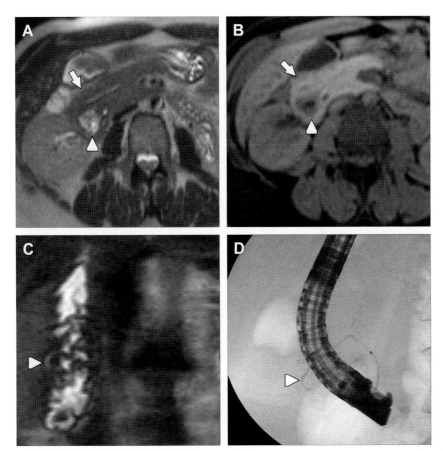

**Fig. 10.** Annular pancreas. (*A*) T2-weighted image shows pancreatic parenchyma and pancreatic duct (*arrow*) encircling the duodenum (*arrowhead*). (*B*) T1-weighted image shows the typical high signal intensity pancreatic parenchyma (*arrow*) encircling the low signal intensity duodenum (*arrowhead*). Diagnosis is easier to make on MR than CT. (*C*) Coronal T2-weighted image shows the pancreatic duct (*arrowhead*) surrounding the duodenum, confirming the presence of an annular pancreas. (*D*) ERCP shows the pancreatic duct (*arrow*) encircling the duodenum.

the late presentation of body and tail masses, a large percentage already have metastases at the time of diagnosis. MR imaging and endoscopic ultrasonography have been shown to have the highest accuracy in detecting pancreatic adenocarcinoma.[40]

Pancreatic adenocarcinomas are best detected using pregadolinium and early gadolinium-enhanced fat-suppressed T1-weighted images (**Fig. 11**).[1,3,41,42] Adenocarcinoma is generally seen as a focal mass of low T1 signal intensity and shows progressive delayed enhancement.[1,3,41] If the mass is located within the pancreatic head, there can sometimes be loss of the normal high T1 signal of the pancreatic body and tail secondary to obstruction of the main pancreatic duct, leading to inflammation, fibrosis, and atrophy. In this situation, the early contrast-enhanced images may show a low signal intensity mass with rim enhancement superimposed on a background of slightly greater enhancing,

chronically inflamed, pancreatic parenchyma. If the mass is located within the pancreatic tail, it is usually well shown on the unenhanced fat-suppressed T1-weighted images.[1]

Diffusion-weighted imaging has been shown to have a high sensitivity (96.2%) and specificity (98.6%) for detecting pancreatic adenocarcinomas and may allow earlier detection of pancreatic adenocarcinoma.[43,44] These tumors show increased signal on diffusion-weighted imaging and relatively low ADC values, because of fibrosis associated with the tumor.[13,43] Diffusion-weighted imaging may also help in detecting liver and lymph node metastases not always readily detected on other sequences. Not every lymph node seen on diffusion-weighted imaging is malignant, because both benign and malignant lymph nodes can show restricted diffusion.[13]

MR criteria of unresectability can vary based on institution but is usually based on the extent of vascular involvement, including the superior

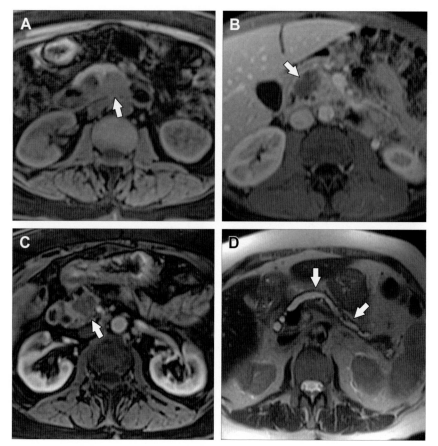

**Fig. 11.** Examples of pancreatic adenocarcinoma in different patients. (*A*) Unenhanced T1-weighted image with fat suppression shows a focal hypointense mass (*arrow*) within the uncinate process. (*B*) Contrast-enhanced T1-weighted image in a different patient shows a hypoenhancing lesion (*arrow*) in the pancreatic head. (*C*) Contrast-enhanced T1-weighted image in a different patient shows a focal hypoenhancing mass (*arrow*) within the pancreatic head. (*D*) T2-weighted image in the same patient as (*C*) shows diffuse pancreatic atrophy and duct dilatation of the pancreatic body and tail upstream from the mass (*arrow*).

mesenteric artery, celiac trunk, or the superior mesenteric vein portal vein confluence or evidence of metastases. Contour deformity, irregularity or obstruction of the vessel, infiltration of the perivascular fat, and contiguity of the tumor with the vessel wall by greater than 180° suggest vascular involvement by tumor.[3] Liver metastases usually show decreased signal on unenhanced T1-weighted fat-suppressed images, increased signal on T2-weighted images, irregular rim enhancement on early phase gadolinium-enhanced images, and restricted diffusion.[1,41] Peritoneal metastases are usually best shown on the delayed postgadolinium images[1] but can also be detected on diffusion-weighted sequences.[45]

## Pancreatic Endocrine Tumors

Also known as islet cell tumors, pancreatic endocrine tumors arise from neuroendocrine cells within the pancreas. The most common pancreatic endocrine tumors are insulinomas, gastrinomas, and nonfunctioning islet cell tumors. If hyperfunctioning, these tumors tend to present when small, because of their early symptoms from hormone production. However, nonhyperfunctioning tumors tend to present when large, usually secondary to symptoms from either mass effect or metastases.[1,46]

These tumors classically present as well-defined T2 hyperintense and T1 hypointense masses with avid arterial enhancement (**Fig. 12**). They are often not classic and can show homogenous, heterogeneous, or rim enhancement.[3,46–48] Sometimes, these masses can appear isointense to the pancreas on all contrast-enhanced and T2-weighted sequences and are depicted only on the unenhanced T1-weighted fat-suppressed images, which have been shown to have the highest sensitivity for detecting pancreatic endocrine

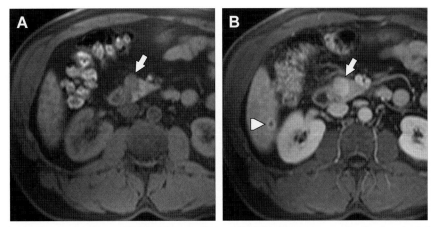

Fig. 12. Endocrine tumor. (*A*) T1-weighted image shows the hypointense mass in the head of the pancreas (*arrow*). (*B*) Contrast-enhanced T1-weighted image shows marked enhancement of the pancreatic head lesion, which is typical for endocrine tumor and helps distinguish this lesion from an adenocarcinoma (*arrow*). Note also the ring-enhancing liver metastasis (*arrowhead*).

tumors.[46–50] Nonhyperfunctioning islet cell tumors tend to present when large and more frequently show cystic, necrotic, or hemorrhagic components as well as calcifications and metastases.[46]

When present, metastases are typically found in the liver and peripancreatic lymph nodes. Liver metastases are usually hypointense on T1-weighted images and mildly hyperintense on T2-weighted images. They usually show prominent enhancement on postgadolinium sequences and can have central necrosis.[46,50]

### Mucinous Cystic Neoplasms

Mucinous cystic neoplasms account for approximately 10% of pancreatic cystic neoplasms.[51] These neoplasms are more common in women in their fourth to sixth decades of life and are usually removed because of malignant potential.[52] Invasive carcinoma has been reported to occur in 6% to 36% of mucinous cystic neoplasms.[53]

Mucinous cystic neoplasms are typically large, multilocular, well-defined cystic-appearing masses, which most commonly arise in the pancreatic body or tail. They tend to have fewer than 6 cysts, with each cyst being larger than 2 cm. Irregular internal septations are also characteristic, and occasionally, capsular or septal calcifications can be present but may not be shown on MR.[3,52]

On MR imaging, these neoplasms typically present as a cystic pancreatic lesion with either a single cyst or a few cysts (**Fig. 13**). A thick wall showing delayed enhancement is typically present. Internally, these neoplasms typically appear similar to simple cysts on both T1-weighted and T2-weighted images, despite their mucin content. Sometimes, they can show intrinsic T1 hyperintensity on unenhanced T1-weighted fat-suppressed

sequences secondary to the presence of hemorrhagic or proteinaceous components. Mildly thickened enhancing septa can be present; however, if there are enhancing soft tissue components, carcinoma should be considered.[51] Likewise, if there is obliteration of the adjacent fat planes, local invasion should be suggested.[52] Diffusion-weighted imaging cannot distinguish mucinous cystic neoplasms from other lesions, because these neoplasms also tend to show high signal intensity on diffusion-weighted images and relatively high ADC values because of T2 shine-through.[13]

### Serous Cystadenomas

Serous cystadenomas, also called microcystic adenomas, are the second most common cystic neoplasm of the pancreas. These tumors are considered benign, often detected incidentally, and tend to affect women older than 60 years.[52] Serous cystadenomas typically present as large tumors with a honeycomb appearance and are made up of at least 6 cysts, which are each smaller than 2 cm. There can be a central stellate scar, dystrophic calcifications, and a thin fibrous pseudocapsule.[3,52]

MR characteristics can be variable, depending on the amount of stromal tissue, size of the cysts, and whether the cysts contain simple or hemorrhagic fluid.[52] Classically, serous cystadenomas typically present as a cluster of small T2 hyperintense cysts with thin fibrous septa, which enhance on delayed gadolinium-enhanced images (**Fig. 14**). As the lesion grows in size, the fibrous tissue can retract and produce a central scar.[51] The central scar shows variable enhancement on gadolinium-enhanced sequences, and if it contains associated coarse calcifications, it may

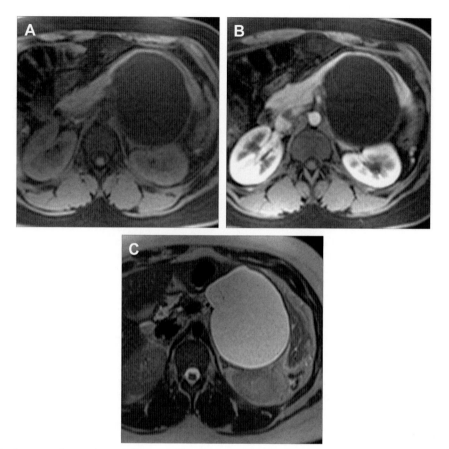

**Fig. 13.** Mucinous cystic neoplasm. A 23-year-old woman presented with abdominal pain. (*A*) T1-weighted image shows 10 × 8 cm hypointense lesion posterior to the pancreatic tail. (*B*) Contrast-enhanced T1-weighted image shows the lesion to be nonenhancing. (*C*) T2-weighted image shows the mass to be cystic. The patient did not have history or symptoms of pancreatitis. The lesion was resected and was a mucinous cystadenoma.

show a signal void.[51,52] These lesions do not communicate with the main pancreatic duct, which helps distinguish them from other cystic lesions of the pancreas.[52] Diffusion-weighted imaging characteristics can vary with these lesions, because of the varying amount of fluid or septa within the lesion. These lesions can show high signal on high b value diffusion-weighted images and relatively lower ADC values compared with nonneoplastic cysts; however, this finding is seen in only some patients.[13]

In contrast to the classic microcystic form of serous cystadenoma, there are also oligocystic and solid variants, which can lead to diagnostic difficulty. In the oligocystic type, there are usually just a few large cysts, which can mimic the potentially malignant mucinous cystadenoma. Solid cystadenomas are less common and are composed of microscopic cysts, which are too small to be depicted by MR imaging. This factor can lead to a solid appearance at imaging and mimic neuroendocrine tumors.[51]

## Intraductal Papillary Mucinous Neoplasms

Intraductal papillary mucinous neoplasms (IPMNs) are tumors characterized by proliferation and mucinous transformation of pancreatic ductal epithelium, leading to production of excess mucin and dilatation of the pancreatic duct. IPMNs can range from noninvasive neoplasms to invasive adenocarcinomas.[3,51] IPMNs occur most commonly between the ages of 60 and 80 years and have a slight male predominance.[3] IPMNs can also occur with increased frequency in patients with pancreatic cancer.[54] IPMNs produce slow progressive distension of the pancreatic duct by hypersecretion of mucin, leading to impairment or obstruction of pancreatic secretion outflow.[3] These neoplasms, unlike mucinous cystic neoplasms, communicate with the pancreatic duct, which can be shown on MRCP sequences.[3]

There are 2 types, branch duct and main duct, or a combination of both. These types can be further subdivided into segmental or diffuse types. The

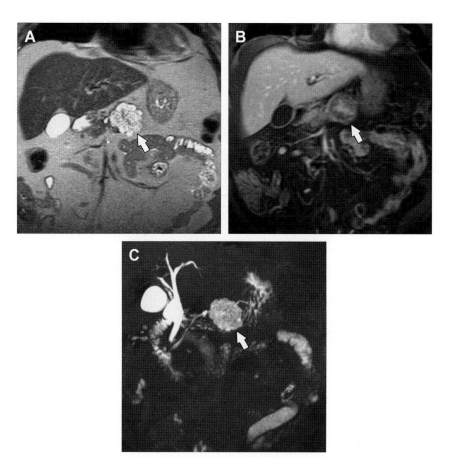

**Fig. 14.** Serous cystadenoma. (*A*) Coronal T2-weighted image shows a lobulated multiseptated cystic mass (*arrow*) with a central stellate scar and small cysts. (*B*) Coronal gadolinium-enhanced T1-weighted image shows enhancement of the central stellate scar (*arrow*). (*C*) MRCP image shows a multiseptated cystic mass with multiple small cysts (*arrow*). Unlike intraductal papillary mucinous neoplasm, the lesion does not communicate with the duct.

branch duct type appears most commonly as cystic dilatation of side branches on T2-weighted and MRCP images (**Fig. 15**).[51] It is often seen as a unilocular or multilocular cyst with lobulated margins and internal septations, usually within the pancreatic head or uncinate process. This appearance can be difficult to distinguish from a cystic pancreatic neoplasm, although showing communication with the pancreatic duct allows distinction. These cystic spaces are composed of dilated branch duct lumen. The mucin-producing tumor is usually not visualized, because it tends to be small and flat. There is typically progressive ductal dilatation with findings of both branch and main duct types. Focal or diffuse pancreatic atrophy may also occur.[3] Small filling defects can be seen, which may be caused by intraluminal mucin or mural nodules.[55,56] Mural nodules enhance after intravenous gadolinium, whereas mucin do not.[56] However, the small size of these filling defects may preclude distinction.

Main duct involvement is more likely to be malignant.[51] Like the branch duct type, the mucin-producing tumor is often small and not visualized. There is moderate to marked dilatation of the main pancreatic duct, with atrophy of the pancreas. At times, there are intraductal calcifications, making it difficult to distinguish from chronic pancreatitis.[3] However, with chronic pancreatitis, there are usually additional findings of chronic pancreatitis, including loss of the normal high T1 signal of the pancreas and delayed enhancement from chronic fibrosis.[51] When diffuse ductal dilatation is present, there is often more involvement of the branch ducts within the pancreatic tail and uncinate process. Bulging of the papilla into the duodenal lumen, which is often seen on ERCP, can sometimes be shown on MR imaging.[3]

MR imaging cannot definitively distinguish between benign and malignant IPMNs. However, features that favor malignancy include main duct type, greater than 15 mm of main duct dilatation,

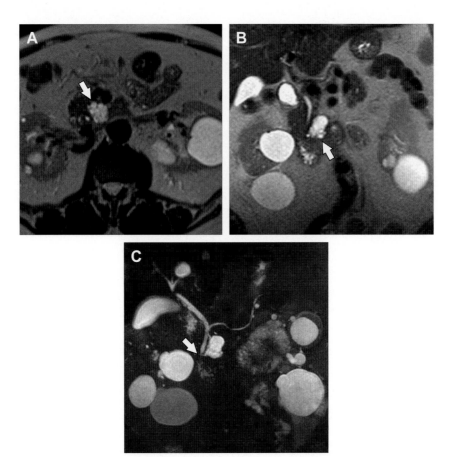

**Fig. 15.** Side branch IPMN confirmed on ERCP. (*A*) Axial and (*B*) coronal T2-weighted image shows a multiseptated cystic mass (*arrow*) in the uncinate process (*arrow*). Appearance is nonspecific and may be from serous cystadenoma or side branch IPMN as well as other causes. (*C*) Rapid acquisition with relaxation enhancement MRCP image shows communication with the pancreatic duct (*arrow*), favoring side branch IPMN over serous cystadenoma. The patient did not have a history of pancreatitis.

or a cystic lesion with a thick wall, solid mural nodules, or filling defects.[52] Other features that suggest malignancy include enhancing soft tissue nodularity and size of the tumor greater than 3.5 cm.[51] It has been postulated that it takes approximately 5 years for an intraductal papillary mucinous adenoma to develop into an invasive carcinoma.[3] Therefore, some people opt for conservative management with close regular follow-up in cases without features suggestive of malignancy.[51] These neoplasms have a better prognosis than adenocarcinomas, likely from earlier detection because of their large noninvasive component when malignant foci are microscopic. These neoplasms do tend to recur after complete resection, so yearly postoperative surveillance is recommended.[3]

### Solid Pseudopapillary Tumor

Previously known as solid and papillary epithelial neoplasms, these tumors are rare and considered low-grade malignancies with a good prognosis. They have been reported to be more common in African American women in their second to fourth decades of life. When occurring in an older population, there is an increased incidence of malignancy. These neoplasms tend to be well defined, large at presentation, and occur typically in the pancreatic tail.[52] The average size at presentation is 9 cm, but can range from 2.5 cm to 17 cm. Hemorrhage is common with these tumors and is secondary to rupture of its poorly supported vasculature.[57] The presence of an encapsulated pancreatic mass with hemorrhage in a younger female should raise this entity as a possibility, because these findings are rarely found in other pancreatic neoplasms.[58,59]

On MR imaging, solid pseudopapillary tumors can have variable imaging appearances based on their internal components (**Fig. 16**). MR imaging can be helpful in the diagnosis, because the presence of hemorrhage suggests the diagnosis.

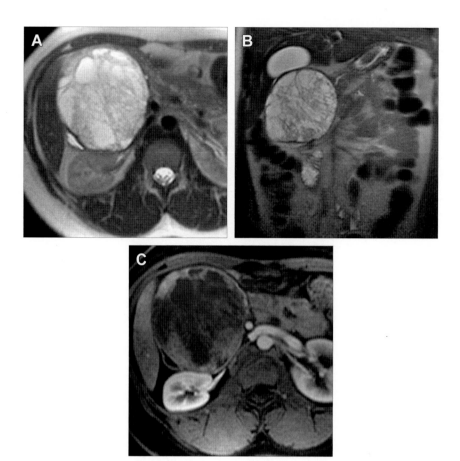

**Fig. 16.** A 25-year-old woman who presented with a palpable mass from solid pseudopapillary epithelial neoplasm. Axial (*A*) and coronal (*B*) T2-weighted image shows a cystic and solid pancreatic mass within the pancreatic head. (*C*) After contrast administration, there is enhancement of the solid components.

Typical findings include a large well-encapsulated mass, with a variable amount of solid and cystic components secondary to hemorrhage and necrosis. On MR imaging, these tumors usually present as a mass with heterogeneous signal intensity on both T1-weighted and T2-weighted images and a thick enhancing fibrous capsule.[59] If they are predominantly solid, these neoplasms tend to show mild increased T2 signal intensity; but if they have large cystic components, they tend to have higher T2 signal intensity areas.[51] Areas of hemorrhage show high T1 signal intensity. In addition, these masses typically show early peripheral heterogeneous enhancement of the solid portions, with progressive fill-in on delayed sequences.[59] Diffusion-weighted imaging findings of these neoplasms can vary, because of differences in their internal composition, which affect the degree of diffusion and the ADC values. Wang and colleagues[13] reported relatively low ADC values in the solid portion of the neoplasm.

Sometimes, small tumors can appear less sharply marginated and unencapsulated with less cystic components. Calcifications, duct obstruction, secondary pseudocyst formation, and invasion through the capsule into adjacent structures can be seen, but rarely. Although these tumors are considered to have a low malignant potential, metastases have been reported in a few cases, usually solitary and to the liver. Rarely, these tumors can metastasize to lymph nodes or the peritoneum.[59]

## Pancreatic Lymphoma

Although the pancreas can be involved in more than 30% of patients with non-Hodgkin lymphoma, primary lymphoma of the pancreas is rare, with less than 2% of extranodal non-Hodgkin lymphoma arising within the pancreas.[60] The pancreas is more commonly involved by direct extension of lymphomatous involvement of peripancreatic lymph nodes.

Lymphoma of the pancreas can present as a focal mass or diffuse infiltration of the pancreatic parenchyma (**Fig. 17**). The focal mass type

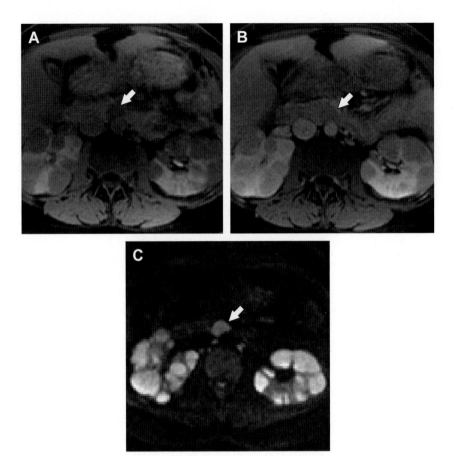

**Fig. 17.** Non-Hodgkin lymphoma of the pancreas and kidneys. A 29-year-old woman who presented with a pelvic mass. (*A*) T1-weighted image shows a subtle hypointense pancreatic lesion in the uncinate process (*arrow*). Multiple solid renal masses are seen. (*B*) Mild enhancement was seen in the pancreatic (*arrow*) and renal masses from lymphoma. (*C*) Diffusion-weighted image (b 800 s/mm²) highlights the mass in the pancreas (*arrow*) and multiple masses in the kidneys from non-Hodgkin lymphoma, because they have restricted diffusion.

presents as a well-defined homogenous low T1 signal intensity mass or masses with mild homogenous enhancement on gadolinium-enhanced images. On T2-weighted images, the mass is usually heterogeneous in appearance and slightly hyperintense relative to the surrounding pancreas. The diffuse infiltrating type usually shows diffuse enlargement of the pancreas, infiltration of the peripancreatic fat, low signal intensity on both T1-weighted and T2-weighted images, and mild to moderate enhancement after gadolinium administration. Usually, only mild pancreatic ductal dilatation is seen, unlike pancreatic adenocarcinoma.[60]

### Pancreatic Metastases

Metastases to the pancreas are rare, with a reported frequency of 2% to 5% in the clinical setting and 1.6% to 11% in autopsy studies of patients with advanced metastatic disease. However, metastases to the pancreas are being seen more frequently in patients with cancer, who are living longer because of advances in therapies. The malignancies that most commonly metastasize to the pancreas are renal cell, lung, breast, ovarian, hepatocellular, thyroid, gastrointestinal, and melanoma. Three patterns of pancreatic involvement have been described, the most common of which is a solitary pancreatic mass. Less commonly, there can be multiple pancreatic masses or diffuse infiltration of the pancreas.[61]

Pancreatic metastases usually have a similar MR appearance to that of the primary malignancy, sometimes allowing for differentiation of metastases from the more common pancreatic adenocarcinoma (**Fig. 18**). Metastases usually show hypointense T1 signal and heterogeneous hyperintense T2 signal.[61] Tsitouridis and colleagues[62] showed that pancreatic metastases usually show peripheral rim enhancement, or less commonly, homogenous enhancement, in contrast to poorly enhancing adenocarcinomas.

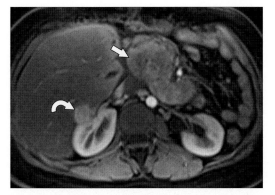

**Fig. 18.** Fibrolamellar hepatocellular carcinoma metastases to the pancreas and hepatic lesion invading the right kidney. T1-weighted fat-suppressed image after contrast administration shows enlargement and heterogeneous enhancement of the pancreas (*arrow*) with multiple conglomerate-appearing masses, enlarged peripancreatic lymph nodes, and hepatic lesion invading the right kidney (*curved white arrow*) in this patient with metastatic fibrolamellar carcinoma.

## SUMMARY

With advances in imaging techniques, including diffusion-weighted imaging, MR imaging is becoming increasingly important and is often the preferred imaging modality to evaluate a variety of pancreatic disease processes. MR imaging with the use of MRCP is particularly useful in evaluating the pancreatic ductal system. In this article, the basics of MR imaging of the pancreas, including the normal appearance of the pancreas on different imaging sequences, as well as inflammatory diseases, congenital abnormalities, and neoplasms of the pancreas, are reviewed.

## REFERENCES

1. Ly JN, Miller FH. MR imaging of the pancreas: a practical approach. Radiol Clin North Am 2002; 40(6):1289–306.
2. Miller FH, Keppke AL, Dalal K, et al. MRI of pancreatitis and its complications: part 1, acute pancreatitis. AJR Am J Roentgenol 2004;183(6):1637–44.
3. Keppke AL, Miller FH. Magnetic resonance imaging of the pancreas: the future is now. Semin Ultrasound CT MR 2005;26(3):132–52.
4. Matos C, Cappeliez O, Winant C, et al. MR imaging of the pancreas: a pictorial tour. Radiographics 2002;22(1):e2.
5. Sica GT, Braver J, Cooney MJ, et al. Comparison of endoscopic retrograde cholangiopancreatography with MR cholangiopancreatography in patients with pancreatitis. Radiology 1999;210(3):605–10.
6. Tanner AR, Dwarakanath AD, Tait NP. The potential impact of high-quality MRI of the biliary tree on ERCP workload. Eur J Gastroenterol Hepatol 2000;12(7):773–6.
7. Sandrasegaran K, Lin C, Akisik FM, et al. State-of-the-art pancreatic MRI. AJR Am J Roentgenol 2010;195(1):42–53.
8. Balci C. MRI assessment of chronic pancreatitis. Diagn Interv Radiol 2011;17(3):249–54.
9. Bali MA, Sztantics A, Metens T, et al. Quantification of pancreatic exocrine function with secretin-enhanced magnetic resonance cholangiopancreatography: normal values and short-term effects of pancreatic duct drainage procedures in chronic pancreatitis. Initial results. Eur Radiol 2005; 15(10):2110–21.
10. Punwani S, Gillams AR, Lees WR. Non-invasive quantification of pancreatic exocrine function using secretin-stimulated MRCP. Eur Radiol 2003;13(2): 273–6.
11. Schneider AR, Hammerstingl R, Heller M, et al. Does secretin-stimulated MRCP predict exocrine pancreatic insufficiency?: a comparison with noninvasive exocrine pancreatic function tests. J Clin Gastroenterol 2006;40(9):851–5.
12. Cappeliez O, Delhaye M, Devière J, et al. Chronic pancreatitis: evaluation of pancreatic exocrine function with MR pancreatography after secretin stimulation. Radiology 2000;215(2):358–64.
13. Wang Y, Miller FH, Chen ZE, et al. Diffusion-weighted MR imaging of solid and cystic lesions of the pancreas. Radiographics 2011;31(3):E47–64.
14. Qayyum A. Diffusion-weighted imaging in the abdomen and pelvis: concepts and applications. Radiographics 2009;29(6):1797–810.
15. Hagmann P, Jonasson L, Maeder P, et al. Understanding diffusion MR imaging techniques: from scalar diffusion-weighted imaging to diffusion tensor imaging and beyond. Radiographics 2006; 26:S205–23.
16. Wang Y, Chen ZE, Yaghmai V, et al. Diffusion-weighted MR imaging in pancreatic endocrine tumors correlated with histopathologic characteristics. J Magn Reson Imaging 2011;33(5):1071–9.
17. Thoeni R. The revised Atlanta classification of acute pancreatitis: its importance for the radiologist and its effect on treatment. Radiology 2012; 262(3):751–64.
18. Morgan DE. Imaging of acute pancreatitis and its complications. Clin Gastroenterol Hepatol 2008; 6(10):1077–85.
19. Sica GT, Miller FH, Rodriquez G, et al. Magnetic resonance imaging in patients with pancreatitis: evaluation of signal intensity and enhancement changes. J Magn Reson Imaging 2002;15(3):275–84.
20. Thomas S, Kayhan A, Lakadamyali H, et al. Diffusion MRI of acute pancreatitis and comparison

with normal individuals using ADC values. Emerg Radiol 2012;19(1):5–9.

21. Xiao B, Zhang XM, Tang W, et al. Magnetic resonance imaging for local complications of acute pancreatitis: a pictorial review. World J Gastroenterol 2010;16(22):2735–42.

22. Xiao B, Zhang XM. Magnetic resonance imaging for acute pancreatitis. World J Radiol 2010;2(8):298–308.

23. Bollen TL. Imaging of acute pancreatitis: update of the revised Atlanta classification. Radiol Clin North Am 2012;50(3):429–45.

24. Morgan DE, Baron TH, Smith JK, et al. Pancreatic fluid collections prior to intervention: evaluation with MR imaging compared with CT and US. Radiology 1997;203(3):773–8.

25. Vege SS, Fletcher JG, Talukdar R, et al. Peripancreatic collections in acute pancreatitis: correlation between computerized tomography and operative findings. World J Gastroenterol 2010;16(34):4291–6.

26. Stamatakos M, Stefanaki C, Kontzoglou K, et al. Walled-off pancreatic necrosis. World J Gastroenterol 2010;16(14):1707–12.

27. Macari M, Finn ME, Bennett GL, et al. Differentiating pancreatic cystic neoplasms from pancreatic pseudocysts at MR imaging: value of perceived internal debris. Radiology 2009;251(1):77–84.

28. Miller FH, Keppke AL, Wadhwa A, et al. MRI of pancreatitis and its complications: part 2, chronic pancreatitis. AJR Am J Roentgenol 2004;183(6):1645–52.

29. Siddiqi AJ, Miller F. Chronic pancreatitis: ultrasound, computed tomography, and magnetic resonance imaging features. Semin Ultrasound CT MR 2007;28(5):384–94.

30. Blasbalg R, Baroni RH, Costa DN, et al. MRI features of groove pancreatitis. AJR Am J Roentgenol 2007;189(1):73–80.

31. Hur BY, Lee JM, Lee JE, et al. Magnetic resonance imaging findings of the mass-forming type of autoimmune pancreatitis: comparison with pancreatic adenocarcinoma. J Magn Reson Imaging 2012;36(1):188–97.

32. Sahani DV, Kalva SP, Farrell J, et al. Autoimmune pancreatitis: imaging features. Radiology 2004;233(2):345–52.

33. Bodily KD, Takahashi N, Fletcher JG, et al. Autoimmune pancreatitis: pancreatic and extrapancreatic imaging findings. AJR Am J Roentgenol 2009;192(2):431–7.

34. Kamisawa T, Tu Y, Egawa N, et al. Can MRCP replace ERCP for the diagnosis of autoimmune pancreatitis? Abdom Imaging 2009;34(3):381–4.

35. Yu J, Turner MA, Fulcher AS, et al. Congenital anomalies and normal variants of the pancreaticobiliary tract and the pancreas in adults: part 2,

pancreatic duct and pancreas. AJR Am J Roentgenol 2006;187(6):1544–53.

36. Manfredi R, Costamagna G, Brizi MG, et al. Pancreas divisum and "santorinicele": diagnosis with dynamic MR cholangiopancreatography with secretin stimulation. Radiology 2000;217(2):403–8.

37. Matos C, Metens T, Devière J, et al. Pancreas divisum: evaluation with secretin-enhanced magnetic resonance cholangiopancreatography. Gastrointest Endosc 2001;53(7):728–33.

38. Chalazonitis NA, Lachanis BS, Laspas F, et al. Pancreas divisum: magnetic resonance cholangiopancreatography findings. Singapore Med J 2008;49(11):951–4.

39. Vitellas KM, Keogan MT, Spritzer CE, et al. MR cholangiopancreatography of bile and pancreatic duct abnormalities with emphasis on the single-shot fast spin-echo technique. Radiographics 2000;20(4):939–57.

40. Balci NC, Semelka RC. Radiologic diagnosis and staging of pancreatic ductal adenocarcinoma. Eur J Radiol 2001;38:105–12.

41. Miller FH, Rini NJ, Keppke AL. MRI of adenocarcinoma of the pancreas. AJR Am J Roentgenol 2006;187(4):W365–74.

42. Birchard KR, Semelka RC, Hyslop WB, et al. Suspected pancreatic cancer: evaluation by dynamic gadolinium-enhanced 3D gradient-echo MRI. AJR Am J Roentgenol 2005;185(3):700–3.

43. Wang Y, Chen ZE, Nikolaidis P, et al. Diffusion-weighted magnetic resonance imaging of pancreatic adenocarcinomas: association with histopathology and tumor grade. J Magn Reson Imaging 2011;33(1):136–42.

44. Ichikawa T, Erturk SM, Motosugi U, et al. High-b value diffusion-weighted MRI for detecting pancreatic adenocarcinoma: preliminary results. AJR Am J Roentgenol 2007;188(2):409–14.

45. Low RN, Sebrechts CP, Barone RM, et al. Diffusion-weighted MRI of peritoneal tumors: comparison with conventional MRI and surgical and histopathologic findings–a feasibility study. AJR Am J Roentgenol 2009;193(2):461–70.

46. Herwick S, Miller FH, Keppke AL. MRI of islet cell tumors of the pancreas. AJR Am J Roentgenol 2006;187(5):W472–80.

47. Owen NJ, Sohaib SA, Peppercorn PD, et al. MRI of pancreatic neuroendocrine tumours. Br J Radiol 2001;74(886):968–73.

48. Semelka RC, Custodio CM, Balci NC, et al. Neuroendocrine tumors of the pancreas: spectrum of appearances on MRI. J Magn Reson Imaging 2000;11(2):141–8.

49. Thoeni RF, Mueller-Lisse UG, Chan R, et al. Detection of small, functional islet cell tumors in the pancreas: selection of MR imaging sequences

for optimal sensitivity. Radiology 2000;214(2): 483–90.

50. Lewis RB, Lattin GE Jr, Paal E. Pancreatic endocrine tumors: radiologic-clinicopathologic correlation. Radiographics 2010;30(6):1445–64.

51. Kalb B, Sarmiento JM, Kooby DA, et al. MR imaging of cystic lesions of the pancreas. Radiographics 2009;29(6):1749–65.

52. Hammond N, Miller FH, Sica GT, et al. Imaging of cystic diseases of the pancreas. Radiol Clin North Am 2002;40(6):1243–62.

53. Testini M, Gurrado A, Lissidini G, et al. Management of mucinous cystic neoplasms of the pancreas. World J Gastroenterol 2010;16(45): 5682–92.

54. Macari M, Eubig J, Robinson E. Frequency of intraductal papillary mucinous neoplasm in patients with and without pancreas cancer. Pancreatology 2010;10(6):734–41.

55. Silas AM, Morrin MM, Raptopoulos V, et al. Intraductal papillary mucinous tumors of the pancreas. AJR Am J Roentgenol 2001;176(1):179–85.

56. Procacci C, Megibow AJ, Carbognin G, et al. Intraductal papillary mucinous tumor of the pancreas: a pictorial essay. Radiographics 1999;19(6):1447–63.

57. Mortele BP, Mortele KJ, Tuncali K, et al. Solid and papillary epithelial neoplasm of the pancreas: MR imaging findings. JBR-BTR 2002;85(6):297–9.

58. Sahni VA, Mortelé KJ. The bloody pancreas: MDCT and MRI features of hypervascular and hemorrhagic pancreatic conditions. AJR Am J Roentgenol 2009;192(4):923–35.

59. Choi JY, Kim MJ, Kim JH, et al. Solid pseudopapillary tumor of the pancreas: typical and atypical manifestations. AJR Am J Roentgenol 2006; 187(2):W178–86.

60. Merkle EM, Bender GN, Brambs HJ. Imaging findings in pancreatic lymphoma: differential aspects. AJR Am J Roentgenol 2000;174(3):671–5.

61. Merkle EM, Boaz T, Kolokythas O, et al. Metastases to the pancreas. Br J Radiol 1998;71(851):1208–14.

62. Tsitouridis I, Diamantopoulou A, Michaelides M, et al. Pancreatic metastases: CT and MRI findings. Diagn Interv Radiol 2010;16(1):45–51.

# MR Imaging of the Kidneys and Adrenal Glands

Amir H. Davarpanah, MD*, Gary M. Israel, MD*

## KEYWORDS

- Magnetic resonance imaging • Genitourinary imaging • Renal mass • Urinary tract • Adrenal mass

## KEY POINTS

- Comprehensive MR imaging of the kidneys can differentiate surgical from nonsurgical lesions in most cases.
- MR imaging can characterize many adrenal masses based on their signal intensities and tissue composition.
- The continued development and growth of MR technology combined with the current trend toward minimally invasive surgery will expand the role of MR imaging in the future.

## INTRODUCTION

MR imaging plays an ever-increasing role in the evaluation of renal and adrenal abnormalities. The excellent soft-tissue contrast resolution combined with a variety of accelerated pulse sequences gives MR imaging an advantage when compared with other imaging modalities in renal and adrenal imaging. The unsurpassed ability of MR imaging in detection of intracellular and extracellular lipid using fat suppression and water-fat separation methods provides for accurate characterization of some renal and adrenal masses.

## MR IMAGING TECHNIQUE

At Yale New Haven Hospital, all abdominal MR imaging examinations are performed using dedicated torso phased array coil, high-field imaging, and a power injector when contrast is administered. The high-field scanners provide higher signal-to-noise ratio (SNR), allowing shorter acquisition times and, therefore, less motion artifact. With lower field strength, the image quality declines due to lower SNR and longer acquisition times, resulting in accentuated motion artifact. Therefore, the field strength of 1.5-T or greater is suggested for abdominal imaging. The use of

abdominal phased array torso coil is preferable because of the improved SNR ratio, which allows for the use of smaller fields of view with concomitant increased spatial resolution. Using parallel imaging techniques, the number of phase-encoding steps could be decreased, with consequent shortening of acquisition time, while maintaining diagnostic image quality and spatial resolution.

Breath-holding or respiratory navigation sequences are used exclusively to minimize artifacts secondary to respiratory motion. Studies may be performed during end-expiration because the position of the abdominal organs is more constant in expiration than in inspiration. This allows optimized image coregistration for subtraction algorithms.

The MR imaging protocol for adrenal or renal imaging is similar. A breath-hold or respiratory-navigated heavily T2-weighted sequence (half-Fourier acquisition single-shot turbo spin-echo [HASTE, Siemens, Erlangen, Germany]) is performed in coronal and axial planes to help provide an anatomic roadmap, characterize cystic lesions of the kidney, and assess for hydronephrosis. A breath-hold dual-echo T1-weighted two-dimensional (2D) gradient-echo (GRE) sequence is implemented in-phase and out-of-phase to detect intracellular lipid, which is present in adrenal

Department of Radiology, Yale-New Haven Hospital, 20 York Street, New Haven, CT 06510, USA
* Corresponding author.
*E-mail addresses:* amir.davarpanah@yale.edu; gary.israel@yale.edu

Radiol Clin N Am 52 (2014) 779–798
http://dx.doi.org/10.1016/j.rcl.2014.02.003
0033-8389/14/$ – see front matter © 2014 Elsevier Inc. All rights reserved.

adenomas and occasionally within clear cell-type RCCs. To differentiate the signal decay from T2* effect from chemical shift, the first echo preferably acquires an image at the opposed-phase and the second echo acquires an image at the in-phase. Both echoes should be obtained in the same breath-hold (dual-echo sequence) to avoid slice misregistration. This sequence, in conjunction with a fat-suppressed sequence, is useful to help detect macroscopic fat within renal (angiomyolipomas [AMLs]) and adrenal masses (myelolipomas).

A baseline unenhanced three-dimensional (3D) fat-suppressed T1-weighted GRE sequence is used to facilitate differentiation of hemorrhage from fat and provide a baseline comparison to postcontrast images to determine presence or absence of tissue enhancement. 3D pulse sequence is advantageous due to increased SNR compared with 2D counterparts, allowing for reduction in acquisition time and implementation of parallel imaging.

As a standard part of a renal mass MR imaging protocol, MR angiography and MR urography (MRU) are also performed to depict the relationship of a renal mass to the renal vasculature and collecting system, which can assist in surgical planning.

At the authors' institution, after administration of intravenous (IV) gadolinium-based contrast, images in arterial and nephrographic phases are obtained. To evaluate the renal vasculature, a high-resolution 3D fat-suppressed T1-weighted fast spoiled gradient echo sequence is performed in conjunction with IV bolus injection of a gadolinium-based contrast agent. This sequence allows fast data acquisition and makes multiplanar reformations and maximum intensity projections rendering possible. Rapid contrast delivery is best achieved by power injecting at a rate of 2 cc per second. The angiographic acquisition can be coordinated with the arrival of the contrast bolus in the aorta at the level of the renal arteries and can be performed using a timing bolus or Care-Bolus (Siemens, Erlangen, Germany). At Yale New Haven Hospital, a 30-second delay is used and found adequate in evaluation of the vascular anatomy as well as a corticomedullary phase of the kidneys. Depiction of renal vascular anatomy and showing its relationship to a renal mass could be used for surgical planning before nephron-saving partial nephrectomy. Following a scanning delay of 2 to 5 minutes, the 3D sequence is repeated and used to evaluate enhancement within a renal mass. It should be noted that postcontrast MR imaging is not necessary in evaluating most adrenal masses because most adrenal masses are adenomas and can be characterized without IV contrast. However, IV contrast would be necessary in evaluating or staging adrenal malignancy or in demonstrating no enhancement within adrenal pseudocysts.

Digital subtraction algorithm enables assessment of enhancement in renal masses and is especially important in masses that are T1 hyperintense or hypovascular. This technique requires optimal precontrast and postcontrast image coregistration and, in case of poor image coregistration, side-by-side comparison or region of interest (ROI) measurements on precontrast and postcontrast images, is necessary to establish or exclude enhancement.[1,2]

MRU sequences are useful in the setting of transitional cell carcinoma (TCC) or a suspicious abnormality in the collecting system. MRU may be performed with unenhanced 2D or 3D heavily T2-weighted turbo spin-echo (Siemens, Erlangen, Germany) sequences, using a thick slab projection technique or with multiple contiguous thin sections (static-fluid MRU).[3] T2-weighted MRU can be conducted independent of renal excretory function, making it applicable in patients with renal failure. Static-fluid MRU is also preferable during pregnancy and in patients with ureteral obstruction, although it is unable to provide functional information regarding the excretory system. Another limitation of T2-weighted MRU is its lower sensitivity for evaluation of nondilated urinary system.

Static-fluid MRU should be performed before administration of IV contrast to avoid T2-shortening effect of excreted contrast into the urine, which causes undesirable signal loss inside the collecting system. Alternatively, a delayed furosemide-enhanced 3D T1-weighted GRE sequence can be performed after IV administration of gadolinium contrast material and 10 to 20 mg of furosemide (excretory MRU).[4] The excretory MRU sequences are obtained in the axial plane at 3 minutes and in the coronal plane at 3 and 7 to 10 minutes. The gadolinium-enhanced MRU techniques provide morphologic and functional information of the excretory system and they can be performed in dilated and nondilated urinary systems. The latter technique is preferable due to higher spatial resolution and near-isotropic voxels although decision about the best-suited MRU sequence largely depends on the renal function and degree of urinary tract dilatation.

## KIDNEYS

Every effort should be made to differentiate surgical from nonsurgical renal lesions based on imaging characteristics thereby preventing unjustified resection of benign lesions. Using a combination of T2-weighted and T1-weighted images with and without fat suppression and with and without contrast, renal lesions can be characterized to surgical and nonsurgical lesions. Presence or absence of fat within a renal mass and enhancement on postcontrast images are the most important aspects in renal lesion characterization.

## Cystic Renal Lesions

Simple renal cysts are routinely encountered in daily practice with higher prevalence in the older population. They are characterized by a hairline thin wall and they appear uniformly hyperintense on T2-weighted images with no contrast enhancement.

The term complex cyst generally refers to any renal cyst that is not simple and may contain hemorrhage, protein, debris, septations, a thickened wall, or neoplastic tissue. It may demonstrate a wide range of signal intensity on T1-weighted and T2-weighted sequences, based on their contents. Demonstration of nodular enhancement within the mass is the most reliable sign in differentiating between benign cystic lesions and cystic renal neoplasms.

The Bosniak classification of renal cystic masses has been in use for more than 25 years and is based on CT scan findings. However, it has been successfully adapted for use with MR imaging[5–8]:

- Category I (simple) cysts demonstrate hypointense signal on T1-weighted images and are uniformly hyperintense on T2-weighted images. These lesions do not enhance after administration of contrast.
- Category II (mildly complicated benign) cysts may contain very thin septa that are best depicted on the T2-weighted images where they appear as thin low signal intensity curvilinear structures against the hyperintense cystic fluid. When these lesions contain hemorrhagic or proteinaceous material, they demonstrate hyperintense signal on the T1-weighted images. MR imaging is an excellent problem-solving modality when a high-attenuating cyst with equivocal enhancement is detected on CT scan and is ideally suited for characterizing hemorrhagic cysts (**Fig. 1**). This is especially true in patients with acquired cystic disease of dialysis or with autosomal dominant polycystic kidney disease, in which hemorrhagic cysts are very common. Using a subtraction algorithm makes it possible to demonstrate that these lesions do not enhance and thereby to characterize them as benign hemorrhagic cysts.

- Category IIF cysts (moderately complicated cystic masses) are thought to be benign but require follow-up examinations because they have some complex features and may contain minimal thickening of the wall and septa or increased number of septations. On the follow-up examinations, interval thickening and enhancement of the wall or septa or the presence of new nodular enhancing tissue indicates progression of the lesion and, in most cases, a surgical evaluation would be necessary. The rate of malignancy in category IIF varies between 5% and 25% in the literature.[9,10] Without exposure to radiation or nephrotoxic contrast material, MR imaging is useful for following these lesions. Some category IIF lesions contain large amounts of calcium. These lesions are difficult to characterize on CT scan because identifying enhancing tissue adjacent to the calcification can be challenging. Because the calcification within these lesions is not well seen on MR imaging, it may be possible to better characterize heavily calcified category IIF lesions previously seen on CT scan with MR imaging.
- Category III lesions (indeterminate masses requiring surgical evaluation) are more complex. They may demonstrate thick enhancing walls and/or thick enhancing septa but do not contain nodular enhancing soft tissue components associated with the wall or septa, which are seen in category IV lesions. The reported rate of malignancy in these lesions has been between 54% and 61% (**Fig. 2**).[10,11] Category III lesions include infectious, hemorrhagic, as well as other benign and neoplastic causes. Pyogenic renal abscesses and infected cysts could be suggested based on clinical features, surrounding inflammation in the perinephric fat, or edema in the renal parenchyma. Another rare benign cystic lesion, the multilocular cystic nephroma (MLCN), characteristically presents in middle-aged women as a septated cystic mass, which tends to occur centrally in the kidney and herniate toward the renal pelvis. The presence of thickened enhancing septa wall in MLCN makes it indistinguishable from cystic renal cell carcinoma (RCC) and, therefore, surgical excision is usually advocated (**Fig. 3**).
- Category IV lesions (cystic neoplasms) are clearly malignant and demonstrate unequivocal enhancing soft tissue components (**Fig. 4**).

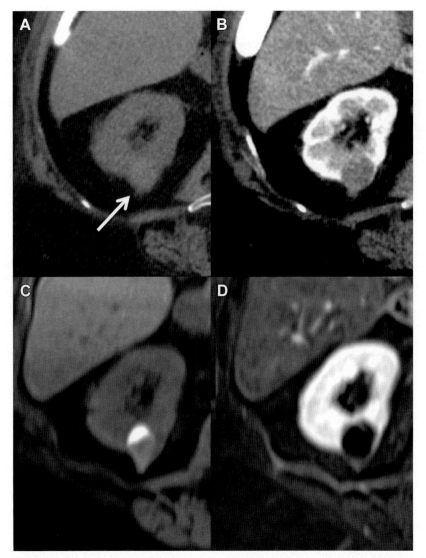

**Fig. 1.** A 37-year-old woman with a right renal hemorrhagic cyst. (*A*) Transverse unenhanced CT scan demonstrates a 2.2-cm slightly high-attenuating lesion (*arrow*) that measures 34 Hounsfield (HU) in the midpole of the right kidney. (*B*) On the transverse contrast-enhanced CT scan, renal lesion measures 54 HU, and there is an apparent 20-HU increase in the attenuation. Therefore, a soft tissue mass is suspected. (*C*) Axial unenhanced T1-weighted MR image with fat-suppression shows a heterogeneous mass with a hemorrhagic component and a fluid-fluid level. (*D*) Transverse subtracted MR image (gadolinium-enhanced fat-suppressed T1-weighted image minus unenhanced fat-suppressed T1-weighted image) shows a single hairline internal septation but no enhancing nodular component within the mass, confirming the diagnosis of a hemorrhagic cyst (Bosniak category II cyst). This case illustrates the usefulness of MR imaging in characterizing renal masses that demonstrate equivocal enhancement on CT.

## Solid Renal Lesions

In general, any solid enhancing renal mass should be considered potentially malignant. However, the differential diagnosis for such a lesion incorporates a wide range of malignant and benign entities. Therefore, once a lesion has been shown to demonstrate enhancement, it is necessary to characterize it as a surgical lesion (RCC, oncocytoma, TCC) or a nonsurgical lesion (metastases, lymphoma, AML, renal pseudotumor).

### RCC

RCC is the most common tumor of the kidney, accounting for 80% to 85% of all malignant renal tumors and 2% to 3% of all malignant diseases in adults.[12] Currently, with the widespread use of cross-sectional imaging, most RCCs are detected incidentally in asymptomatic patients. When symptomatic, the most common presentations include hematuria, flank pain, and palpable mass although this classic triad is only seen in 10% of

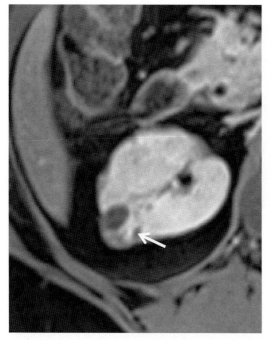

Fig. 2. A 61-year-old man with a category III cystic renal mass in the midpole of the right kidney. Transverse gadolinium-enhanced fat-suppressed T1-weighted MR image shows a 2 cm cystic renal mass that contains thick enhancing septa (*arrow*) consistent with a Bosniak category III lesion. A partial nephrectomy was performed and a clear cell RCC was diagnosed at pathologic examination.

the patients and it usually indicates advanced disease.

The role of imaging is central to detection, staging, and treatment of the RCC. Improved equipment and pulse sequence techniques has resulted in similar accuracy of MR imaging in detecting and staging of RCCs compared with those of CT scanning.[13] MR imaging offers inherently exquisite tissue contrast, which allows characterization of hemorrhage, fat, and subtle enhancement, making it particularly useful when ultrasonography or CT are inconclusive. It can be also used as an alternative modality when iodinated contrast medium is contraindicated or tumor thrombus is suspected.

The imaging approach to RCC focuses on demonstrating enhancement within a renal mass. The presence of enhancement can be assessed subjectively or by the means of subtraction algorithms when the tumor is hypovascular or T1-hyperintense. RCC is often slightly hypointense on T1-weighted images and isointense to slightly hyperintense on the T2-weighted images compared with the background renal parenchyma. However, their MR imaging signal characteristics can be variable depending on their content of fluid and hemorrhagic material. The three most common subtypes of RCC, including clear cell (70%), papillary (10%–15%), and chromophobe (6%–11%) carcinomas, may demonstrate distinct MR imaging characteristics.[14] Clear cell RCCs tend to exhibit heterogeneously increased signal on T2-weighted sequences and may contain intracytoplasmic lipid vacuoles, resulting in signal drop on opposed-phase T1-weighted images. Papillary carcinomas characteristically demonstrate homogenously lower signal on T2-weighted sequences. Contrast-enhanced MR imaging can also be helpful for the determination of the histologic subtype in RCC. Clear cell carcinomas are usually hypervascular and demonstrate greater enhancement, whereas chromophobe and papillary tumors exhibit intermediate and the lowest percentage enhancement, respectively.[15,16]

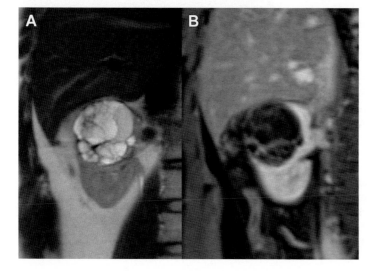

Fig. 3. MLCN in a 47-year-old woman. (*A*) Coronal T2-weighted MR image of the right kidney shows a 5.2 cm multiseptated cystic mass, some of the septa appear thickened. (*B*) Corresponding gadolinium-enhanced fat-suppressed T1-weighted image shows enhancement of the septa, compatible with Bosniak category III lesion. A MLCN was diagnosed at pathologic examination.

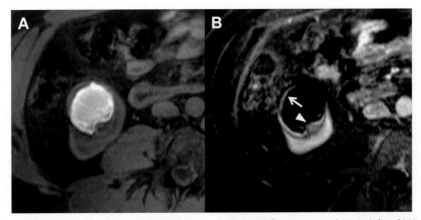

**Fig. 4.** Cystic RCC in a 54-year-old woman. (*A*) Transverse unenhanced fat-suppressed T1-weighted MR image of the right kidney shows a 5.2 cm hemorrhagic lesion in the right kidney. (*B*) Transverse subtracted MR image (gadolinium-enhanced fat-suppressed T1-weighted image minus unenhanced fat-suppressed T1-weighted image) shows enhancement within the wall of the lesion that is thickened (*arrow*) and nodular enhancement (*arrowhead*) posteriorly, consistent with a Bosniak category IV lesion. A cystic RCC was diagnosed at pathologic examination.

Determination of the extent of tumor is critical for selection of optimal therapy and surgical approach, particularly in case of nephron-sparing surgery. The multiplanar capability of MR imaging and its ability to differentiate enhancing tumor thrombus from bland thrombus within the renal vein and inferior vena cava (IVC) makes it an accurate tool for the staging of RCC (**Fig. 5**).[17] Assessment for retroperitoneal lymphadenopathy is performed in similar fashion to a CT scan, with lymph nodes greater than 1 cm in short axis considered suspicious for metastatic disease.

After surgery, gadolinium-enhanced MR imaging may be used to evaluate for early postoperative complications, including hemorrhage or urinary leak, in those patients who undergo partial nephrectomy (**Fig. 6**). In addition, MR imaging is useful in the routine postoperative surveillance for recurrent neoplasm or metachronous lesion for which these patients are at increased risk.

### Angiomyolipoma

Angiomyolipoma (AML) accounts for 2.0% to 6.4% of all renal tumors.[18] It is composed of varying amounts of blood vessels, smooth muscle, and adipose tissue. Although 90% of AMLs occur sporadically and are often solitary, nearly 50% of patients with tuberous sclerosis develop AMLs, which tend to be multiple and bilateral.[19] These lesions occur more commonly in women than men.

Patients are usually asymptomatic and AMLs are usually incidentally discovered when the patient is imaged for another reason. However, when large, AMLs may exert mass effect on the adjacent organs and cause symptoms. In addition,

patients with large AMLs may present with acute flank pain caused by spontaneous hemorrhage. This may be life-threatening and require emergent embolization or nephrectomy.

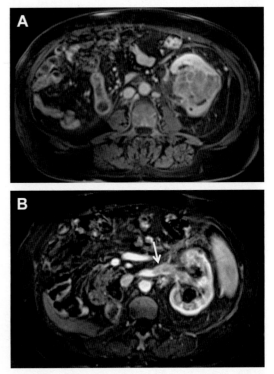

**Fig. 5.** RCC and tumor thrombus in a 76-year-old man. (*A*) Axial gadolinium-enhanced fat-suppressed three-dimensional T1-weighted acquisition shows a 7.8 cm heterogeneously enhancing left renal mass consistent with RCC. (*B*) Enhancing tumor thrombus extends into the left renal vein (*arrow*) up to the level of the aorta.

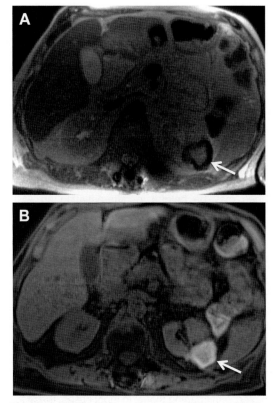

**Fig. 6.** A postsurgical hematoma in a 59-year-old man with history of recent left partial nephrectomy for a RCC. Follow-up ultrasound showed a lesion in the upper pole of the left kidney. (*A*) Axial T2-weighted MR image shows a 3.5 cm mass (*arrow*) in the postoperative bed of the superior pole of the left kidney. The mass has a dark rim, suggesting hemosiderin. (*B*) Unenhanced fat-suppressed T1-weighted imaging demonstrates uniform hyperintense signal within the mass (*arrow*), consistent with hemorrhage in the postoperative bed. Follow-up imaging showed resolution of the hemorrhage.

AML may be characterized based on its tissue composition and signal characteristics. The MR imaging appearance of AMLs depends on the relative composition of all three histologic elements. The diagnosis of AML rests on demonstrating the presence of macroscopic fat within the lesion. When an AML is predominately composed of fatty tissue, it will demonstrate hyperintense signal on the T1-weighted images (**Fig. 7**). However, other renal masses, including hemorrhagic cysts, may show similar signal characteristics. Therefore, it is necessary to compare the T1-weighted images with fat-suppressed T1-weighted images, which will differentiate the fat seen in AMLs from other renal masses containing hemorrhage or proteinaceous material.

AML may also be diagnosed with the use of chemical shift imaging (CSI) techniques.[20]

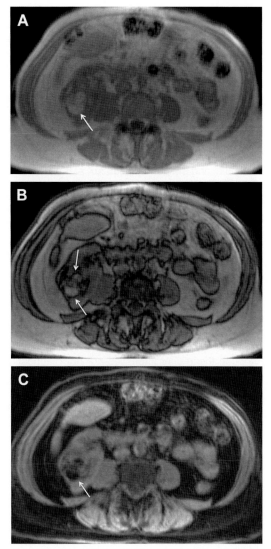

**Fig. 7.** A renal AML in a 50-year-old woman. (*A*) Axial in-phase T1-weighted GRE image shows a 4.0 cm right renal mass (*arrow*) that is heterogeneous in signal but contains regions that are T1 hyperintense. These are nonspecific and could be hemorrhage or fat. (*B*) Axial opposed-phase T1-weighted GRE image at the same level demonstrates the India ink artifact at the interface of the kidney and the mass (*arrows*), diagnostic of fat containing lesion (AML). (*C*) Axial T1-weighted GRE image obtained with frequency-selective fat suppression demonstrates signal loss within the T1 hyperintense position of the mass (*arrow*), diagnostic of macroscopic fat, confirming the diagnosis of AML.

Acquiring images at different echo times enables exploitation of the difference in resonance frequency between water and fat. This technique provides images when fat and water signal are in-phase (additive) or out-of-phase (destructive). This produces the characteristic India ink artifact on the T1-weighted out-of-phase images, manifested as a low signal intensity rim at any soft tissue (water) and fat interface. Hemorrhagic cysts and AMLs may be hyperintense on T1-weighted in-phase images and may be indistinguishable from each other. However, they are readily differentiated on the T1-weighted out-of-phase images. For AMLs, the India ink artifact appears at the interface of the mass (fat) with the kidney (water) or at the interface at the fatty and nonfatty portions of the mass (see **Fig. 7**). For hemorrhagic cysts, the India ink artifact occurs at the interface of the cyst (fluid) and the perirenal fat, not at the interface of the cyst and the kidney (**Fig. 8**).

In some instances, AMLs may not contain enough fat to be diagnosed on imaging and are referred to as AML with minimal fat.[21] These masses have typical imaging characteristics. On MR imaging, they are homogeneously hypointense on T2-weighted images due to the presence of a large amount of smooth muscle within them[22] and they homogeneously enhance with IV contrast. On unenhanced CT, these masses are typically high in attenuation compared with the renal parenchyma, similar to that of muscle. Although these characteristics are not diagnostic

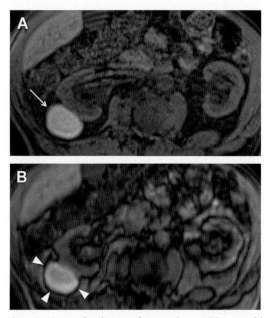

**Fig. 8.** Hemorrhagic renal cyst in a 70-year-old woman. (*A*) Axial fat-suppressed T1-weighted image shows a 5.0 cm right renal mass (*arrow*) with homogenous hyperintense signal indicating a hemorrhagic cyst. (*B*) Axial opposed-phase T1-weighted GRE image demonstrates India ink artifact at the interface of the lesion and the retroperitoneal fat (*arrowheads*), indicating a hemorrhagic cyst. The India ink artifact at the interface of the lesion and the kidney would indicate that the lesion contained fat, consistent with an AML.

of AML with minimal fat, they are suggestive of that diagnosis. Therefore, when a solid mass is encountered that has these imaging characteristics a biopsy is suggested to confirm an AML.[22] It has been shown that clear cell RCC may contain intracellular lipid and may show signal loss on opposed-phase images. Therefore, caution should be used in diagnosing a renal mass as an AML if it only loses signal on out-of-phase imaging.[23] AML should only be diagnosed when macroscopic fat is present within a renal mass. Loss of signal on opposed-phase images may be seen with AML but is not diagnostic. T2-weighted images may be helpful in differentiating an AML with minimal fat from a clear cell carcinoma because AML with minimal fat should be hypointense, whereas clear cell RCC should be hyperintense or heterogeneous.[22]

### Oncocytoma

Oncocytoma is the second most common benign renal neoplasm after AML, accounting for 5% of all renal tumors.[24] Although, the classic central scar and spoke-wheel pattern of enhancement have been described (**Fig. 9**), these features are not pathognomonic and may also be seen in RCCs. Therefore, oncocytomas cannot be diagnosed with imaging alone. In most cases, these tumors are removed and are suspected to be RCC. When the characteristic imaging features are present (scar with spoke-wheel enhancement), a renal mass biopsy can be considered but may not be diagnostic in all cases.

## Infiltrative Renal Masses

Some renal masses have an infiltrative growth pattern and they are not well defined. Infiltrative neoplasms of the kidney include some cases of lymphoma, invasive TCC, RCC, and metastatic disease. See later discussion for a review of invasive TCC.

### Lymphoma

Lymphoma of the kidneys may be found in patients with known lymphoma, more frequently in non-Hodgkin lymphoma. Renal involvement could be via hematogenous spread, in which a single mass or multiple bilateral masses are present, or by direct extension of retroperitoneal lymphoma, which can invade the renal sinus and infiltrate the renal parenchyma. The MR imaging appearance of lymphoma is nonspecific; however, the most common appearance is that of multiple homogeneous solid masses that may be well defined but tend to have infiltrative margins with the kidney. Renal lymphoma is characteristically hypovascular and often demonstrates modest homogenous

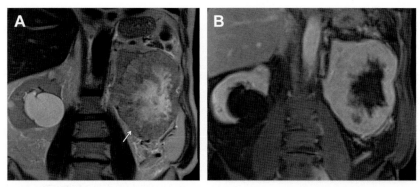

**Fig. 9.** An oncocytoma in a 67-year-old man. (*A*) Coronal T2-weighted image shows a large mass arising from the inferior pole of the left kidney (*arrow*) with central T2 hyperintense signal and a suggestion of a spoke-wheel appearance. (*B*) The corresponding gadolinium-enhanced coronal T1-weighted GRE MR image shows enhancement within the mass. Although the mass has features suggesting oncocytoma, this diagnosis could not be made with certainty at imaging. A nephrectomy was performed and oncocytoma was diagnosed at pathologic examination.

enhancement, a differentiating property from clear cell RCC, which is typically hypervascular. Other distinguishing features from RCC include relatively decreased mass effect on the kidney for the size of the mass and lack of necrosis or vascular invasion. When lymphoma diffusely infiltrates a kidney, the kidney enlarges but maintains its reniform shape.[25]

Generally, most patients with renal lymphoma have systemic involvement and, therefore, the diagnosis should not be difficult given the appropriate clinical history. In these cases when imaging characteristics of lymphoma is present, systemic treatment of lymphoma should be instituted. On the other hand, percutaneous biopsy may be indicated for instances when the renal mass is not responsive to systemic treatment, the imaging characteristic of renal lymphoma is not present, or in rare cases when a renal mass with imaging characteristics of lymphoma is detected in a patient with no known history of lymphoma.

### Metastases

The most common tumor to metastasize to the kidney is carcinoma of the lung, followed by breast carcinoma and melanoma.[26,27] Renal metastases frequently occur in the setting of widespread metastatic disease and tend to be multiple and bilateral and involve the renal cortex. Although they have nonspecific MR imaging features, renal metastases may demonstrate infiltrative growth patterns. With the proper clinical history, the diagnosis should be obvious. However, in a patient with a history of malignancy (without other metastases) and a solitary renal mass, the renal mass is more likely to represent RCC, and not a metastasis.[28] Nevertheless, it is possible that a single

renal metastasis could occur, and differentiation from RCC may not be obvious. In this situation, a renal biopsy is indicated to determine the exact cause of the lesion.

### Renal Mass Mimickers

The renal mass mimicker group of lesions includes non-neoplastic causes, usually inflammatory or vascular processes that may mimic renal neoplasm.

#### Pyelonephritis

Occasionally, focal pyelonephritis can have a mass-like appearance on imaging. However, with the appropriate clinical history, the correct diagnosis usually becomes apparent. In some cases, the diagnosis may not be obvious. In these instances, it is useful to obtain a follow-up examination after treatment to ensure resolution of the abnormality in the kidney. A complication of untreated or incompletely treated pyelonephritis is the formation of pyogenic renal abscess, which can mimic a cystic renal neoplasm, especially in a subacute or chronic setting (**Fig. 10**).

#### Vascular causes

Vascular anomalies, such as renal artery aneurysm and arteriovenous fistula (AVF), can manifest as an enhancing renal mass, especially when the contrast bolus is suboptimal or the scan is performed during the excretory phase. These lesions are usually centrally located and the observation that the mass follows the blood pool on all phases of enhancement is the clue to the diagnosis. In addition, a renal artery aneurysm or AVF may also demonstrate a flow void on T2-weighted images.

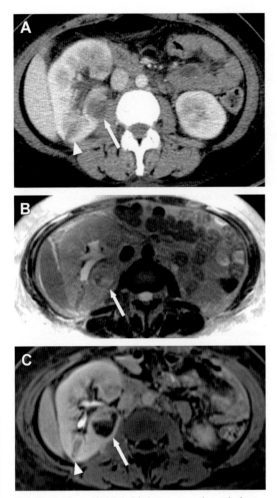

**Fig. 10.** Pyelonephritis with intraparenchymal abscess in a 36-year-old woman with sepsis and positive urinalysis. (*A*) Axial contrast-enhanced CT image demonstrates right renal enlargement with associated focal region of linear decreased enhancement posteriorly (*arrowhead*), which can be seen in pyelonephritis. A rounded heterogeneous hypodense mass is seen medially (*arrow*). It is possible that this is a neoplasm or a focal abscess. (*B, C*) Axial T2-weighted and gadolinium-enhanced fat-suppressed T1-weighted MR images again demonstrate the focal region of linear decreased enhancement posteriorly (*arrowhead*) with a predominately nonenhancing mass (*arrow*) suggesting an abscess. The patient was thought to have pyelonephritis with an abscess and was treated with antibiotics. Follow-up study demonstrated resolution of the imaging findings, confirming a renal abscess.

## EXCRETORY SYSTEM

Recent advances in modern MR imaging technology have affected MR applications in the urinary excretory system with the indications for MRU encompassing a wide range of urinary tract disorders in adults and children, making it an alternative to CT urography (**Figs. 11** and **12**).

### Urothelial Neoplasms

Transitional cell carcinomas (TCCs) account for 90% of urothelial tumors, followed by squamous cell carcinoma (9%) and mucinous adenocarcinoma (1%).[29] TCC is a malignant tumor arising from the transitional epithelial cells lining the urinary tract and occur three times more commonly in men than in women, typically during the sixth to seventh decades of life. They are associated with tobacco use as well as industrial carcinogen exposure. Due to the high incidence of synchronous or metachronous tumors of the collecting system, these patients undergo full urothelial and bladder screening at the time of diagnosis.[30]

Most (85%) upper tract TCCs are superficial neoplasms growing in an expansile papillary fashion. On MRU, the primary urothelial mass appears as polypoid filling defect within the collecting system, with secondary findings, such as calyceal obliteration, occasionally present (**Fig. 13**). A smaller percentage of TCCs (15%) have an infiltrating pattern and tends to behave more aggressively with invasion into the renal sinus and kidney parenchyma at diagnosis (**Fig. 14**). These have a poor prognosis, often presenting with lymph node metastases. They appear as a centrally situated mass arising from the collecting system with invasion into the renal parenchyma.

Because TCCs are nearly isointense to the renal parenchyma on T1-weighted and T2-weighted images,[31] performing gadolinium-enhanced imaging is necessary for complete evaluation of the urinary system. This results in higher diagnostic efficacy of MR imaging for detection of primary urothelial lesions and it could improve identification of possible renal sinus or parenchymal invasion, calyceal obliteration, and periureteral involvement.[32]

Despite the superior tissue contrast, MRU suffers from poorer spatial resolution than CT urography and a variety of artifacts, including flow-related and motion artifacts, which make detection of small tumors of urothelium less likely. In a report by Takahashi and colleagues,[33] MRU has shown a sensitivity of 74% for detection of small (less than 2 cm) urothelial carcinomas, whereas CT urography has a reported sensitivity of 96%.[34] Therefore, CT urography remains the test of choice when evaluating patients with hematuria for urothelial neoplasms. Future advancements in hardware technology may help overcome current limitations.

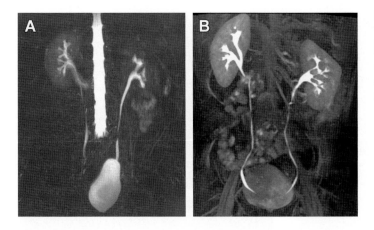

Fig. 11. MRU techniques in two patients. (*A*) Maximum intensity projection (MIP) image of heavily T2-weighted sequence (Static-fluid MRU). (*B*) MIP image of gadolinium-enhanced T1-weighted 3D GRE sequence (Excretory MRU).

## ADRENAL GLANDS

Similar to the increased detection of asymptomatic renal masses, the detection of incidental adrenal lesions has increased with the widespread use of cross-sectional imaging. Benign and malignant lesions of the adrenal glands are common and characterization of these lesions is of great clinical importance.

Adrenal lesions can be broadly classified as cystic versus solid lesions or functional versus nonfunctional lesions. More commonly, adrenal masses are characterized by their tissue composition, including adenoma, myelolipoma, hematoma, and cyst.

### Adrenal Adenoma

Adrenal adenoma is a common benign tumor arising from the cortex of the adrenal gland with an incidence of 2% to 8%.[35] The adrenal gland is the most common site of metastasis per unit weight of any organ.[36] Therefore, within the oncologic population, it is common to find an adrenal mass. A frequent clinical problem is determining the cause of such a lesion. MR imaging can accurately distinguish an adenoma from a metastasis in most cases. This allows more accurate staging of patients with cancer, decreases the number of adrenal biopsies, and allows the appropriate treatment regimen to be instituted sooner.

Identifying microscopic fat within an adrenal mass has remained the mainstay of characterizing an adrenal lesion as an adenoma. In a meta-analysis of the literature, Boland and colleagues[37] showed that a density cut-off of 10 Hounsfield units (HU) on noncontrast CT (NCCT) yields a sensitivity of 71% and specificity of 98% for diagnosing adrenal adenomas. The optimal density of 10 HU was chosen by the investigators because of its high accuracy for characterizing adrenal lesions below this threshold as adenomas. However, adrenal masses with density measurements greater than 10 HU can be seen in metastases as well as in adenomas that are not lipid rich.

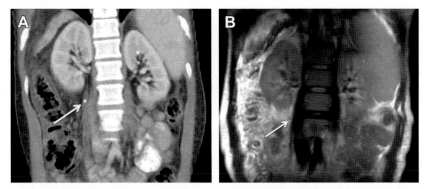

Fig. 12. Ureterolithiasis in a 34-year-old man. (*A*) Coronal reformatted CT image shows a 2 mm calculus in the proximal right ureter. (*B*) Coronal T2-weighted image shows a very subtle 2-mm filling defect in the right ureter (*arrow*), compatible with nonobstructing stone. This illustrates a limitation of MR imaging in the evaluation of renal stones and colic. In most cases, renal or ureteral stones will not be identified on MR imaging.

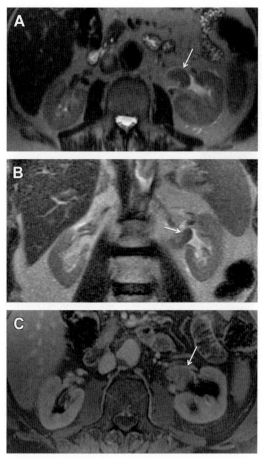

Fig. 13. TCC in a 78-year-old man. (*A*) Axial and (*B*) coronal T2-weighted MR images show a polypoid mass (*arrows*) within the left renal pelvis. Although it is nonspecific and could represent a blood clot, this is concerning for a neoplasm. (*C*) Axial gadolinium-enhanced fat-suppressed T1-weighted image demonstrates enhancement within the mass (*arrow*), which excludes the diagnosis of a blood clot. At pathologic examination, this represented a TCC.

Chemical-shift imaging (CSI) is a fast and reliable technique that rests on demonstrating lipid within the mass (lipid-rich adenoma) to diagnose an adrenal adenoma (**Fig. 15**).[38] The presence of intracellular lipid and water protons within the same imaging voxel accounts for signal dropout on opposed-phase images. Although NCCT and CSI are used in clinical practice for differentiating adenoma from malignancy, some investigators have reported that between 62% and 100% of adenomas with attenuation of greater than 10 HU on NCCT can be characterized confidently as lipid-rich adenomas using CSI.[39,40] Therefore, CSI may be preferable in characterizing adrenal lesions as adenomas because it has better sensitivity for intracellular lipid and does not expose the patient to radiation.

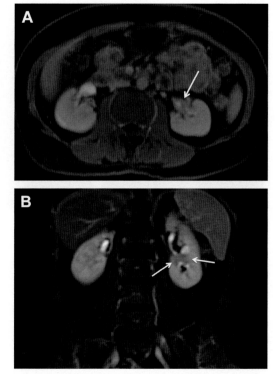

Fig. 14. TCC in a 57-year-old man. (*A*) Axial and (*B*) coronal gadolinium-enhanced fat-suppressed T1 weighted images obtained during the excretory phase show circumferential thickening of the renal pelvis (*arrow* in *A*) and a soft tissue mass centered in the lower pole infundibulum (*arrow* in *B*), highly suggestive of TCC, which was confirmed after nephroureterectomy.

Usually, subjective identification of signal loss on opposed-phase imaging suffices. However, there are equivocal cases in which the signal loss is subtle and not readily apparent. In these cases, objective comparison of signal from adrenal mass and an internal standard is warranted. In general, the liver is not a reliable standard secondary to the possibility of coexisting steatosis. Therefore, the spleen can be used as an internal standard for analysis of signal loss.[41] Typically, a relative adrenal-to-spleen signal dropout ratio of less than 0.7 establishes diagnosis of lipid-rich adenoma.[42] Alternatively, in the case of iron deposition in the spleen, muscle, and renal cortex could serve as internal reference. It is crucial to note other lesions, such as adrenal cortical carcinoma (ACC), pheochromocytoma, clear cell renal cell cancer metastasis, and hepatocellular carcinoma metastasis, may show signal loss on out-of-phase sequences, similar to adenomas.[43] Differentiating a cortical carcinoma from adenoma should not be difficult because most cortical carcinomas are large at presentation

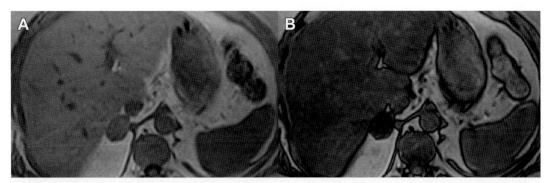

**Fig. 15.** Adrenal adenoma in a 50-year-old woman. (*A*) Axial T1-weighted (in-phase) GRE image demonstrates a 2.8-cm a right adrenal mass, which is slightly higher in signal intensity when compared with the spleen. (*B*) Opposed-phase axial T1-weighted GRE image shows the adrenal mass is now hypointense in signal when compared with the spleen, diagnostic of an adrenal adenoma. Diffuse signal loss throughout the liver on opposed-phase image is compatible with fatty infiltration.

and most adenomas are small. Pheochromocytomas can be differentiated from adenomas by demonstrating excess catecholamine production in patients with pheochromocytomas. In patients with RCC or hepatocellular carcinoma who also have an adrenal nodule in which the primary neoplasm and adrenal nodule lose signal on CSI, the diagnosis of adrenal adenoma should be made with caution. If other metastases are not present, biopsy of the adrenal nodule may be warranted.

A minority of adrenal adenomas does not contain sufficient quantities of lipid to be diagnosed at MR imaging (lipid-poor adenomas) and will not lose signal on opposed-phase imaging. Therefore, these lesions are indeterminate and are especially troublesome in the oncologic patient because a metastasis cannot be excluded. It has been demonstrated that these lipid-poor adenomas can be characterized by means of their washout characteristics on a CT scan.[44–47] Metastatic lesions usually enhance rapidly and often show a slower washout of contrast when compared with adenomas. In a recent study, Choi and colleagues[48] showed adrenal metastases from hypervascular primary malignancies could show washout similar to that of adenomas. Therefore, caution should be taken in interpreting adrenal lesions with rapid washout in patients with primary malignancies, such as such as clear cell RCC or hepatocellular carcinoma. In these instances, close imaging surveillance or pathologic correlation is needed.

Adrenal adenomas may also be classified as hyperfunctioning or, more commonly, as non-hyperfunctioning. Hyperfunctioning adrenal adenomas may produce aldosterone (Conn syndrome), cortisol (Cushing syndrome), or androgens (hyperandrogenism). Because intracellular lipid may be present in hyperfunctioning and non-hyperfunctioning adenomas, it is not possible to differentiate them with MR imaging and correlation with the appropriate laboratory values is necessary. In a patient with an adrenal adenoma, the observation that the contralateral adrenal gland is atrophic could be a hint that the adenoma is functioning, producing cortisol. The excess cortisol produced by the adenoma will cause the hypothalamus to limit corticotrophin-releasing hormone, which can result in subsequent adrenal atrophy.

## Myelolipoma

Adrenal myelolipoma is an uncommon benign neoplasm that contains a variable amount of adipose tissue and myeloid components.[28] In general, myelolipomas are unilateral and asymptomatic, incidentally diagnosed at imaging; however, they may become symptomatic if they hemorrhage or are large enough to exert mass effect on the adjacent organs.

The diagnosis of myelolipoma rests on the demonstration of macroscopic fat within an adrenal mass. With MR imaging, the fatty portion of the lesion would be hyperintense on T1-weighted images. This is nonspecific and can be seen in any lesion that contains hemorrhage. Therefore, as in diagnosing a renal AML, it is necessary to perform a frequency-selective fat-suppressed T1-weighted sequence and compare it to the nonfat-suppressed T1-weighted sequence. The fatty portion of the lesion should lose signal on the fat-suppressed sequence and, therefore, would be diagnostic of a myelolipoma (**Fig. 16**). Myelolipomas may also be diagnosed with CSI by identifying the India ink artifact at the interface of the bulk fat and soft tissue components of the lesion.

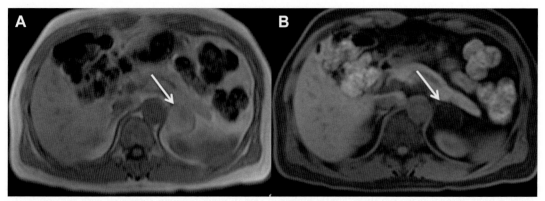

**Fig. 16.** Myelolipoma in a 49-year-old man. (*A*) Axial T1-weighted MR images obtained without fat suppression demonstrates a 3.5 cm left adrenal mass (*arrow*) that has portions that are hyperintense, possibly secondary to fat or hemorrhage. (*B*) Fat-suppressed T1-weighted image demonstrates loss of signal within the mass (*arrow*), diagnostic of fat within the mass and a myelolipoma.

When a predominately fatty adrenal myelolipoma becomes large and exerts mass effect on the adjacent organs, it may become difficult to ascertain that it arises from the adrenal gland. In this instance, a myelolipoma may be confused with other masses that may contain macroscopic fat, including a liposarcoma or exophytic renal AML. By viewing images in multiple planes, an AML can be excluded if it is clearly shown that the mass does not arise from the kidney by demonstrating that the mass has a smooth interface with the kidney and that there is no defect in the renal parenchyma. A liposarcoma would be expected to engulf or displace the adrenal gland. Therefore, if a normal adrenal gland is identified, a myelolipoma may be excluded. An adrenal gland that contains a large myelolipoma would be expected to be stretched around the periphery of the tumor or, if the tumor is large enough, not be seen at all (**Fig. 17**).

## ACC

ACC is a rare malignant tumor of the adrenal cortex, with a reported incidence of 1 to 2 cases per million. It most commonly occurs in the fourth to fifth decades of life with equal prevalence in men and women. ACCs are typically large at presentation and may have metastasized at the time of diagnosis. These lesions may contain varying degrees of hemorrhage and necrosis, and may contain calcium. Some ACCs are hyperfunctioning and,

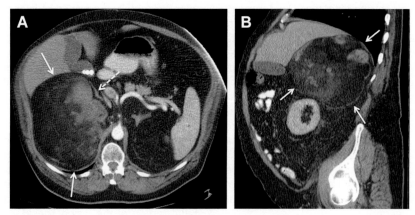

**Fig. 17.** Large myelolipoma in a 75-year-old man. (*A*) Axial contrast-enhanced CT image demonstrates a large predominantly lipomatous retroperitoneal mass (*solid arrows*) with areas of soft-tissue attenuation within the mass. The mass is in close proximity to the right adrenal gland (*dotted arrow*) and appears separate from it. (*B*) Sagittal CT image shows the mass (*arrows*) is separate from the right kidney and displacing it inferiorly and anteriorly. The patient underwent surgical resection of the mass because a retroperitoneal liposarcoma was suspected. At surgical pathologic examination, an exophytic myelolipoma arising from the adrenal gland with areas of hemorrhage within it was diagnosed.

therefore, could present earlier and at a smaller size, compared with non-hyperfunctioning tumors. The most common hormone produced is cortisol, which manifests as Cushing syndrome.[35,49]

The signal intensity of ACC is variable and they generally is heterogeneous, with areas of high signal intensity on T1-weighted and T2-weighted sequences, representing blood products and areas of necrosis within these lesions, respectively. After the administration of gadolinium, the viable portion of the tumor will enhance (**Fig. 18**). Because this neoplasm originates from the adrenal cortex, it may contain foci of intracytoplasmic lipid, resulting in loss of signal intensity on out-of-phase images, similar to an adenoma.[50] Although, in most cases, differentiation from an adenoma should not be difficult, one should be cautious to not diagnose a small ACC as an adenoma. Smaller ACCs may have regions of necrosis and they may be poorly marginated. Previous examinations demonstrating stability over time are very helpful in this differentiation when the classic imaging findings are not present. Laparoscopic adrenalectomy can be performed in equivocal cases in which radiologic differentiation is not possible.[51]

ACCs may directly invade adjacent organs, including the kidney, liver, spleen, pancreas, and diaphragm. At times, it may be difficult to determine the exact organ of origin, especially when a normal adrenal gland cannot be identified. ACC has a known predilection to spread via venous tumor thrombus into the renal vein on the left and IVC, and extend cephalad toward the heart. Gadolinium-enhanced MR imaging can clearly demonstrate the venous extension of the tumor. It is critical to include a pheochromocytoma in the differential diagnosis because their imaging features may be identical and failure to do so may result in a hypertensive crisis in the operating room.

## Pheochromocytoma

Pheochromocytomas, the most common adrenal medullary neoplasms, are hormonally active in 90% of cases and secrete catecholamines. They occur with equal frequency in men and women, and most commonly occur during the third and fourth decades of life. Pheochromocytomas follow the rule of 10s: 10% bilateral, 10% extraadrenal, and 10% malignant. Although most commonly sporadic, pheochromocytomas may be inherited

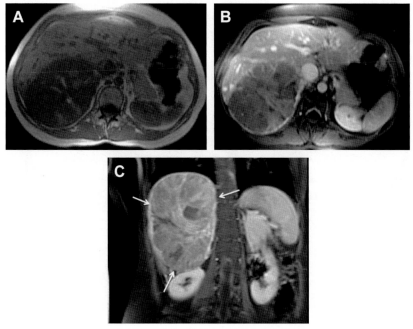

**Fig. 18.** ACC in an 18-year-old woman with Cushing syndrome. (*A*) Axial unenhanced in-phase T1-weighted GRE image without fat-suppression demonstrates a large heterogeneous mass with areas of high T1 signal (consistent with hemorrhage) in the right retroperitoneum abutting the liver and marked mass effect on the posterior hepatic lobe. (*B*) Axial gadolinium-enhanced fat-suppressed MR image shows heterogenous enhancement within the mass. In the axial plane, it can be difficult to differentiate a large adrenal mass from an exophytic renal mass arising from the upper pole of the kidney. (*C*) A coronal gadolinium-enhanced T1-weighted fat-suppressed GRE image shows the enhancing mass (*arrows*) displacing the kidney inferiorly and, therefore, likely arising from the adrenal gland, which could not be identified. At pathologic examination, ACC was confirmed.

in the form of syndromes, including multiple endocrine neoplasia types IIa and IIb, von Hippel-Lindau disease, and neurofibromatosis type 1. Although patients may be symptomatic, the symptoms are nonspecific and include palpitations, headache, sweating, and hypertension. Hypertension could be episodic or refractory and even though it is one of the more common presentations, pheochromocytoma is present in only 0.1% to 0.9% of patients with hypertension.[52]

Pheochromocytomas have been shown to have variable T1 and T2 signal, especially when larger than 5 cm. The classic intense light bulb T2 bright appearance occurs in fewer than half of the cases.[53] Pheochromocytomas are highly vascular tumors that show avid arterial enhancement and may have a salt-and-pepper pattern on unenhanced imaging that reflects signal voids of the tumor vessels.[54]

Due to considerable overlap in the imaging appearance, MR imaging is more useful in identifying an adrenal mass in a patient who is clinically thought to have a pheochromocytoma, than in characterizing an adrenal mass as a pheochromocytoma (Fig. 19). On the other hand, if an asymptomatic adrenal mass with characteristic features of pheochromocytoma is detected, additional endocrine investigation is warranted. Furthermore,

MR imaging is useful in identifying extraadrenal pheochromocytomas (paragangliomas) in the retroperitoneum along the paraspinal muscles. Confirmation with nuclear medicine studies (such as MIBG scan) may be useful in equivocal cases.

## Metastases

The adrenal gland is the fourth most common site of metastatic involvement, after lung, liver, and bone. The most common primary sites are lung, breast, skin, kidney, thyroid, and colon. Most adrenal metastases are asymptomatic; however, extensive metastatic involvement may lead to adrenal insufficiency. Adrenal metastases can be easily distinguished from fat-containing adenomas based on signal loss on CSI in adenomas. Metastases usually appear hypointense on T1-weighted images and hyperintense on T2-weighted images, with the exception of hemorrhagic and melanoma metastases, which are T1 hyperintense. Morphologic features suggestive of malignancy on MR imaging include irregular margins, heterogeneity, and interval growth on close follow-up examination.

## Adrenal Cysts, Pseudocysts

Adrenal cystic lesions are rare with an incidence of less than 1%.[55] They are usually incidentally

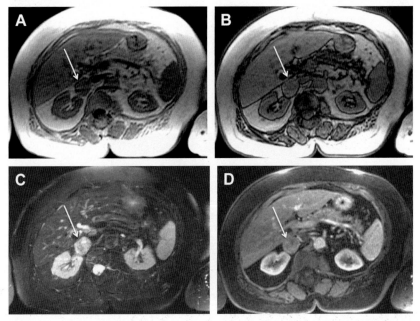

**Fig. 19.** Pheochromocytoma in a 62-year-old woman with increased blood pressure, palpitations, and laboratory value consistent with pheochromocytoma. (*A*) Axial GRE T1-weighted in-phase and (*B*) out-of-phase MR images show a 3.2 cm right adrenal mass (*arrow*) with no evidence loss of signal intensity on the out-of-phase sequence. (*C*, *D*) The mass (*arrow*) exhibits moderately bright signal on axial T2-weighted image and enhancement of post-gadolinium image. In this case, the imaging findings are nondiagnostic. However, the mass most likely represents a pheochromocytoma given the clinical scenario. Diagnosis of pheochromocytoma was confirmed at pathologic examination.

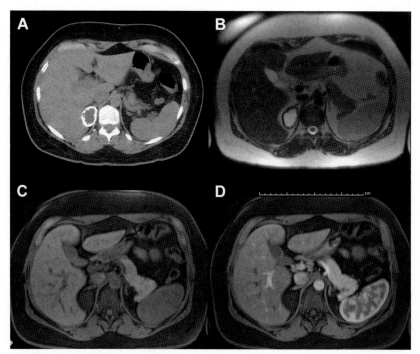

**Fig. 20.** Adrenal pseudocyst. (A) Axial unenhanced CT image of a 2.8 cm hypoattenuating right adrenal mass with thick irregular peripheral rim calcification. (B) Axial T2-weighted sequence shows a hyperintense cystic right adrenal mass, with a hypointense rim. (C) Axial 3D fat-suppressed GRE unenhanced T1-weighted image shows a hypointense mass, (D) with no enhancement on postgadolinium image, compatible with adrenal pseudocyst.

detected during radiological investigation. Patients with these lesions are usually asymptomatic unless the lesion is large enough to produce a mass effect on adjacent organs. The adrenal cysts have been categorized into four main categories based on their pathologic origin:

- Endothelial cysts are lined with a single layer of endothelial cells and can be further subdivided into hemangiomatous or lymphangiomatous subtypes based on their origin (ectatic blood vs lymphatic vessels).

- Pseudocysts (the most common adrenal cyst) are lined with fibrous capsule and are usually the result of hemorrhage within the normal gland, and could have a posttraumatic or postinfectious cause (**Fig. 20**). These lesions are typically hyperintense on fat-suppressed T1-weighted images and do not enhance with contrast. They may contain calcification that can be thick and irregular, which would be better appreciated with CT.

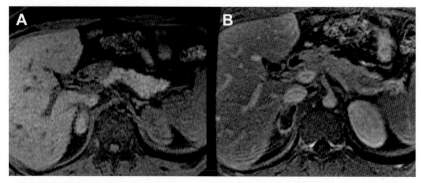

**Fig. 21.** Adrenal hematoma in a 17-year-old man after trauma to the right flank. (A) Axial unenhanced fat-suppressed GRE T1-weighted image shows a 3 cm uniformly hyperintense right adrenal mass. (B) Subtracted gadolinium-enhanced image at the same level shows no enhancing components within the mass. These findings are diagnostic for adrenal hematoma.

- Epithelial cysts are rare and represent (glandular) retention cysts, or arise from adrenal cortical adenoma and embryonal cyst.
- Parasitic (hydatid) cysts are also rare and can occur in cases of disseminated echinococcal infestation. The pathognomonic honeycomb appearance with internal floating membrane and multiple daughter cysts is diagnostic.

## Adrenal Hematoma

Rich adrenal arterial supply predisposes to adrenal hemorrhage and may occur in response to catecholamines a result of physiologic stress, trauma, or a coagulopathic state. Adrenal hematomas appear as mass-like enlargements and demonstrate signal hyperintensity on precontrast T1-weighted sequences. The absence of solid component can be best shown by lack of enhancement on subtracted images, a differentiating property from hemorrhagic solid lesions (**Fig. 21**). Most hematomas resolve completely. Occasionally, however, a pseudocyst may develop because of liquefaction.

## SUMMARY

MR imaging has proven to be a versatile modality in evaluation of the kidneys, collecting system, and adrenal glands. By performing a comprehensive MR examination, it is not only possible to accurately characterize cystic and solid lesions of the kidneys, as well as urothelial masses, but also to provide important preoperative information to the surgeon. In addition, MR imaging can characterize many adrenal lesions and can frequently obviate biopsy. The continued development and growth of MR technology combined with the current trend toward minimally invasive surgery will expand the role of MR imaging in the future.

## REFERENCES

1. Ho VB, Allen SF, Hood MN, et al. Renal masses: quantitative assessment of enhancement with dynamic MR imaging. Radiology 2002;224(3): 695–700.
2. Hecht EM, Israel GM, Krinsky GA, et al. Renal masses: quantitative analysis of enhancement with signal intensity measurements versus qualitative analysis of enhancement with image subtraction for diagnosing malignancy at MR imaging. Radiology 2004;232(2):373–8.
3. Aerts P, Van Hoe L, Bosmans H, et al. Breath-hold MR urography using the HASTE technique. AJR Am J Roentgenol 1996;166(3):543–5.
4. Nolte-Ernsting CC, Bucker A, Adam GB, et al. Gadolinium-enhanced excretory MR urography after low-dose diuretic injection: comparison with conventional excretory urography. Radiology 1998; 209(1):147–57.
5. Bosniak MA. The current radiological approach to renal cysts. Radiology 1986;158(1):1–10.
6. Bosniak MA. Difficulties in classifying cystic lesions of the kidney. Urol Radiol 1991;13(2):91–3.
7. Bosniak MA. The use of the Bosniak classification system for renal cysts and cystic tumors. J Urol 1997;157(5):1852–3.
8. Israel GM, Hindman N, Bosniak MA. Evaluation of cystic renal masses: comparison of CT and MR imaging by using the Bosniak classification system. Radiology 2004;231(2):365–71.
9. Israel GM, Bosniak MA. Follow-up CT of moderately complex cystic lesions of the kidney (Bosniak category IIF). AJR Am J Roentgenol 2003;181(3): 627–33.
10. Smith AD, Remer EM, Cox KL, et al. Bosniak category IIF and III cystic renal lesions: outcomes and associations. Radiology 2012;262(1):152–60.
11. Harisinghani MG, Maher MM, Gervais DA, et al. Incidence of malignancy in complex cystic renal masses (Bosniak category III): should imaging-guided biopsy precede surgery? AJR Am J Roentgenol 2003;180(3):755–8.
12. Motzer RJ, Hutson TE, Tomczak P, et al. Overall survival and updated results for sunitinib compared with interferon alfa in patients with metastatic renal cell carcinoma. J Clin Oncol 2009;27(22): 3584–90.
13. Walter C, Kruessell M, Gindele A, et al. Imaging of renal lesions: evaluation of fast MRI and helical CT. Br J Radiol 2003;76(910):696–703.
14. Prasad SR, Humphrey PA, Catena JR, et al. Common and uncommon histologic subtypes of renal cell carcinoma: imaging spectrum with pathologic correlation. Radiographics 2006;26(6):1795–806 [discussion: 1806–10].
15. Vargas HA, Chaim J, Lefkowitz RA, et al. Renal cortical tumors: use of multiphasic contrast-enhanced MR imaging to differentiate benign and malignant histologic subtypes. Radiology 2012; 264(3):779–88.
16. Pedrosa I, Alsop DC, Rofsky NM. Magnetic resonance imaging as a biomarker in renal cell carcinoma. Cancer 2009;115(Suppl 10):2334–45.
17. Laissy JP, Menegazzo D, Debray MP, et al. Renal carcinoma: diagnosis of venous invasion with Gd-enhanced MR venography. Eur Radiol 2000;10(7): 1138–43.
18. Lopez-Beltran A, Scarpelli M, Montironi R, et al. 2004 WHO classification of the renal tumors of the adults. Eur Urol 2006;49(5):798–805.
19. Helenon O, Merran S, Paraf F, et al. Unusual fat-containing tumors of the kidney: a diagnostic dilemma. Radiographics 1997;17(1):129–44.

20. Israel GM, Hindman N, Hecht E, et al. The use of opposed-phase chemical shift MRI in the diagnosis of renal angiomyolipomas. AJR Am J Roentgenol 2005;184(6):1868–72.

21. Jinzaki M, Silverman SG, Tanimoto A, et al. Angiomyolipomas that do not contain fat attenuation at unenhanced CT. Radiology 2005;234(1):311 [author reply: 311–2].

22. Silverman SG, Mortele KJ, Tuncali K, et al. Hyperattenuating renal masses: etiologies, pathogenesis, and imaging evaluation. Radiographics 2007; 27(4):1131–43.

23. Outwater EK, Bhatia M, Siegelman ES, et al. Lipid in renal clear cell carcinoma: detection on opposed-phase gradient-echo MR images. Radiology 1997;205(1):103–7.

24. Rosenkrantz AB, Hindman N, Fitzgerald EF, et al. MRI features of renal oncocytoma and chromophobe renal cell carcinoma. AJR Am J Roentgenol 2010;195(6):W421–7.

25. Pickhardt PJ, Lonergan GJ, Davis CJ Jr, et al. From the archives of the AFIP. Infiltrative renal lesions: radiologic-pathologic correlation. Armed Forces Institute of Pathology. Radiographics 2000;20(1): 215–43.

26. Bracken RB, Chica G, Johnson DE, et al. Secondary renal neoplasms: an autopsy study. South Med J 1979;72(7):806–7.

27. Nathanson L, Hall TC, Farber S. Biological aspects of human malignant melanoma. Cancer 1967; 20(5):650–5.

28. Bosniak MA. Problems in the radiologic diagnosis of renal parenchymal tumors. Urol Clin North Am 1993;20(2):217–30.

29. Guinan P, Vogelzang NJ, Randazzo R, et al. Renal pelvic cancer: a review of 611 patients treated in Illinois 1975–1985. Cancer Incidence and End Results Committee. Urology 1992; 40(5):393–9.

30. Vikram R, Sandler CM, Ng CS. Imaging and staging of transitional cell carcinoma: part 1, lower urinary tract. AJR Am J Roentgenol 2009;192(6): 1481–7.

31. Browne RF, Meehan CP, Colville J, et al. Transitional cell carcinoma of the upper urinary tract: spectrum of imaging findings. Radiographics 2005;25(6): 1609–27.

32. Obuchi M, Ishigami K, Takahashi K, et al. Gadolinium-enhanced fat-suppressed T1-weighted imaging for staging ureteral carcinoma: correlation with histopathology. AJR Am J Roentgenol 2007; 188(3):W256–61.

33. Takahashi N, Kawashima A, Glockner JF, et al. Small (<2-cm) upper-tract urothelial carcinoma: evaluation with gadolinium-enhanced three-dimensional spoiled gradient-recalled echo MR urography. Radiology 2008;247(2):451–7.

34. Caoili EM, Cohan RH, Inampudi P, et al. MDCT urography of upper tract urothelial neoplasms. AJR Am J Roentgenol 2005;184(6):1873–81.

35. Fishman EK, Deutch BM, Hartman DS, et al. Primary adrenocortical carcinoma: CT evaluation with clinical correlation. AJR Am J Roentgenol 1987;148(3):531–5.

36. Katz RL, Shirkhoda A. Diagnostic approach to incidental adrenal nodules in the cancer patient. Results of a clinical, radiologic, and fine-needle aspiration study. Cancer 1985;55(9): 1995–2000.

37. Boland GW, Lee MJ, Gazelle GS, et al. Characterization of adrenal masses using unenhanced CT: an analysis of the CT literature. AJR Am J Roentgenol 1998;171(1):201–4.

38. Outwater EK, Siegelman ES, Radecki PD, et al. Distinction between benign and malignant adrenal masses: value of T1-weighted chemical-shift MR imaging. AJR Am J Roentgenol 1995;165(3): 579–83.

39. Israel GM, Korobkin M, Wang C, et al. Comparison of unenhanced CT and chemical shift MRI in evaluating lipid-rich adrenal adenomas. AJR Am J Roentgenol 2004;183(1):215–9.

40. Haider MA, Ghai S, Jhaveri K, et al. Chemical shift MR imaging of hyperattenuating (>10 HU) adrenal masses: does it still have a role? Radiology 2004; 231(3):711–6.

41. Korobkin M, Lombardi TJ, Aisen AM, et al. Characterization of adrenal masses with chemical shift and gadolinium-enhanced MR imaging. Radiology 1995;197(2):411–8.

42. Fujiyoshi F, Nakajo M, Fukukura Y, et al. Characterization of adrenal tumors by chemical shift fast low-angle shot MR imaging: comparison of four methods of quantitative evaluation. AJR Am J Roentgenol 2003;180(6):1649–57.

43. Blake MA, Cronin CG, Boland GW. Adrenal imaging. AJR Am J Roentgenol 2010;194(6):1450–60.

44. Inan N, Arslan A, Akansel G, et al. Dynamic contrast enhanced MRI in the differential diagnosis of adrenal adenomas and malignant adrenal masses. Eur J Radiol 2008;65(1):154–62.

45. Chung JJ, Semelka RC, Martin DR. Adrenal adenomas: characteristic postgadolinium capillary blush on dynamic MR imaging. J Magn Reson Imaging 2001;13(2):242–8.

46. Krestin GP, Freidmann G, Fishbach R, et al. Evaluation of adrenal masses in oncologic patients: dynamic contrast-enhanced MR vs CT. J Comput Assist Tomogr 1991;15(1):104–10.

47. Caoili EM, Korobkin M, Francis IR, et al. Delayed enhanced CT of lipid-poor adrenal adenomas. AJR Am J Roentgenol 2000;175(5):1411–5.

48. Choi YA, Kim CK, Park BK, et al. Evaluation of adrenal metastases from renal cell carcinoma and

hepatocellular carcinoma: use of delayed contrast-enhanced CT. Radiology 2013;266(2): 514–20.

49. Dunnick NR, Heaston D, Halvorsen R, et al. CT appearance of adrenal cortical carcinoma. J Comput Assist Tomogr 1982;6(5):978–82.

50. Siegelman ES. MR imaging of the adrenal neoplasms. Magn Reson Imaging Clin N Am 2000; 8(4):769–86.

51. Kebebew E, Siperstein AE, Duh QY. Laparoscopic adrenalectomy: the optimal surgical approach. J Laparoendosc Adv Surg Tech A 2001;11(6): 409–13.

52. Sutton MG, Sheps SG, Lie JT. Prevalence of clinically unsuspected pheochromocytoma. Review of a 50-year autopsy series. Mayo Clin Proc 1981; 56(6):354–60.

53. Elsayes KM, Narra VR, Leyendecker JR, et al. MRI of adrenal and extraadrenal pheochromocytoma. AJR Am J Roentgenol 2005;184(3):860–7.

54. Blake MA, Kalra MK, Maher MM, et al. Pheochromocytoma: an imaging chameleon. Radiographics 2004;24(Suppl 1):S87–99.

55. Rozenblit A, Morehouse HT, Amis ES Jr. Cystic adrenal lesions: CT features. Radiology 1996;201(2): 541–8.

# MR Enterography for Assessment and Management of Small Bowel Crohn Disease

Brian C. Allen, MD*, John R. Leyendecker, MD

## KEYWORDS

- Enterography • Crohn • Inflammatory bowel disease • Magnetic resonance

## KEY POINTS

- Advantages of magnetic resonance enterography include excellent soft tissue contrast resolution, potential for dynamic assessment of the small bowel, and lack of ionizing radiation.
- Crohn disease may be classified as primarily inflammatory, penetrating, or fibrostenotic, and each type of disease is treated differently.
- Bowel wall thickening and edema, mucosal hyperenhancement, mesenteric vascular engorgement, and lymphadenopathy are signs of active inflammation.
- Magnetic resonance enterography has similar diagnostic efficacy to computed tomography for small bowel Crohn disease and correlates well with endoscopic and surgical findings.

## INTRODUCTION

Before computed tomography (CT) existed, radiologic imaging of the small bowel consisted primarily of barium fluoroscopic examinations. CT enterography (CTE), performed with low Hounsfield value enteric contrast, has been shown to be accurate in the radiologic diagnosis of small bowel Crohn disease and associated complications.[1–4] Because of this, there has been a significant increase in the number of CTE examinations performed in the evaluation of Crohn disease, with an associated decrease in the number of fluoroscopic small bowel studies.[5] CT accounts for approximately 16% of the diagnostic imaging studies in patients with Crohn disease and 77% of diagnostic radiation exposure, and effective doses may be up to 5 times higher with CT when compared with barium fluoroscopic examinations.[5,6] There has been much investigation and success in lowering radiation dose with CTE, using a variety of techniques.[7–10] Even so, because

many patients with inflammatory bowel disease are young, there is concern that cumulative radiation dose may have detrimental effects.[11]

Magnetic resonance enterography (MRE) has played an increasing role in the evaluation of small bowel Crohn disease over the last several years. MRE has been shown to have a diagnostic effectiveness similar to that of CTE.[12,13] Advantages of MRE include lack of ionizing radiation, the ability to image the small bowel dynamically, and improved soft tissue contrast resolution compared with CT. Limitations of MRE include higher cost, lower spatial resolution, greater susceptibility to motion-related blurring and artifacts, and a smaller pool of experienced readers. Typical indications for MRE include evaluation of inflammatory bowel disease, low-grade partial small bowel obstruction, chronic abdominal pain and diarrhea, and small bowel neoplasms.

The purpose of this article is to review imaging protocols for MRE, normal small bowel anatomy and imaging appearance, and the findings

The authors have nothing to disclose.
Abdominal Imaging, Department of Radiology, Wake Forest Baptist Medical Center, Wake Forest University School of Medicine, Medical Center Boulevard, 3rd Floor MRI, Winston-Salem, NC 27157-1088, USA
* Corresponding author.
*E-mail address:* bcallen2@wakehealth.edu

Radiol Clin N Am 52 (2014) 799–810
http://dx.doi.org/10.1016/j.rcl.2014.02.001
0033-8389/14/$ – see front matter © 2014 Elsevier Inc. All rights reserved.

radiologic.theclinics.com

of small bowel Crohn disease that affect patient management.

## IMAGING PROTOCOLS

Optimal MRE requires adequate bowel distention, fast sequences, use of a large field-of-view surface coil, administration of an intravenous contrast agent, and a moderate degree of patient cooperation.

Several types of enteric contrast have been used to study the small bowel with MR imaging. Negative enteric contrast agents are of low signal intensity on both T1-weighted and T2-weighted imaging and include ferumoxsil oral suspension. Negative enteric contrast agents provide the ability to visualize the higher signal intensity bowel wall against dark luminal contents.[14] Positive enteric contrast agents are of high signal intensity on both T1-weighted and T2-weighted imaging and are based on substances such as gadolinium chelates, manganese, and various food ingredients, such as blueberry juice and milk. Positive enteric contrast agents can mask bowel wall abnormalities, but allow for assessment of enteric contrast progression through the bowel.[14] Biphasic enteric contrast agents are typically low signal on T1-weighted images and high signal on T2-weighted images and include water, polyethylene glycol, diatrizoate meglumine, mannitol, and locust bean gum solutions, as well as methylcellulose and low-density barium suspensions. The biphasic contrast agents provide excellent contrast between the bowel lumen and the bowel wall on most sequences without obscuring enhancement of the bowel wall with gadolinium-based contrast agents on T1-weighted images.[14]

Having patients fast for 6 hours before imaging may improve compliance with and tolerance for the ingestion of a large volume of enteric contrast, and fasting helps decrease the amount of food residue and debris that can be mistaken for mass lesions or polyps.

Optimal distention of the small bowel is paramount to adequate imaging, although opinions differ as to how best to achieve this for routine clinical imaging. A typical protocol begins with oral ingestion of 1350 mL of a commercially available dilute barium sulfate solution in 3 aliquots over a 45- to 60-minute period, as investigation has shown that an ingested volume of 1350 mL is preferable to either 900 mL or 1800 mL.[15] Alternatively, enteroclysis may be performed via injection of a large volume (1350–2000 mL) of enteric contrast through an enterojejunal tube with an MR-compatible pump at a rate of 80–150 mL/min. MR enteroclysis is time intensive and requires a

dedicated team of technologists, nurses, and radiologists for optimal performance, and this has resulted in a decline in favor of MR enterography, particularly considering that the improved distension of enteroclysis does not necessarily translate to better diagnostic effectiveness.[16,17] A study comparing MR enterography to MR enteroclysis, evaluating only small bowel distension, showed no significant difference between the methods for ileal distension, but did find that proximal small bowel distension was better with enteroclysis.[18] Another study comparing MR enterography to MR enteroclysis showed improved luminal distension in the proximal and distal small bowel with enteroclysis, which resulted in better sensitivity for the evaluation of superficial abnormalities, but found no difference for the identification of transmural inflammation or penetrating disease.[19]

Once oral contrast has been administered, a multichannel surface coil is placed over the abdomen and pelvis and a single-shot fast/turbo spin-echo (ssFSE/ssTSE or HASTE) sequence is performed to encompass the entire abdomen and pelvis in the coronal plane, providing an anatomic overview and preliminary assessment of bowel distention (**Box 1**). Such long echo train sequences are susceptible to artifacts, caused by the bulk motion of intraluminal fluid, that simulate masses and filling defects but provide high contrast between the bowel lumen, bowel wall,

---

**Box 1**
**MR imaging protocol: sequences for MR enterography**

Single-shot fast spin echo (ssFSE, ssTSE, HASTE) in the coronal plane as an anatomic overview

Multiphase SSFP (True FISP or FIESTA) in the coronal plane viewed as a cine clip to assess bowel motility, stenoses, segmental dilatation, and adhesions

Fat-suppressed T1-weighted imaging following intravenous contrast administration in the coronal plane in multiple vascular phases to assess bowel wall enhancement, vasculature, lymph nodes, enteric fistulas, and abscesses

Fat-suppressed T1-weighted imaging following intravenous contrast administration in the axial plane for multiplanar correlation and to demonstrate fistulas not well displayed in the coronal plane

Fat-suppressed T2-weighted imaging in the axial plane to assess for bowel wall and mesenteric edema and fluid

DWI (optional) to demonstrate active inflammation and detect abscesses

and adjacent fluid collections (**Fig. 1**). Next, fast imaging with steady-state free precession (SSFP, TrueFISP, or FIESTA) images are obtained in the coronal plane. Generally, 15 to 25 phases per level are acquired during free breathing, which can be displayed as a cine loop to assess bowel motility and to detect fixed stenoses, segmental dilatation, or adhesions. These sequences can be limited by susceptibility artifact when the bowel lumen is distended by gas, but provide high contrast between the bowel wall and lumen and clearly demonstrate mesenteric vessels and lymph nodes.

Fat-suppressed 3-dimensional T1-weighted breath-hold gradient-echo images of the abdomen and pelvis are then performed in the coronal plane before and after the intravenous administration of 0.1 mmol/kg of a gadolinium-based contrast agent at 2 mL/s followed by a 20-mL saline flush at 2 mL/s. Several breath-held enhanced phases are typically imaged, with the first set of postcontrast images obtained 25 seconds after the intravenous administration of contrast. To reduce bowel motility during this and subsequent imaging, many sites administer an antiperistaltic agent, such as glucagon, intramuscularly or intravenously before gadolinium-based contrast administration. Although subjective image quality may be reduced without an antiperistaltic agent, studies have shown that diagnostic accuracy remains adequate.[20,21]

Axial fat-suppressed T2-weighted images are useful to evaluate for bowel wall edema and intra-abdominal fluid collections (**Figs. 2** and **3**). Fat suppression is critical to enhance the conspicuity of bowel wall edema and inflammatory changes in the adjacent fat. Some sites include diffusion-weighted imaging (DWI) at multiple b values in their protocol. However, the clinical utility of diffusion-weighted small bowel imaging is not clearly defined and remains an area of active investigation. Apparent diffusion coefficient values are typically decreased in active inflammatory disease, and quantitative dynamic contrast-enhanced imaging and DWI have been combined to potentially improve sensitivity.[22,23] DWI can also aid in differentiating small abscesses from surrounding bowel, because abscesses will manifest as focal areas of diffusion restriction (see **Fig. 3**).

Additional imaging can be performed in alternate imaging planes depending on preference. The authors routinely include single-shot fast spin-echo and postcontrast fat-suppressed 3D T1-weighted breath-hold gradient-echo images of the abdomen and pelvis in the axial plane for multiplanar correlation and to demonstrate fistulae and strictures not optimally displayed in the coronal plane.

## NORMAL ANATOMY AND MR IMAGING APPEARANCE OF SMALL BOWEL

Knowledge of the normal small bowel anatomy is imperative when evaluating for pathologic changes. A study assessing 65 subjects with no

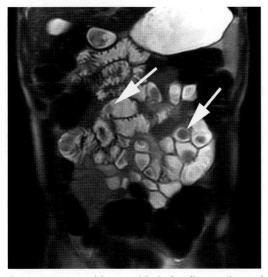

**Fig. 1.** A 17-year-old man with Crohn disease. Coronal single-shot fast-spin echo image demonstrates ovoid filling defects (*arrows*) within the small bowel, artifacts likely related to gas pockets and motion induced signal loss within the small bowel.

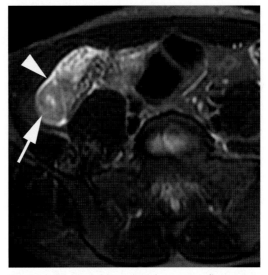

**Fig. 2.** A 21-year-old man with active inflammatory Crohn disease. Axial fat-suppressed T2-weighted image through the pelvis demonstrates a thick-walled, edematous terminal ileum (*arrow*) with surrounding fluid (*arrowhead*).

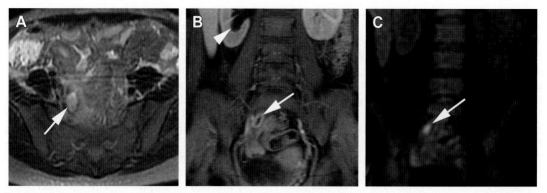

**Fig. 3.** A 19-year-old woman with active, penetrating Crohn disease. (*A*) Axial fat-suppressed T2-weighted image through the pelvis demonstrates a small loculated fluid collection (*arrow*). (*B*) Coronal contrast-enhanced fat-suppressed T1-weighted image shows that the fluid collection has a thick, enhancing wall (*arrow*). Note that there is associated right hydronephrosis (*arrowhead*). (*C*) Coronal DWI (b500) shows the fluid collection to be hyperintense (*arrow*).

known small bowel disease before MRE, or for 3 years following the examination, evaluated normal measurements throughout the small bowel.[24] Mean diameters of the duodenum, jejunum, proximal ileum, distal ileum, and terminal ileum measure approximately 2.5, 2.5, 2.0, 1.9, and 1.9 cm, respectively. Wall thickness is similar throughout the length of the small bowel, measuring between 0.1 and 0.2 cm. Folds per 2.5 cm vary from 4.6 in the jejunum to 1.5 in the terminal ileum, and fold thickness decreases from 0.2 cm in the duodenum to slightly less than 0.2 cm in the terminal ileum. Investigation into peak bowel wall enhancement in normal patients has shown that enhancement plateaus approximately 70 seconds after intravenous contrast administration.[25] Because of the increased surface area, the jejunum enhances more than the ileum (**Fig. 4**). Inflamed segments enhance to a greater extent than normal bowel segments on dynamic contrast-enhanced images.[26] Also, CTE studies have shown that collapsed bowel appears more enhanced when compared with adjacent distended bowel (see **Fig. 4**).[27,28]

## IMAGING FINDINGS/PATHOLOGY

Crohn disease is an idiopathic, inflammatory disease of the gastrointestinal tract that affects between 400,000 and 600,000 patients in North America.[29] Crohn disease is a chronic illness with a peak age of onset in the second to fourth decades of life and an unpredictable course marked by relapses and remissions.[29] Crohn disease affects any portion of the digestive tract, but the small bowel, particularly the terminal ileum, is the most common site of disease. Inflammation manifests as ulceration, ranging from superficial

aphthoid lesions to deep linear ulcers, with areas of inflammation separated by regions of normal mucosa (skip areas). Crohn disease is often a transmural process that leads to penetrating or stricturing disease complicated by bowel obstruction, fistula formation, and abscess.

Crohn disease is typically classified as primarily active inflammatory (without fistulas or stenosis), penetrating (with fistulas and/or abscesses), or fibrostenotic disease (with stricturing).[30,31] However, Crohn disease is best conceptualized as a

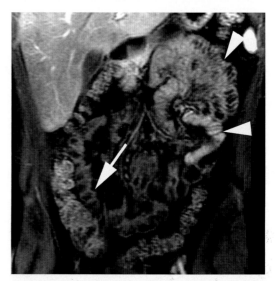

**Fig. 4.** An 18-year-old man with chronic diarrhea, but no proven inflammatory bowel disease. Coronal contrast-enhanced fat-suppressed T1-weighted image demonstrates that the jejunum (*arrowheads*) appears to enhance more than the ileum (*arrow*). Also note that collapsed jejunum appears to enhance more than distended jejunum.

spectrum from active inflammation to fibrosis and from ulceration to penetrating disease and abscess formation, with multiple stages frequently coexisting in the same patient or bowel segment.[32]

## Active Inflammation

Active inflammatory disease manifests on MRE as mucosal hyperenhancement, which may be seen with or without bowel wall thickening (**Box 2**). Involved segments of bowel appear hypervascular compared with adjacent loops of bowel from a similar level. Deep fissuring ulcers result in submucosal edema, which is hyperintense on T2-weighted imaging.[33,34] In general, discrete ulcers require dedicated high-resolution imaging to be evident on MRE.[35,36]

A stratified appearance of active inflammation has been described, in which mucosal and serosal hyperenhancement, along with submucosal edema, leads to a layered appearance on fat-suppressed T1-weighted postcontrast images (**Fig. 5**).[37,38] In many cases, however, active inflammation manifests simply as mucosal hyperenhancement with mural thickening/edema (**Figs. 6** and **7**). Some authors have suggested that transmural enhancement, without stratification, may be more common in the early stages of Crohn disease and in children with Crohn disease, whereas the stratified appearance may be more common with long-standing disease.[39]

Associated extraenteric findings of active inflammatory bowel disease include increased mesenteric vascularity adjacent to the inflamed loop of bowel (see **Box 2**). This engorgement of the vasa recta, or "comb sign," is best visualized on SSFP or postcontrast T1-weighted fat-suppressed imaging (see **Figs. 6** and **7**; **Fig. 8**).[38,40] These sequences also show reactive mesenteric lymphadenopathy well. The enhancement pattern

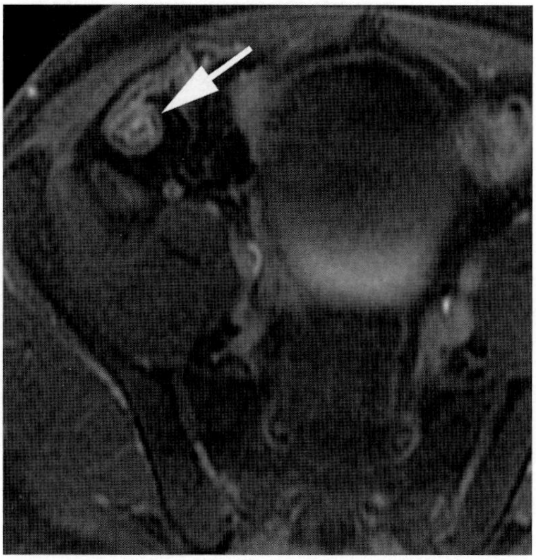

Fig. 5. A 52-year-old man with active inflammatory Crohn disease. Axial contrast-enhanced fat-suppressed T1-weighted image demonstrates a stratified appearance of the terminal ileum (*arrow*), with hyperenhancement of terminal ileal mucosa and serosa.

and morphology of lymph nodes in Crohn disease have been studied, but it remains unclear if this evaluation adds value in confirming the presence of active inflammation.[41] Edema, fluid, and enhancement in the soft tissues adjacent to an inflamed loop of bowel are additional secondary findings of acute inflammation (see **Fig. 2**).

Wall thickness, degree and pattern of enhancement, submucosal edema, and mesenteric vascularity are all independent predictors of pathologic inflammation in both endoscopic and surgical series.[42,43] DWI can also distinguish inflamed from normal bowel, but the added value of DWI over standard T2-weighted and dynamic contrast-enhanced imaging is not firmly established (see **Fig. 7**).[22,23] When present, active inflammatory disease without penetrating disease is generally treated medically with immunosuppressants and steroids. Patients with bowel obstruction are sometimes given a trial of medical therapy when the obstruction is thought to be predominately related to active inflammation.

## Penetrating Disease

Deep ulceration leads to transmural inflammation. Transmural inflammation can progress to stricturing or sinus tract/fistula formation and abscess (see **Box 2**). One benefit of MRE over CTE is that multiphase cine imaging allows a dynamic assessment of bowel motility and the distinction between a fixed stricture and transient luminal narrowing. Upstream bowel dilatation helps confirm

---

**Box 2**
**Diagnostic criteria: signs of active inflammation**

Submucosal edema—wall thickening with hyperintense bowel wall on T2-weighted images

Mucosal hyperenhancement on T1-weighted postcontrast imaging

Mesenteric vascular engorgement—Comb sign

Mesenteric lymphadenopathy

Mural diffusion restriction

Fistulas, sinus tracts, and abscesses (signs of penetrating disease component)

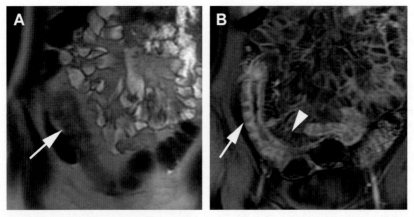

**Fig. 6.** A 19-year-old woman with active inflammatory Crohn disease of the terminal ileum. (*A*) Coronal single-shot fast-spin echo image demonstrates a thick-walled terminal ileum (*arrow*). (*B*) Coronal contrast-enhanced, fat-suppressed T1-weighted image demonstrates mucosal hyperenhancement of the terminal ileum (*arrow*) and engorged vasa recta in the mesentery "comb sign" (*arrowhead*).

the functional significance of a narrowed segment (**Fig. 9**). When an obstructing stricture is present distal to a fistula, the fistula is unlikely to close as long as the stricture persists.

In general, there seems to be an association between the presence of stricturing disease and fistula formation.[44] Fistulas may form between an actively inflamed segment of bowel and other loops of small bowel, and to colon, stomach, the urinary bladder, or the skin. Clues to fistula formation include angulated and inflamed small bowel fixed to an adjacent structure. Linear enhancement extending from the inflamed loop to the adjacent structure or a stellate arrangement of small bowel loops is often seen (**Figs. 10** and **11**). An enterovesical fistula manifests as focal bladder wall thickening at the site of intimate contact with an inflamed loop of small bowel with or without urinary bladder gas.

Abscesses are organized mesenteric fluid collections that may contain gas, typically located adjacent to an inflamed loop of bowel or connected to a bowel loop via a sinus tract (see **Fig. 3**). Abscesses can often be managed percutaneously, provided a safe approach is present. Generally, penetrating Crohn disease is treated with antibiotics or biologics, not steroids.

## Fibrostenosing Disease

Chronic inflammation leads to mural fibrosis; fibrosis leads to stricture formation, and stricturing can lead to bowel obstruction. Strictures manifest as fixed segments of narrowing on cine SSFP

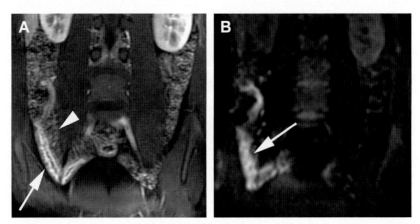

**Fig. 7.** A 21-year-old man (same as **Fig. 2**) with active inflammatory Crohn disease of the terminal ileum. (*A*) Coronal contrast-enhanced, fat-suppressed T1-weighted image demonstrates mucosal hyperenhancement of the terminal ileum (*arrow*) and engorged vasa recta in the mesentery "comb sign" (*arrowhead*). (*B*) Coronal DWI (b500) demonstrates signal hyperintensity in the bowel wall (*arrow*).

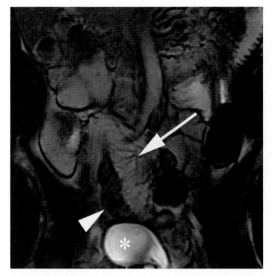

**Fig. 8.** A 55-year-old man with active inflammatory Crohn disease of the terminal ileum. Coronal fast imaging with SSFP demonstrates a thick-walled terminal ileum (*arrowhead*) with engorged vasa recta in the mesentery "comb sign" (*arrow*). The urinary bladder is seen at the lower part of the image (*asterisk*).

images, sometimes accompanied by mural thickening. Chronic fibrotic strictures are hypointense on both T1-weighted and T2-weighted sequences, lack edema and surrounding hyperemia, and enhance less than segments of active inflammation (**Fig. 12**). When associated with superimposed active inflammation, mucosal hyperenhancement may be present. Bowel dilatation proximal to a fixed, narrowed segment implies obstruction. Obstructing bowel strictures are generally treated surgically, with either stricturoplasty or resection,

unless contributing active inflammation coexists that might respond to medical therapy.

## Crohn Colitis

Because MRE is most often performed for evaluation of the small bowel, there is a paucity of data regarding evaluation of the colon with MRE. One study evaluating MRE without specific colonic preparation for colonic Crohn disease found that sensitivity was related to pathologic disease severity: 27% for mild inflammation, 58% for moderate inflammation, and 88% for severe inflammation.[20] The addition of a biphasic contrast enema to MRE improves sensitivity of colonic disease from 38% to 79%.[45] In the setting of active inflammatory colonic Crohn disease, mural thickening with hyperenhancement, bowel edema, and mesenteric vascular engorgement (**Fig. 13**) is expected to be seen.

## Other Findings

Perianal Crohn with anal and perianal fistulas with associated complications are seen in up to 36% of patients with Crohn disease.[46] Although perianal disease may be seen on standard imaging of the abdomen and pelvis as linear sinus tracts and fistulas, dedicated high-resolution imaging is necessary for accurate anatomic delineation of perianal Crohn disease before intervention.

## UTILITY OF MRE

MRE can assess disease activity and detect complications in patients with known small bowel Crohn disease and has utility in monitoring disease

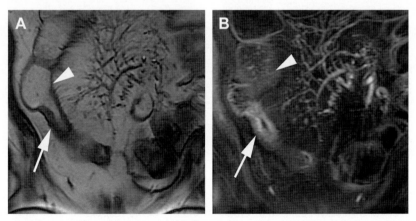

**Fig. 9.** A 60-year-old man with active transmural inflammation with stricturing. (*A*) Coronal true fast imaging with steady-state precession image demonstrates a fixed, thick-walled loop of ileum (*arrow*) with upstream dilatation (*arrowhead*). Note the engorged vasa recta "comb sign." (*B*) Coronal contrast-enhanced, fat-suppressed T1-weighted image demonstrates hyperenhancement of this thick-walled loop of ileum (*arrow*), suggesting a component of active inflammation. Upstream dilatation persists (*arrowhead*).

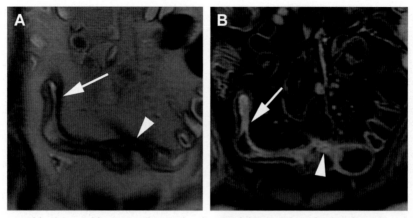

**Fig. 10.** A 34-year-old woman with penetrating Crohn disease. (*A*) Coronal single-shot fast spin-echo image demonstrates a long segment of terminal ileal wall thickening (*arrow*) and a fistulous tract between 2 fixed loops of small bowel (*arrowhead*). (*B*) Coronal contrast-enhanced, fat-suppressed T1-weighted image demonstrates a long segment of mucosal hyperenhancement (*arrow*) with an enhancing fistula (*arrowhead*) to an adjacent segment of mildly dilated small bowel.

activity following therapy. When compared with optical ileocolonoscopy, MRE shows an overall sensitivity of 85% for active inflammatory disease, with calculated area under the curve from receiver operating characteristic analysis of up to 0.950.[12] Individual signs of active inflammation have varying sensitivity and specificity, but mural thickening and edema, mucosal hyperenhancement, mesenteric engorgement, and mesenteric adenopathy are typical findings.[20] MRE also correlates well with surgical findings of stricture, abscess, and

fistula, with sensitivities of 95, 92, and 72%, respectively, and specificities of 72, 90, and 76%, respectively.[47] MRE has been shown to have a significant impact on patient care, by influencing therapy in up to 61% of patients with Crohn disease.[48]

## MRE Versus CTE

There have been several studies comparing the effectiveness of MRE and CTE for detecting active

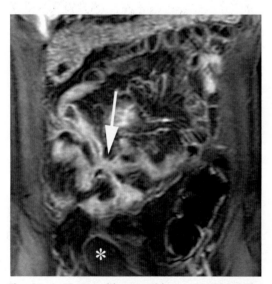

**Fig. 11.** A 45-year-old man with penetrating Crohn disease. Coronal contrast-enhanced, fat-suppressed T1-weighted image demonstrates complex enteroenteric fistulas (*arrow*) and active inflammatory disease. The urinary bladder is present at the lower part of this image (*asterisk*).

**Fig. 12.** A 48-year-old woman with fibrostenosing Crohn disease of the proximal small bowel. Coronal fast imaging with SSFP demonstrates a hypointense, thick-walled segment of bowel (*arrow*) with marked upstream dilatation (*arrowhead*). This stricture was treated surgically.

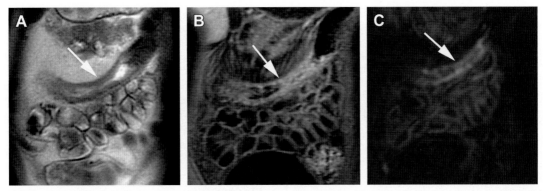

**Fig. 13.** A 17-year-old woman with Crohn colitis. (*A*) Coronal single-shot fast spin-echo image demonstrates mild hyperintensity and wall thickening of the transverse colon (*arrow*). (*B*) Coronal contrast-enhanced fat-suppressed T1-weighted image demonstrates wall thickening and hyperenhancement of the transverse colon (*arrow*). (*C*) Coronal DWI demonstrates signal hyperintensity within the transverse colon (*arrow*).

inflammatory disease. Two studies have shown that MRE image quality is inferior to that of CTE, related to many more potential artifacts in MRE, but that sensitivity and diagnostic yields are not significantly different.[49,50] Other studies have shown no significant difference in the sensitivity and specificity between MRE and CTE with regard to localizing Crohn disease, bowel wall thickening, and bowel wall enhancement.[12,50,51] Some studies have shown that MRE outperforms CTE in the evaluation of strictures and fistulas, but other studies showed no significant difference.[13,51,52] Both modalities are equally sensitive for extraintestinal complications.[12] A study evaluating interobserver agreement between CTE and MRE for active inflammatory bowel disease suggested that agreement was better for CTE, but went on to suggest that having adequate clinical experience with small bowel Crohn disease and the specific imaging modality are important for accurate evaluation.[49]

## PITFALLS

Appropriate patient management requires familiarity with common interpretive pitfalls of MRE.[32] In Crohn disease, dilated small bowel does necessarily equate with obstruction, and not all small bowel obstructions relate to fibrotic strictures. With transmural inflammation and prior surgery, adhesions are common and may cause bowel obstructions. Signs of adhesive disease include

---

**Box 3**
**Pearls and pitfalls of the MR evaluation of Crohn disease**

*Pearls:*

The primary utility of MRE in patients with known or suspected small bowel Crohn disease is to guide management

Active inflammation often coexists with fibrostenosing or fistulizing disease. The dominant feature, in conjunction with clinical presentation, determines management

SSFP images viewed in cine mode can help distinguish normal peristaltic contractions from abnormal mural thickening and strictures

DWI is useful for distinguishing bowel loops from abscess

*Pitfalls:*

Not all small bowel obstructions in Crohn disease are related to strictures; adhesive disease is also common

Not all dilated segments of bowel indicate obstruction; stricturoplasty sites also manifest as dilated segments of bowel

Collapsed loops of bowel can appear thickened and hyperenhancing; correlate with other sequences to confirm fixed, rather than transient, wall thickening

Not all thickened, hyperenhancing small bowel is Crohn disease; the differential diagnosis includes normal collapsed bowel, infectious and ischemic enteritis, radiation-induced enteritis, and vasculitis

---

**Box 4**
**Differential diagnosis of enteritis**

Inflammatory bowel disease including Crohn disease and ulcerative colitis with backwash ileitis

Infectious (bacterial or viral) enteritis

Small bowel ischemia or vasculitis

Radiation-induced enteritis

---

Box 5
**What the referring physician needs to know: Crohn disease**

Relative contribution of active inflammation, penetrating disease, and fibrostenosing disease to patient's symptoms and clinical presentation

Length and location of involved segments of bowel

Presence of bowel obstruction and cause (eg, active inflammation, stricture, adhesions)

Extramural complications such as fistula and abscess

---

angled or tethered loops of bowel, an abrupt transition point, and absence of mural thickening or abnormal enhancement. SSFP or other fast sequences assessed in cine mode can also be helpful to identify adhesions.[53,54] Knowledge of the surgical history is important, as sites of stricturoplasty may appear as focally dilated segments of bowel (**Box 3**).

Not all small bowel wall thickening and hyperenhancement are secondary to Crohn disease. Collapsed segments of normal small bowel may appear thickened and hyperenhancing compared with adjacent loops but will often show normal peristalsis and wall thickness when distended on cine SSFP images. Such normal loops will also lack edema or other secondary signs of inflammation. When true inflammation of the bowel is present in the absence of a known diagnosis of Crohn disease, the differential diagnosis should also include other entities, such as radiation-induced enteritis, infectious enteritis, vasculitis, and intestinal ischemia (**Box 4**).

Submucosal fat deposition can simulate mural edema on non-fat-suppressed T2-weighted sequences, and true submucosal edema on T2-weighted images can be seen proximal to intestinal obstruction in the absence of active inflammation. When submucosal edema is secondary to bowel obstruction rather than active inflammation, other findings, such as mucosal or mural hyperenhancement, are typically lacking.

## SUMMARY

Radiologic imaging of the small bowel has progressed from fluoroscopic imaging toward CT and MR imaging. Using fast sequences and a large volume of orally administered enteric contrast, MR enterography has become a primary imaging modality for the evaluation of Crohn disease. Biphasic enteric contrast and dynamic contrast-enhanced imaging allow excellent visualization of the bowel wall and assessment of transmural and extraenteric processes.

Active inflammatory bowel disease is characterized by bowel wall edema and thickening and hyperenhancement. Engorged mesenteric vasculature and mesenteric lymphadenopathy are typical extraluminal findings of active inflammatory disease. Strictures, fistula tracts, and abscesses are well delineated with MR imaging, and their correct identification has significant therapeutic implications (**Box 5**).

## REFERENCES

1. Wold PB, Fletcher JG, Johnson CD, et al. Assessment of small bowel Crohn disease: noninvasive peroral CT enterography compared with other imaging methods and endoscopy–feasibility study. Radiology 2003;229(1):275–81.
2. Hara AK, Alam S, Heigh RI, et al. Using CT enterography to monitor Crohn's disease activity: a preliminary study. AJR Am J Roentgenol 2008;190(6): 1512–6.
3. Hara AK, Leighton JA, Heigh RI, et al. Crohn disease of the small bowel: preliminary comparison among CT enterography, capsule endoscopy, small-bowel follow-through, and ileoscopy. Radiology 2006;238(1):128–34.
4. Vogel J, da Luz Moreira A, Baker M, et al. CT enterography for Crohn's disease: accurate preoperative diagnostic imaging. Dis Colon Rectum 2007; 50(11):1761–9.
5. Desmond AN, O'Regan K, Curran C, et al. Crohn's disease: factors associated with exposure to high levels of diagnostic radiation. Gut 2008;57(11): 1524–9.
6. Jaffe TA, Gaca AM, Delaney S, et al. Radiation doses from small-bowel follow-through and abdominopelvic MDCT in Crohn's disease. AJR Am J Roentgenol 2007;189(5):1015–22.
7. Allen BC, Baker ME, Einstein DM, et al. Effect of altering automatic exposure control settings and quality reference mAs on radiation dose, image quality, and diagnostic efficacy in MDCT enterography of active inflammatory Crohn's disease. AJR Am J Roentgenol 2010;195(1):89–100.
8. Kambadakone AR, Chaudhary NA, Desai GS, et al. Low-dose MDCT and CT enterography of patients with Crohn disease: feasibility of adaptive statistical iterative reconstruction. AJR Am J Roentgenol 2011;196(6):W743–52.
9. Lee SJ, Park SH, Kim AY, et al. A prospective comparison of standard-dose CT enterography and 50% reduced-dose CT enterography with and without noise reduction for evaluating Crohn disease. AJR Am J Roentgenol 2011; 197(1):50–7.

10. O'Neill SB, Mc Laughlin PD, Crush L, et al. A prospective feasibility study of sub-millisievert abdominopelvic CT using iterative reconstruction in Crohn's disease. Eur Radiol 2013;23(9):2503–12.

11. Brenner DJ, Hall EJ. Computed tomography–an increasing source of radiation exposure. N Engl J Med 2007;357(22):2277–84.

12. Lee SS, Kim AY, Yang SK, et al. Crohn disease of the small bowel: comparison of CT enterography, MR enterography, and small-bowel follow-through as diagnostic techniques. Radiology 2009;251(3): 751–61.

13. Schmidt S, Guibal A, Meuwly JY, et al. Acute complications of Crohn's disease: comparison of multidetector-row computed tomographic enterography with magnetic resonance enterography. Digestion 2010;82(4):229–38.

14. Fidler JL, Guimaraes L, Einstein DM. MR imaging of the small bowel. Radiographics 2009;29(6): 1811–25.

15. Kuehle CA, Ajaj W, Ladd SC, et al. Hydro-MRI of the small bowel: effect of contrast volume, timing of contrast administration, and data acquisition on bowel distention. AJR Am J Roentgenol 2006; 187(4):W375–85.

16. Negaard A, Paulsen V, Sandvik L, et al. A prospective randomized comparison between two MRI studies of the small bowel in Crohn's disease, the oral contrast method and MR enteroclysis. Eur Radiol 2007;17(9):2294–301.

17. Schreyer AG, Geissler A, Albrich H, et al. Abdominal MRI after enteroclysis or with oral contrast in patients with suspected or proven Crohn's disease. Clin Gastroenterol Hepatol 2004;2(6):491–7.

18. Lawrance IC, Welman CJ, Shipman P, et al. Small bowel MRI enteroclysis or follow through: which is optimal? World J Gastroenterol 2009;15(42): 5300–6.

19. Masselli G, Casciani E, Polettini E, et al. Comparison of MR enteroclysis with MR enterography and conventional enteroclysis in patients with Crohn's disease. Eur Radiol 2008;18(3):438–47.

20. Grand DJ, Kampalath V, Harris A, et al. MR enterography correlates highly with colonoscopy and histology for both distal ileal and colonic Crohn's disease in 310 patients. Eur J Radiol 2012;81(5): e763–9.

21. Grand DJ, Beland MD, Machan JT, et al. Detection of Crohn's disease: comparison of CT and MR enterography without anti-peristaltic agents performed on the same day. Eur J Radiol 2012;81(8): 1735–41.

22. Oto A, Zhu F, Kulkarni K, et al. Evaluation of diffusion-weighted MR imaging for detection of bowel inflammation in patients with Crohn's disease. Acad Radiol 2009;16(5):597–603.

23. Oto A, Kayhan A, Williams JT, et al. Active Crohn's disease in the small bowel: evaluation by diffusion weighted imaging and quantitative dynamic contrast enhanced MR imaging. J Magn Reson Imaging 2011;33(3):615–24.

24. Cronin CG, Delappe E, Lohan DG, et al. Normal small bowel wall characteristics on MR enterography. Eur J Radiol 2010;75(2):207–11.

25. Lauenstein TC, Ajaj W, Narin B, et al. MR imaging of apparent small-bowel perfusion for diagnosing mesenteric ischemia: feasibility study. Radiology 2005;234(2):569–75.

26. Knuesel PR, Kubik RA, Crook DW, et al. Assessment of dynamic contrast enhancement of the small bowel in active Crohn's disease using 3D MR enterography. Eur J Radiol 2010;73(3):607–13.

27. Booya F, Fletcher JG, Huprich JE, et al. Active Crohn disease: CT findings and interobserver agreement for enteric phase CT enterography. Radiology 2006;241(3):787–95.

28. Baker ME, Walter J, Obuchowski NA, et al. Mural attenuation in normal small bowel and active inflammatory Crohn's disease on CT enterography: location, absolute attenuation, relative attenuation, and the effect of wall thickness. AJR Am J Roentgenol 2009;192(2):417–23.

29. Loftus EV Jr, Schoenfeld P, Sandborn WJ. The epidemiology and natural history of Crohn's disease in population-based patient cohorts from North America: a systematic review. Aliment Pharmacol Ther 2002;16(1):51–60.

30. Gasche C, Scholmerich J, Brynskov J, et al. A simple classification of Crohn's disease: report of the Working Party for the World Congresses of Gastroenterology, Vienna 1998. Inflamm Bowel Dis 2000;6(1):8–15.

31. Maglinte DD, Gourtsoyiannis N, Rex D, et al. Classification of small bowel Crohn's subtypes based on multimodality imaging. Radiol Clin North Am 2003;41(2):285–303.

32. Leyendecker JR, Bloomfeld RS, DiSantis DJ, et al. MR enterography in the management of patients with Crohn disease. Radiographics 2009;29(6): 1827–46.

33. Maccioni F, Bruni A, Viscido A, et al. MR imaging in patients with Crohn disease: value of T2- versus T1-weighted gadolinium-enhanced MR sequences with use of an oral superparamagnetic contrast agent. Radiology 2006;238(2):517–30.

34. Udayasankar UK, Martin D, Lauenstein T, et al. Role of spectral presaturation attenuated inversion-recovery fat-suppressed T2-weighted MR imaging in active inflammatory bowel disease. J Magn Reson Imaging 2008;28(5):1133–40.

35. Kitazume Y, Satoh S, Hosoi H, et al. Cine magnetic resonance imaging evaluation of peristalsis of small bowel with longitudinal ulcer in Crohn

disease: preliminary results. J Comput Assist To-mogr 2007;31(6):876–83.

36. Sinha R, Rajiah P, Murphy P, et al. Utility of high-resolution MR imaging in demonstrating transmural pathologic changes in Crohn disease. Radiographics 2009;29(6):1847–67.

37. Del Vescovo R, Sansoni I, Caviglia R, et al. Dynamic contrast enhanced magnetic resonance imaging of the terminal ileum: differentiation of activity of Crohn's disease. Abdom Imaging 2008;33(4):417–24.

38. Malago R, Manfredi R, Benini L, et al. Assessment of Crohn's disease activity in the small bowel with MR-enteroclysis: clinico-radiological correlations. Abdom Imaging 2008;33(6):669–75.

39. Paolantonio P, Ferrari R, Vecchietti F, et al. Current status of MR imaging in the evaluation of IBD in a pediatric population of patients. Eur J Radiol 2009;69(3):418–24.

40. Meyers MA, McGuire PV. Spiral CT demonstration of hypervascularity in Crohn disease: "vascular jejunization of the ileum" or the "comb sign". Abdom Imaging 1995;20(4):327–32.

41. Gourtsoyianni S, Papanikolaou N, Amanakis E, et al. Crohn's disease lymphadenopathy: MR imaging findings. Eur J Radiol 2009;69(3):425–8.

42. Zappa M, Stefanescu C, Cazals-Hatem D, et al. Which magnetic resonance imaging findings accurately evaluate inflammation in small bowel Crohn's disease? A retrospective comparison with surgical pathologic analysis. Inflamm Bowel Dis 2011;17(4):984–93.

43. Rimola J, Rodriguez S, Garcia-Bosch O, et al. Magnetic resonance for assessment of disease activity and severity in ileocolonic Crohn's disease. Gut 2009;58(8):1113–20.

44. Oberhuber G, Stangl PC, Vogelsang H, et al. Significant association of strictures and internal fistula formation in Crohn's disease. Virchows Arch 2000;437(3):293–7.

45. Friedrich C, Fajfar A, Pawlik M, et al. Magnetic resonance enterography with and without biphasic contrast agent enema compared to conventional ileocolonoscopy in patients with Crohn's disease. Inflamm Bowel Dis 2012;18(10):1842–8.

46. Rankin GB, Watts HD, Melnyk CS, et al. National Cooperative Crohn's Disease Study: extraintestinal manifestations and perianal complications. Gastroenterology 1979;77(4 Pt 2):914–20.

47. Pozza A, Scarpa M, Lacognata C, et al. Magnetic resonance enterography for Crohn's disease: what the surgeon can take home. J Gastrointest Surg 2011;15(10):1689–98.

48. Hafeez R, Punwani S, Boulos P, et al. Diagnostic and therapeutic impact of MR enterography in Crohn's disease. Clin Radiol 2011;66(12):1148–58.

49. Jensen MD, Ormstrup T, Vagn-Hansen C, et al. Interobserver and intermodality agreement for detection of small bowel Crohn's disease with MR enterography and CT enterography. Inflamm Bowel Dis 2011;17(5):1081–8.

50. Siddiki HA, Fidler JL, Fletcher JG, et al. Prospective comparison of state-of-the-art MR enterography and CT enterography in small-bowel Crohn's disease. AJR Am J Roentgenol 2009;193(1):113–21.

51. Fiorino G, Bonifacio C, Peyrin-Biroulet L, et al. Prospective comparison of computed tomography enterography and magnetic resonance enterography for assessment of disease activity and complications in ileocolonic Crohn's disease. Inflamm Bowel Dis 2011;17(5):1073–80.

52. Ippolito D, Invernizzi F, Galimberti S, et al. MR enterography with polyethylene glycol as oral contrast medium in the follow-up of patients with Crohn disease: comparison with CT enterography. Abdom Imaging 2010;35(5):563–70.

53. Lang RA, Buhmann S, Hopman A, et al. Cine-MRI detection of intraabdominal adhesions: correlation with intraoperative findings in 89 consecutive cases. Surg Endosc 2008;22(11):2455–61.

54. Buhmann-Kirchhoff S, Lang R, Kirchhoff C, et al. Functional cine MR imaging for the detection and mapping of intraabdominal adhesions: method and surgical correlation. Eur Radiol 2008;18(6):1215–23.

# MR Imaging of the Prostate

Joseph H. Yacoub, MD[a],*, Aytekin Oto, MD[b], Frank H. Miller, MD[c]

## KEYWORDS

- Prostate cancer • Prostate MR imaging • Multiparametric MR imaging • Pelvic MRI • Male Pelvis
- MRI techniques

## KEY POINTS

- Magnetic resonance (MR) imaging of the prostate is playing an increasing role in the detection, staging, and localization of prostate cancer.
- Multiparametric MR is the accepted standard for prostate imaging. It consists of T2-weighted imaging in combination with other functional techniques: diffusion-weighted imaging, dynamic contrast-enhanced MR imaging, or MR spectroscopic imaging.
- A systematic approach in reporting prostate MR imaging constitutes identifying abnormal regions and grading each region on the degree of suspicion for cancer based on its features on multiparametric sequences.
- Central gland tumors are more challenging and are approached differently than the more common peripheral zone lesions.
- Emerging and potential indications of prostate MR imaging include tumor localization, guiding biopsy, guiding focal therapy, assessing aggressiveness, selecting and monitoring patients for active surveillance, and posttreatment follow-up.

## INTRODUCTION

Prostate cancer is the most common nonskin cancer and the second most common cause of cancer death in US men, accounting for 28% of new cancer cases and 10% of cancer deaths in 2013.[1] One in 6 men are clinically diagnosed with prostate cancer.[2] Since the widespread use of serum prostate-specific antigen (PSA) for screening, prostate cancer is often diagnosed at an early stage, with an estimated 82% of new cases being clinically localized at diagnosis. Screening for prostate cancer consists of measuring the PSA and performing a digital rectal examination. PSA is increased in most, but not all, prostate cancers. It is also increased in benign prostate diseases such as prostatitis or benign prostatic hypertrophy (BPH). Digital rectal examination is inherently insensitive for localized prostate cancer. Screening for prostate cancer has long been a controversial subject with differing and changing recommendations.[3] The most recent statement by the US preventive services task force recommended against PSA-based screening for prostate cancer.[4] This recommendation marks a significant shift from the commonly used recommendation of the American Cancer Society of PSA screening individuals aged more than 50 years. A commonly used threshold PSA for biopsy is 4.0 ng/mL.

At present, the diagnosis of prostate cancer is based on transrectal ultrasonography (TRUS)–guided biopsy (TRUS GB). In TRUS GB,

Disclosures: J.H. Yacoub, F.H. Miller: None; A. Oto: Research support from Philips and Invivo.
[a] Department of Radiology, Stritch School of Medicine, Loyola University Chicago, 2160 South 1st Avenue, Maywood, IL 60153, USA; [b] Department of Radiology, University of Chicago, 5841 South Maryland Avenue, MC 2026, Chicago, IL 60637, USA; [c] Department of Radiology, Feinberg School of Medicine, Northwestern University, Northwestern Memorial Hospital, 676 North Saint Clair Street, Suite 800, Chicago, IL 60611, USA
* Corresponding author.
E-mail address: jyacoub@lumc.edu

6, 8, 10, or 12 core biopsies are performed in a systematic fashion to sample the different regions of the prostate that are likely to contain the suspected malignancy rather than targeting a specific lesion.[5–8] The cores are obtained from the peripheral zone of the prostate, which has the highest chance of harboring malignancy. For each core, the most common pattern of cancer is assigned a Gleason grade[1–5] and similarly the second most common pattern is also assigned a Gleason grade. The sum of the most and second most common pattern grades is called the Gleason score. An overall Gleason score of 7 may either represent Gleason 4 + 3 or Gleason 3 + 4, the former of which is higher in grade.

The current diagnostic paradigm has several limitations:

- Serum PSA has a low specificity for diagnosis of prostate cancer, leading to many unnecessary biopsies.
- The accepted threshold for PSA of 4 ng/mL may miss clinically significant disease with lower PSA values.[9]
- TRUS GB offers unreliable information about the volume, extent, and aggressiveness of the prostate cancer. It may lead to overestimation or underestimation of the Gleason score.[10,11]
- Certain regions of the prostate, such as the anterior gland and the apex, are undersampled on TRUS, with increasing evidence that they may harbor clinically significant tumors.[12–14]
- The current paradigm is limited in its ability to locally stage the prostate cancer, which can have a bearing on treatment planning.

## TREATMENT

Multiple treatment options are available for patients with localized prostate cancer. The selection between these options may depend in part on the staging and risk assessment of the disease, but it is also subject to the preference of the patient and the availability of these techniques. Nomograms have been developed to risk stratify the disease and to determine the appropriate treatment and prognosis of the patient.[15] These nomograms are based on the combination of PSA level, digital rectal examination findings, and systematic random biopsy–based Gleason score. The treatment options include:

- Radical prostatectomy. This can be performed through open retropubic, laparoscopic, or robotically assisted approaches.
- Radiation therapy. This can be offered as external beam radiotherapy or as brachytherapy. A newer technique of external bean radiotherapy known as intensity-modulated radiotherapy is becoming more commonly used in prostate cancer treatment.
- Active surveillance. This refers to the close monitoring of patients with favorable-risk prostate cancer using typically annual PSA, digital rectal examination, and TRUS GB with appropriate treatment provided to patients who show evidence of disease progression.
- Focal therapy. These are new emerging techniques such as cryoablation, high-intensity focused ultrasonography (HIFU), and laser ablation of tumors focally in the prostate under image guidance rather than treating the entire gland.

## ANATOMY

The prostate gland is divided into the following major zones:

- Peripheral zone. This zone is located in the posterior, lateral, and apical portions of the prostate and it constitutes 70% of the glandular tissue. On T2-weighted MR images, it shows high signal intensity. Around 70% of prostate cancer occurs in the peripheral zone.[12,16–18]
- Central zone. This zone is located superiorly just posterior to the proximal urethra. It is defined anatomically as the region of the prostate surrounding the ejaculatory ducts from the prostatic base to the verumontanum.[19] Around 5% of prostate cancers occur in the central zone.[16–18,20]
- Transitional zone. This zone is located just anterior and lateral to the proximal urethra superior to the verumontanum. The transitional zone harbors 25% of prostate cancer.[16–18]
- Periurethral zone. In addition to these 3 zones there is a ring of periurethral tissue that has low signal intensity on T2-weighted images and that surrounds the urethra, which is located in the anterior aspect of the prostate.
- Anterior fibromuscular stroma. This is a region of nonglandular tissue located in the most anterior aspect of the prostate and that has a low T2 signal intensity.

The transitional and central zones are together referred to as the central gland (CG). They show lower T2-weighted signal intensity and less contrast enhancement compared with the peripheral zone. In a recent article by Vargas and colleagues[19] the central zone could be distinguished from the other zones in 81% to 84% of patients, challenging the widespread notion that the transitional and central zones are indistinguishable. In that article, the transitional zone was described to have homogeneous low signal intensity on T2-weighted images and apparent diffusion coefficient (ADC) maps, and symmetric appearance on either side of the verumontanum.

Surrounding the prostate is an outer band of concentric fibromuscular tissue that is inseparable from the prostatic stroma.[21] This outer band is referred to as the capsule, although it is not a true capsule and is made up of pure stroma.[17,21] This capsule is best seen on T2-weighted images as a thin layer of dark tissue most apparent posteriorly and posterolaterally.

The seminal vesicles are paired organs located superior and posterior to the prostate and drain via the ejaculatory ducts into the urethra. The ejaculatory ducts course through the central zone of the gland and open in the urethra at the level of verumontanum. **Figs. 1** and **2** show the normal anatomy and signal intensity of the prostate gland on T2-weighted images. **Fig. 3** shows the appearance of the central zone of the prostate.

## IMAGING PROTOCOL
### Preparation

Hemorrhage from recent biopsy significantly limits the diagnostic performance of prostate MR imaging. Therefore, MR imaging should be performed at least 6 to 8 weeks after prostate biopsy.[22–25] Because ejaculation can affect the perfusion and diffusion of the gland as well as the distention of the seminal vesicles, the patients should be asked to refrain from ejaculation for 48 to 72 hours before the study.

### Choice of the Scanner and Coils

Prostate MR imaging can be performed on 1.5- or 3-T MR imaging scanners; 3-T MR imaging allows higher signal/noise ratio and faster scan time, both of which can enhance the quality of the MR imaging significantly. When using 1.5-T MR imaging, the use of an endorectal coil in combination with an external phased array coil is considered to be the best method to evaluate the prostate.[26–28] The need for an endorectal coil when imaging at 3 T remains a subject of controversy. Using 3-T MR imaging, one study has reported comparable image quality for an external phased array coil compared with imaging at 1.5 T using an endorectal coil.[28] However, another study reported that 3-T MR imaging with an external phased array coil is inferior in image quality and delineation of prostate cancer compared with imaging at 1.5 T with endorectal and external coils.[29] Comparing the use of endorectal coils with external phased array coils alone on 3-T imaging, Heijmink and colleagues[26] concluded that using an endorectal coil improves image quality and diagnostic performance for localization and staging. Turkbey and colleagues[30] similarly showed higher sensitivity and positive predictive value for prostate cancer using an endorectal coil compared with not using an endorectal coil on 3 T. Although some centers have shifted to performing all the prostate imaging on 3-T scanners using endorectal coils, other centers prefer the use of external phased array coils only on 3-T imaging in the interest of patients' comfort and acceptability. The European consensus article by Barentz and colleagues[25] presents a shortened protocol for detection for which the use of endorectal coil is optional, whereas, for the longer staging protocol, the use of an endorectal coil is preferred. When using an endorectal coil on 3-T scanners, the coil should be distended with barium or liquid perfluorocarbon and care should be taken to eliminate as much air as possible from the coil to avoid artifact related to gas.

### Multiparametric Sequences

Multiparametric MR is the accepted standard for prostate imaging. It consists of high-resolution T2-weighted imaging in combination with all or some of the functional sequence such as diffusion-weighted imaging (DWI), dynamic contrast-enhanced MR imaging (DCE-MR imaging), and MR spectroscopic imaging (MRSI). The importance of DWI has increased recently, whereas most centers have stopped performing MRSI as a part of their routine prostate MR imaging protocols.

### T2-weighted Imaging Technique

High-resolution T2-weighted imaging provides the best depiction of the prostate zonal anatomy and it allows detection, localization, and staging of prostate cancer. T2-weighted turbo spin echo (TSE) images are obtained in 3 orthogonal planes with a slice thickness of 3 mm and an in-plane resolution of 0.3 to 0.5 mm on 3 T or 0.5 to 0.7 mm on 1.5 T. The European consensus articles[25,31] describe a shorter protocol to be used for detection as opposed to staging, in which only 2 planes of imaging are required (axial and sagittal) and the in-plane resolution is 0.5 to 0.7 mm.

Three-dimensional (3D) T2-weighted techniques have recently been described in prostate imaging. Using these techniques the data can be acquired in the axial plane using a slice thickness of 1 mm

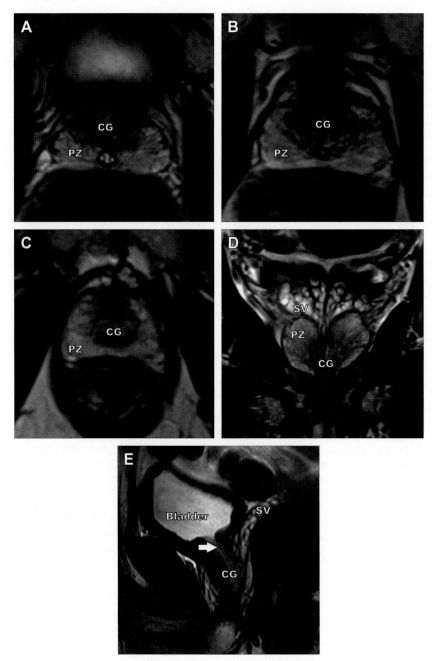

**Fig. 1.** Normal prostate anatomy. T2-weighted images show the normal appearance of the prostate in the axial plane at the base (*A*), midgland (*B*), and apex (*C*), as well as the in the coronal plane (*D*) and the sagittal plane (*E*). In the normal prostate, the peripheral zone (PZ) constitutes about 70% of the volume, whereas the central gland (CG) constitutes the remainder and contains the central zone and transitional zone. The seminal vesicles (SV) are a paired organ located superior and posterior to the prostate. The prostatic urethra (*arrow*) is located in the CG.

and near-isovolumetric voxels and then it can be reconstructed in all 3 planes yielding a significant time saving. Early small reports of 3D T2 techniques showed similar image quality and accuracy in evaluating prostate cancer and extracapsular extension compared with standard T2 TSE[32,33]; however, many centers continue to find two-dimensional (2D) sequences to be of better image quality. Using the standard T2 TSE acquiring 3 planes of images exceeds 11 minutes, whereas using 3D T2 sequences the acquisition time can be reduced to 4 to 5 minutes.

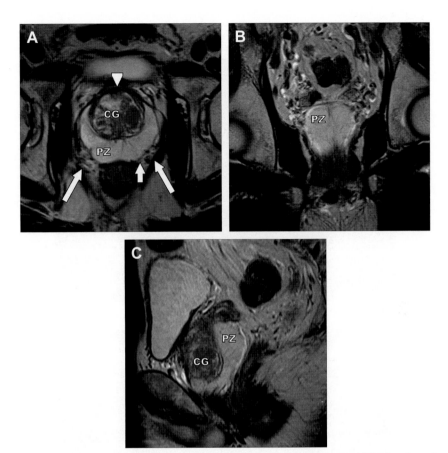

Fig. 2. Normal high T2 signal of peripheral zone. Axial (*A*), coronal (*B*), and sagittal (*C*) T2 turbo spin echo (TSE) images show the intrinsic high T2 signal of the peripheral zone (PZ). The central gland (CG) shows a heterogeneous appearance with low-signal nodular areas representing BPH resulting in mild enlargement of the CG and the overall size of the prostate. The thin layer of low T2 signal surrounding the prostate is known as the capsule (*short arrow*). In the anteriormost aspect of the gland there is a thickened band of low T2 signal (*white arrowhead*) known as the anterior fibromuscular stroma. The neurovascular bundle is noted posterolateral to the peripheral zone (*long arrows*).

## DWI Technique

DWI is usually acquired in the axial plane with an ultrafast echo planar imaging sequence using parallel imaging. The in-plane resolution is about 1 to 1.5 mm on 3 T (1.5–2 mm on 1.5 T). A range of b values of 0 to 2000 s/mm$^2$ are obtained. The ADC value is calculated from these different b-value diffusion-weighted images. In qualitatively evaluating the diffusion data, the ADC maps and the high-b-value DWI should be reviewed together. The use of higher b values of 1500 and 2000 s/mm$^2$ has been reported to increase the conspicuity of prostate cancer relative to the bright peripheral zone[34–37] as well as to suppress the effects of hemorrhage, improving the diagnostic capability of DWI in hemorrhagic peripheral zones.[38] Larger b values provide better contrast, and less T2 shine-through effect, but they have lower signal/noise ratio and more

motion artifact owing to longer acquisition times. There are no established threshold ADC values to determine the presence of malignancy because of the wide range of reported mean ADC values in the malignant regions as well as in healthy peripheral zones and the overlap with other conditions, including prostatitis. Reported ADCs in the literature ranged from $0.93 \times 10^{-3}$ mm$^2$/s to $1.58 \times 10^{-3}$ mm$^2$/s for cancerous regions and from $1.61 \times 10^{-3}$ mm$^2$/s to $2.61 \times 10^{-3}$ mm$^2$/s for healthy peripheral zone tissue.[39] **Fig. 4** shows the normal appearance of the prostate gland on diffusion-weighted images.

## DCE-MR Imaging Technique

DCE-MR imaging refers to the acquisition of a series of T1-weighted gradient echo sequences covering the prostate at regular intervals after the intravenous injection of the contrast bolus at a

A

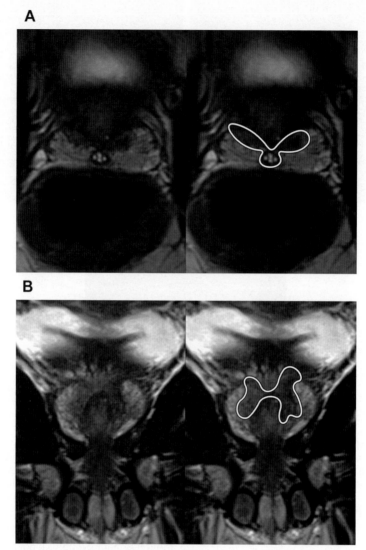

B

Fig. 3. Central zone of the prostate. The central zone is defined anatomically as the region of the prostate surrounding the ejaculatory ducts from the prostatic base to the verumontanum. Axial (*A*) and coronal (*B*) T2 TSE images show the central zone to have homogeneous low signal intensity (outlined on the images on the *right*) with symmetric appearance on either side of the midline.

rate of 2 to 4 mL/s. The total volume of the prostate is scanned every 3 to 12 seconds for a minimum of 5 minutes.[25,31,40] Some investigators recommend a temporal resolution of 5 seconds or less, especially for quantitative DCE-MR imaging analysis using the Tofts model.[40] A longer temporal resolution could be adequate for semiquantitative or qualitative analysis but it should not exceed 15 seconds.[25,31,40] The generated sequences can be reviewed on Picture Archiving and Communication system (PACS) or on commercially available software that can calculate dynamic enhancement parameters and subtraction images and also allow display of other sequences (T2 and

DWI) with image coregistration. Prostate cancer typically enhances and washes out early compared with normal peripheral zone.

There are generally 3 ways of evaluating the DCE data (**Fig. 5**):

- The DCE data can be evaluated qualitatively by looking for areas of early hyperenhancement and washout seen typically in prostate cancer relative to the normal prostate.[41–45] Subtraction images may be helpful for this purpose.
- The DCE data can be evaluated semiquantitatively by evaluating the enhancement curve

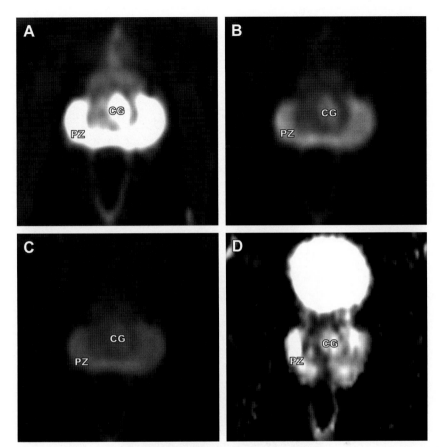

**Fig. 4.** DWI of the prostate; b values 50 s/mm² (*A*), 500 s/mm² (*B*), and 800 s/mm² (*C*) showing a bright signal in the normal peripheral zone relative to the CG. The signal of the peripheral zone decrease with the higher b values. The ADC map shows a bright signal in the peripheral zone (*D*). In evaluating the peripheral zone the ADC is most helpful in identifying foci of relative restricted diffusion to suggest cancer in the peripheral zone, which appears dark relative the background.

for a region of interest. The enhancement curve can be categorized into 3 types: type 1, persistent increase; type 2, plateau; and type 3, initial upslope and then decline. The type 3 curve is the most suspicious for prostate cancer. Additional semiquantitative parameters can be calculated from these curves, such as peak enhancement, time to peak, slope of the wash-in portion of the curve, and slope of the washout portion of the curve.[42–45] The wash-in rate (represented by the slope of or the area under the initial rise of the enhancement curve) has recently been reported to have high sensitivity, specificity, and accuracy of 83%, 97%, and 91%, respectively.[44] The inherent limitation of the semiqualitative methods is their dependence on various factors such as hardware, sequence parameters, and contrast dose.

- The DCE data can be evaluated quantitatively using pharmacokinetic models to summarize DCE data in terms of parameters that relate to underlying vascular anatomy and physiology. Using the 2-compartment model, which refers to the extravascular extracellular space and the intravascular compartment, 3 basic parameters can be calculated: $K^{trans}$, $K_{ep}$, and $V_e$. $K^{trans}$ is the transfer constant of the contrast from the intravascular to the extravascular extracellular space. $K_{ep}$ is the reverse reflux rate constant between extracellular space and plasma. High $K^{trans}$ and $K_{ep}$ are more suspicious for cancer. $V_e$ is the extravascular extracellular volume, which is equal to $K^{trans}/K_{ep}$.

The analyzed DCE data, whether semiquantitative or quantitative, can be displayed as colored maps and superimposed on the T2 images.

## MR Spectroscopic Imaging

MRSI can assess tumor metabolism by displaying the relative concentrations of citrate, choline,

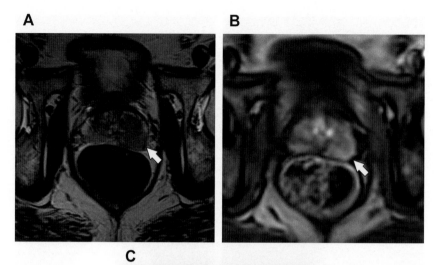

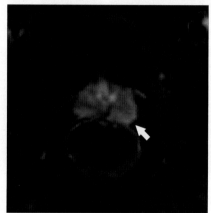

**Fig. 5.** Dynamic contrast enhancement analysis. Prostate cancer lesion is identified on a T2 TSE image (*A*) as a region of low T2 signal in the peripheral zone (*arrow*). On qualitative analysis of the DCE a representative T1 gradient echo image (*B*) obtained about 30 seconds after contrast injection shows early hyperenhancement of the lesion (*arrow*). Subtraction image (*C*) is generated by subtracting image (*A*) from the precontrast T1 gradient echo image (not shown) and shows early hyperenhancement of the lesion more clearly (*arrow*). On semiquantitative analysis, the enhancement curve generated from the region of interest placed within the lesion shows a type 3 curve (*D*) with early hyperenhancement and washout. The area under the early enhancement curve can also be displayed as a color map overlaid on the T2 images (*E*) and again shows the lesion in the peripheral zone (*arrow*). Quantitative analysis of the DCE data yields values such as $K_{ep}$ (the reverse reflux rate constant between extracellular space and plasma), $K^{trans}$ (the transfer constant of the contrast from the intravascular to the extravascular extracellular space), and $V_e$. The $K_{ep}$ is the most commonly used value displayed as color map overlaid on the T2 images (*F*) with red showing areas of suspicious enhancement kinetics and blue showing normal enhancement kinetics. The lesion in the peripheral zone is shaded as red on the $K_{ep}$ color map (*arrow*).

creatinine, and polyamines. The normal prostate is rich in citrate, whereas prostate cancers have a characteristic loss of the citrate peak and gain in the choline/creatine peak. MRSI of the prostate is typically performed with a combination of point-resolved spectroscopy volume localization and 3D chemical shift imaging rather than the traditional single-voxel or 2D MRSI technique used in brain imaging.[46] For quantitative analysis, the choline + creatine/citrate ratio is calculated and compared with the mean value. Establishing and running a successful MRSI protocol involves more attention to detail and technical knowledge than do most MR imaging sequences and is more time consuming,[46] which may have led many clinical centers to prefer the use of the other multiparametric sequences, namely DWI and DCE MR imaging instead of MRSI. In addition, the ACRIN (American College of Radiology Imaging Network) multicenter trial results[47] showing no incremental benefit of MRSI for localizing prostate cancer compared with standard anatomic imaging present a challenge to the reported benefit of MRSI.[48,49]

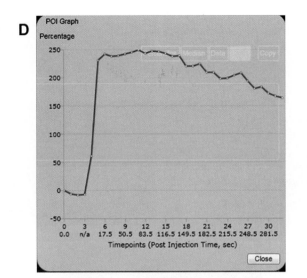

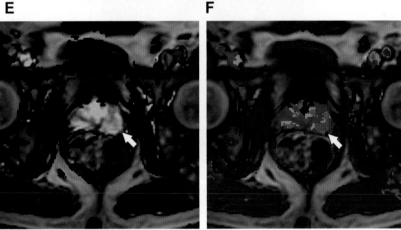

Fig. 5. (*continued*)

## T1-weighted Imaging Technique

A T1-weighted spin echo sequence is typically acquired as a part of the prostate imaging protocol. This sequence is useful for detection of hemorrhage in the prostate, evaluation of bones for metastatic disease, and evaluation of the contour of the prostate and the neurovascular bundle. In addition to small field of view sequences focusing on the prostate, a large field of view sequence covering the pelvis from the level of the aortic bifurcation to the symphysis pubis should be added to the prostate MR imaging protocol for optimal evaluation of the pelvic bones and lymph nodes.

## INTERPRETATION OF PROSTATE MR IMAGING

Prostate MR imaging interpretation can be a challenging task for the beginner and there is a steep learning curve. Studies have shown that experienced readers were significantly more accurate than the nonexperienced.[50–52] Efforts for standardization of interpretation and reporting of prostate MR imaging are underway. The basic principle of proposed scoring systems constitutes identifying abnormal regions and then grading each region on the degree of suspicion for prostate cancer based on the features of that region on multiparametric MR imaging. The European Society of Urogenital Radiology recently published a standardized structured reporting system referred to as PI-RADS (Prostate Imaging Reporting and Data System).[25] Although this system has not yet achieved wide adoption, the underlying principle for the scoring system can be helpful in approaching prostate MR imaging. In the PI-RADS system, lesions are scored on a 5-point scale that reflects the likelihood of cancer. Early validation studies of the PI-RADS are promising.[53,54] In the study

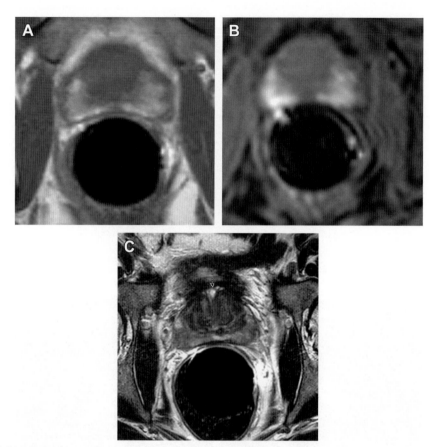

**Fig. 6.** Peripheral zone hemorrhage. Axial T1 TSE (*A*) and precontrast axial T1 gradient echo (*B*) images show high signal in the peripheral zone consistent with postbiopsy hemorrhage, which limits the evaluation of the T2 TSE sequences (*C*) for prostate lesions. *Small arrow* indicates and incidental cyst in the prostate.

by Rosenkrantz and colleagues,[53] radiologists using PI-RADS generally performed better in assessment of the peripheral zone than in assessment of the transitional zone and had higher sensitivity for detection of tumors with a primary Gleason grade of greater than 3. However, the agreement between the 3 readers in the study was only moderate.

Serum PSA level, date and result of most recent TRUS GB, and history of previous treatment are important clinical information that can help the radiologist in the interpretation of prostate MR imaging. In addition to the peripheral zone and CG of the prostate, extraprostatic extension, tumor involvement of the neurovascular bundles, seminal vesicles, lymph nodes, and pelvic bones need to be evaluated on the prostate MR imaging report.

### Peripheral Zone Cancer

In evaluating the peripheral zone, the T1-weighted images are reviewed to exclude the presence of hemorrhage, which can obscure tumors, especially on T2-weighted images, and makes the findings difficult to evaluate (**Fig. 6**). Postbiopsy hemorrhage has been reported in 28% to 95% of patients in the literature.[22,23,55] The T2-weighted sequence is then evaluated for the presence of suspicious lesions and provides the highest resolution for visualization of tumors, zonal anatomy, capsule, neurovascular bundles, anterior fibrous stroma, and seminal vesicles.[56] In the peripheral zone, prostate cancer appears as a discrete nodule with low T2 signal (**Fig. 7**) against the intrinsic high signal of the peripheral zone. Higher Gleason components of 4 and 5 were shown to have lower T2 signal intensity than lower Gleason components of 3.[57] Tumors with low Gleason score and small tumors are more difficult to detect compared with large and high-Gleason prostate cancers. Sparse tumors (cancers intermixed with normal prostate tissue) have also been reported to be undetectable on T2-weighted sequences compared with dense tumors.[58] These sparse tumors are often of lower Gleason score.

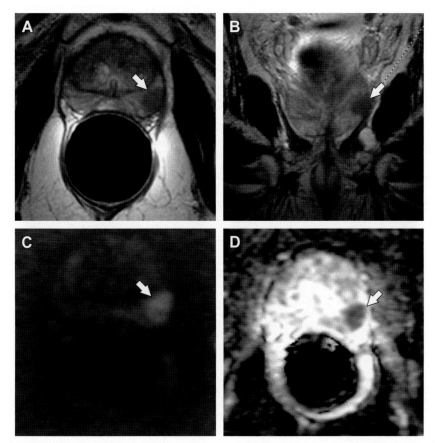

**Fig. 7.** Peripheral zone lesion. Patient with PSA 6.2 ng/mL and prostate cancer on TRUS biopsy. Axial T2 TSE (*A*) and coronal T2 TSE (*B*) images show a well-defined T2 hypointense lesion in the peripheral zone (*arrow*) with corresponding high signal on DWI (*C*) and low signal on the ADC map (*D*). Biopsy of this region was positive for Gleason 4 + 3 prostate cancer.

More recently the hemorrhage exclusion sign has been evaluated, whereby prostate tumors are outlined by postbiopsy hemorrhagic changes on T1-weighted images. The degree of hemorrhage has been shown to be significantly lower in regions of positive biopsy findings than in regions of negative biopsy findings,[55] likely because of the lower citrate content of prostate cancer relative to the normal prostate. Barrett and colleagues[23] showed that the presence of excluded hemorrhage on T1-weighted imaging in conjunction with a corresponding area of homogeneous low signal intensity at T2-weighted imaging is highly accurate for cancer identification, with a positive predictive value of 95%. **Fig. 8** shows the hemorrhage exclusion sign.

There are other causes of low T2 signal in the peripheral zone that may be confused with tumor, including hemorrhage, prostatitis, atrophy, and posttreatment changes including scarring from radiation, cryotherapy, and hormonal therapy. **Fig. 9** shows an example of prostatitis, which can be difficult to distinguish from prostate cancer.

In evaluating the peripheral zone, the currently accepted standard is to evaluate the T1-weighted and T2-weighted sequences in conjunction with the multiparametric techniques. The addition of DWI, DCE-MR imaging, and MRSI separately or in various combinations improved the diagnostic performance compared with T2 alone.[37,59–62] Low ADC value was the best-performing single variable in multiparametric analysis.[59–61] Multiparametric MR imaging may also enable the evaluation of the peripheral zone with postbiopsy hemorrhage with reasonable diagnostic accuracy.[55] The ADC value was particularly useful in distinguishing prostate cancer from postbiopsy hemorrhage.[63] In evaluating the DWI sequences, the presence of a focal area of reduced ADC is sufficient to increase the suspicion for prostate cancer even if the area is isointense on the high-b-value image ($\geq$b800 s/mm$^2$). The presence of a corresponding hyperintensity on the high-b-value image ($\geq$b800 s/mm$^2$) makes the lesion highly likely to be cancer (see **Fig. 7**).

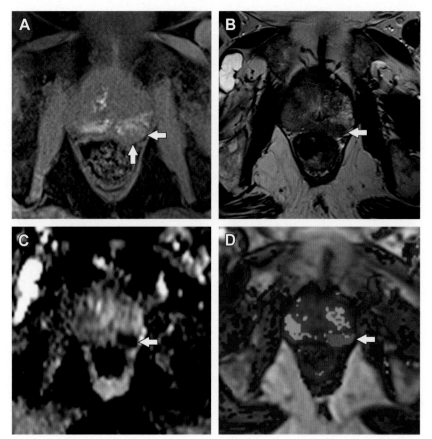

**Fig. 8.** Hemorrhage exclusion sign. Axial T1 fat-suppressed image (*A*) shows hemorrhage exclusion sign where there is well-defined area of low signal intensity surrounded by areas of high signal intensity from hemorrhage (*arrows*). The areas of low signal intensity are from tumor surrounded by the high-signal blood. Axial T2-weighted image (*B*) shows low signal intensity from the tumor (*arrow*). ADC map (*C*) shows abnormal low signal intensity from restricted diffusion at the site of prostatic cancer (*arrow*). DCE-MR imaging color map (*D*) shows abnormal perfusion kinetics (*arrow*).

## Evaluation for Extracapsular Extension and Neurovascular Bundle Invasion

Detection for extracapsular extension is one of the most important contributions of MR imaging to the work-up of patients with prostate cancer. Extension of the tumor through the prostate capsule upgrades the tumor stage to T3a. This upgrading has significant implications on the choice and approach to treatment and on the outcomes.

MR imaging has been reported to have a wide range of sensitivities (13%–95%) and specificities (49%–97%) for detection of extracapsular extension.[17,27,64–67] Multiple signs have been described to assess for extracapsular extensions:

- Breach of the capsule with evidence of direct measurable tumor extension
- Tumor encasing the neurovascular bundle
- Bulging prostate contour with loss of capsule

- Obliteration of the rectoprostatic angle
- Capsular retraction or irregularity
- Asymmetric neurovascular bundles
- A tumor-capsular interface greater than 1 cm

Although MR imaging can detect substantial extracapsular extension, its ability for detection of microscopic invasion is limited. However, it can still be used in guiding the surgeon in the selection of excision margin around the prostate. **Fig. 10** shows extracapsular extension with neurovascular bundle invasion.

## Evaluation of Seminal Vesicle Invasion

Seminal vesicle invasion (SVI) upgrades the staging to stage T3b and is associated with larger and more aggressive tumors with higher Gleason scores and with increased risk of tumor recurrence in patients treated for prostate cancer, and therefore it has important implications

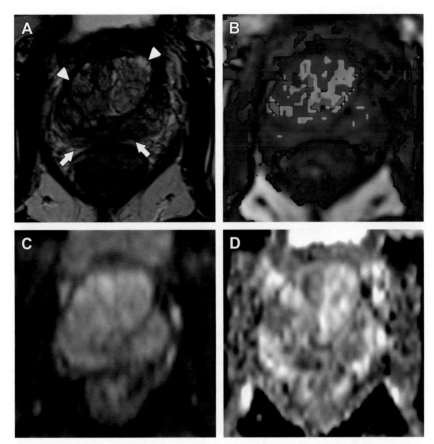

**Fig. 9.** Prostatitis. Axial T2 TSE image (*A*) shows a diffuse low-T2 signal in the peripheral zone (*arrows*). The CG is enlarged and contains multiple well-defined, T2-hyperintense, heterogeneous nodules consistent with BPH nodules (*arrowheads*). The color map from the DCE (*B*) analysis shows no suspicious enhancement kinetics in the peripheral zone. There are no lesions of high signal on the DWI b-800 image (*C*). The ADC map (*D*) shows a heterogeneous appearance with no discrete area of significant restricted diffusion. The patient had a PSA of 2.5 ng/mL. Targeted biopsy of this region as well as 12 systematic biopsies of the remainder of the peripheral zone showed chronic and acute inflammation with no evidence of prostate cancer. This case is an example of the difficulty in distinguishing prostate cancer from prostatitis. It was reasonable to the raise the question of prostate cancer on this study, but the lack of convincing restricted diffusion and suspicious enhancement kinetics should have lowered the suspicious for a high-grade prostate cancer.

for treatment and prognosis.[68,69] Endorectal MR imaging has been shown to be accurate in showing seminal vesicle invasion.[70] For detection of seminal vesicle invasion it has reported specificities of 81% to 99%, but has a range of reported sensitivities from 23% to 80%.[17,27,71,72]

MR criteria have been developed to evaluate for SVI on T2-weighted sequences:

- Demonstration of direct tumor extension from the base of the prostate into and around the seminal vesicle
- Disruption or loss of normal architecture of the seminal vesicles
- Focal low signal in the seminal vesicle (without corresponding high signal intensity on T1-weighted images at the same location)
- Enlarged low-signal-intensity seminal vesicle
- Asymmetric thickening or irregularity of the seminal vesicle wall
- Obliteration of the angle between the prostate and seminal vesicle

Enhancement and restricted diffusion can further improve the accuracy of MR imaging for detection of SVI. Soylu and colleagues[71] reported improved specificity and positive predictive value with the addition DWI. In that study DCE-MR imaging did not add incremental value to T2-weighted images and DWI and low sensitivity remained an issue even for multiparametric MR imaging. **Fig. 11** shows SVI.

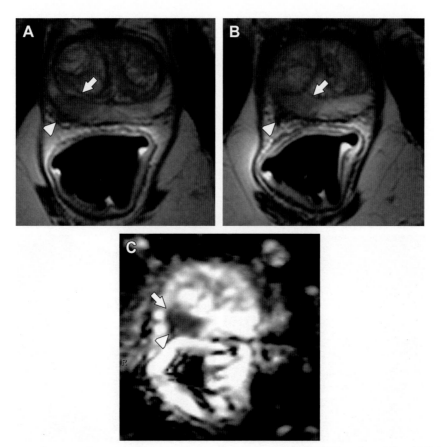

Fig. 10. Extracapsular extension and neurovascular bundle invasion. Axial T2 TSE at the midlevel (*A*) shows a T2 hypointense lesion in the right peripheral zone (*white arrow*). The overlying capsule appears irregular with a focal bulge that is suspicious for extracapsular extension (*arrowhead*). Additional axial T2 TSE more inferiorly (*B*) shows the same lesion (*white arrow*) with a capsular bulge with loss of the adjacent fat surrounding the right neurovascular bundle (*arrowhead*) suggesting neurovascular bundle invasion and further confirming the extracapsular extension of the tumor. The ADC map (*C*) obtained at the same level of the more inferior T2 image (*B*) showed restricted diffusion in the lesion (*white arrow*) that extends beyond the capsule to the neurovascular bundle (*arrowhead*). Pathology results from prostatectomy show a Gleason score of 4 + 5 prostate cancer with extracapsular extension.

## CG Cancer

CG carcinoma constitutes about 30% of all prostate cancers.[16,18] Although most CG tumors tend to show low aggressiveness,[73] the potential for disease progression remains substantial. Tumor detection in the CG is more challenging than in the peripheral zone owing to the overlap in the MR appearance between prostate cancer lesions and BPH nodules, particularly the stromal hyperplasia. The typical appearance of BPH nodules is described as organized chaos, whereas multiple nodules are present in an enlarged CG, each of which has a well-defined margin but a heterogeneous T2 signal (**Fig. 12**). In contrast, prostate cancer lesions have uniform low signal intensity on T2-weighted images (sensitivity, 76%–78%; specificity, 78%–87%) with irregular margins (sensitivity, 76%–78%; specificity, 78%–89%).[16,74,75] This appearance is described as the erased-charcoal sign (**Fig. 13**). If the lesion has a lenticular (water-drop) shape, it is more specific for prostate cancer (sensitivity, 48%–56%; specificity, 85%–98%).[16,25,74,76] Extension of the lesion in the anterior fibromuscular stroma or in the anterior horn of the peripheral zone makes the lesion highly likely to be a prostate cancer (see **Fig. 13**).

The role of multiparametric technique in the CG remains to be completely defined. Although few articles found DWI to be helpful in tumor detection in the CG,[77,78] multiple articles have found no improvement in diagnostic performance in the CG with the addition of DWI or DCE,[37,59,76,79] because of overlap in findings

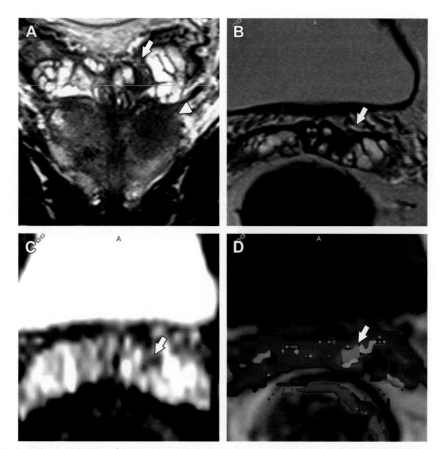

**Fig. 11.** SVI. A patient with PSA of 5.9 ng/mL. Coronal T2 TSE image (*A*) shows a lesion in the left base consistent with prostate cancer (*arrowhead*). The seminal vesicles are well distended with fluid aiding the evaluation. There is small lesion of low T2 signal in the left seminal vesicle (*arrow*) near the junction with the base of the prostate and within close proximity to the suspicious lesion in the left base of the prostate. Axial T2 TSE (*B*) shows the same lesion in the left seminal vesicle. Corresponding ADC map (*C*) shows restricted diffusion (*arrow*). Color map from DCE-MR imaging (*D*) shows suspicious enhancing kinetics displayed in red (*arrow*). Pathology results from prostatectomy showed Gleason 4 + 5 prostate cancer with SVI.

with BPH nodules. Based on these reports, T2-weighted imaging remains the most important sequence for evaluating CG cancers and distinguishing them from benign hyperplasia. The ADC map and, to a lesser extent, the DCE parameters can improve the sensitivity by highlighting areas of suspicion that should be further scrutinized on the T2-weighted imaging; however, the likelihood of cancer is best assessed on T2-weighted images. Using an ultrahigh b value of 2000 s/mm$^2$, Katahira and colleagues[37] showed the sensitivity, specificity, and accuracy for CG tumor detection to increase. Therefore, the use of ultrahigh b values (>1000 s/mm$^2$) could be of particular help in characterizing CG tumors.

The overlap in appearance between CG cancer and some BPH nodules was further examined in a study by Oto and colleagues[75] in which CG cancer foci were compared with stromal hyperplasia and glandular hyperplasia. Glandular hyperplasia had a different appearance on T2 and minimal overlap in ADC values with cancer foci; however, there was a significant overlap between stromal hyperplasia and cancer foci based on their T2 appearance and ADC values.

## Quantitative Approach and Computer-aided Diagnosis

Commercial software tools are now available that are capable of calculating the DCE parameters and displaying the DCE data and the ADC values in a fashion that allows for correlation of lesions across different sequences. The DCE pattern is often displayed as a color map that can be superimposed on or correlated with other sequences. These software tools can facilitate the interpretation of multiparametric prostate MR imaging and can ease the evaluation of regions of interest across different sequences.

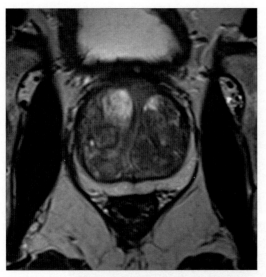

Fig. 12. BPH; organized chaos. Axial T2 TSE image shows enlargement of the CG with multiple well-defined nodules in the CG showing variable T2 signal intensities.

More recently there have been efforts in applying computer-aided diagnosis (CAD) techniques in the evaluation of prostate MR imaging.[80,81] The quantitative nature of CAD analysis can help achieve standardization of diagnostic criteria and improve the reproducibility of prostate MR imaging interpretation. In a recent article by Peng and colleagues,[80] multiple parameters including the 10th percentile pixelwise ADC, average ADC, and T2-weighted signal intensity skewness were effective in the differentiation of prostate cancer from normal peripheral zone. The 10th percentile ADC, average ADC, and $K^{trans}$ correlated moderately with the Gleason score. CAD can help radiologists to analyze the overwhelming amount of data from various MR sequences and also provide the standardization of the interpretation of prostate MR imaging.

## CLINICAL INDICATIONS
### Staging

Staging represents the most widely accepted indication for prostate MR imaging. Conventional methods of staging based on digital rectal examination, PSA, and TRUS findings result in significant levels of clinical understaging (59%) and some overstaging (5%).[82] In a meta-analysis by Engelbrecht and colleagues,[27] the use of MR imaging for cancer staging (cT2 vs cT3) had a joint maximum sensitivity and specificity of 71%. The addition of DCE-MR imaging to T2-weighted image yields improved assessment of ECE and better results for prostate cancer.[83] Although the older literature showed a wide range of accuracies in local staging, more recently Heijmink and colleagues[26] reported sensitivity of 73% to 80% and specificity of 97% to 100%. Bloch and colleagues[84] reported staging accuracy, sensitivity, and specificity of 86%, 75%, and 92%, respectively. Most recently the American College of Radiologists appropriateness criteria stated that staging for organ-confined versus extracapsular disease shows consistent accuracies of about 90%.[70] The detection of microscopic ECE and SVI remain problematic. In addition to the staging of local disease, MR imaging is useful for evaluation of pelvic lymphadenopathy in patients with high risk of disease spread.[85,86]

### Detection

The current paradigm for detection of prostate cancer has significant limitations. About 25% of cancers are missed on the initial TRUS biopsy.[87] The low diagnostic yield of TRUS biopsies leads to repeat biopsies, which have a lower detection rate than the initial biopsy.[88,89] Furthermore, the Gleason score on the TRUS biopsy matched the final Gleason score on the prostatectomy specimen in only 30% to 58%.[90,91]

Because of this current inefficient diagnostic algorithm, there is increased interest in the use of MR imaging for prostate cancer detection. MR imaging may be helpful in the evaluation of patients with increasing PSA and negative prostate biopsies.[70,92] MR imaging may be particularity useful in the diagnosis of anterior and apical tumors, which are commonly missed on the TRUS-guided biopsy.[92,93] MR imaging can help in targeting the repeat biopsies in those cases.

The data from prospective studies on the detection of prostate cancer for MR imaging are difficult to compare owing to differences in methodologies. There is a broad range of sensitivities and specificities reported using MR imaging, which ranged from 53% to 95%, and 63% to 97%, respectively.[59,94] However, these values can be significantly different between peripheral zone tumors and transition zone tumors, which is one reason for the broad range of reported values. For instance, Delongchamps and colleagues[59] reported a sensitivity and specificity of 80% and 97% respectively in the peripheral zone but only 53% and 83% in the transition zone.

Multiparametric MR imaging has been shown to be sensitive to underlying histologic changes.[75,95,96] Langer and colleagues[95] identified significant relationships between most the MR imaging parameters (quantitative T2, ADC, $K^{trans}$, and $V_e$) and tissue composition (percentage

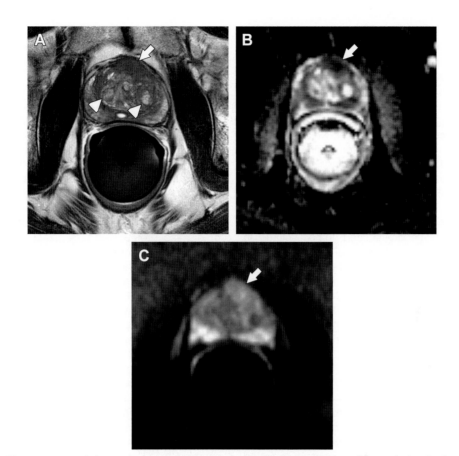

**Fig. 13.** CG tumor; erased-charcoal appearance. Axial T2 TSE (*A*) shows a T2-hypointense lesion in the anterior-most apex of the CG (*arrow*). The lesion has poorly defined margins and has a homogeneous low-T2 signal with the characteristic erased-charcoal appearance. This appearance is in contrast with the BPH nodules (*arrowhead*), which typically have well-defined margins. ADC map (*B*) shows corresponding dark signal (*arrow*) and DWI (*C*) shows a bright signal indicating restricted diffusion (*arrow*).

areas of nuclei, cytoplasm, stroma, and luminal space) and observed significant differences in MR imaging and tissue component values between prostate cancer and normal prostate tissue. It has been reported that there are fundamental histologic differences between detected and missed prostate tumors using MR imaging.[96] The histologic features that were different included size, Gleason score, and solid growth. These findings may provide reasons for the low detection rate in some studies and may also explain in part the overlap in findings between malignancy and other benign conditions of the prostate. Multiple studies have shown a significant difference in detection rates based on size[47,97,98] and Gleason score.[97–99] Tumors less than 5 mm are difficult to detect, whereas tumors larger than 10 mm are more readily detectable. Tumors of Gleason 3 + 3 are less likely to be detected than tumors of Gleason greater than or equal to 4 + 3. An additional factor that lowers

the detection rate of prostate cancer is a subset of prostate cancer that is described as sparse tumors, in which the prostate cancer is intermixed with normal tissue and there tends to be similar ADC and T2 values to those of normal peripheral zone tissue.[58]

## Localization

MR techniques can provide useful information about the location and size of prostate cancer. Accurate localization offers the potential for targeted biopsy, improves and supports focused intensity-modulated radiation therapy planning of the dominant prostatic lesion, and assists guidance of minimally invasive focal therapies.

As with the other indication for prostate MR imaging, the sensitivity and specificity of endorectal T2-weighted MR imaging prostate cancer localization vary, ranging from 54% to 91% and 27% to 91%, respectively.[79,100–102] The values at the higher end of the range reflect studies in which multiparametric techniques were used and showed improved localization; however, there are also conflicting results from other studies in which multiparametric techniques were not shown to improve the localization performance.[39,47,102]

Multiparametric MR imaging may also have a role in assessing tumor volume, which may have prognostic implications as well as affecting treatment choice. Nakashima and colleagues[103] showed a good correlation of the tumor diameter between MR imaging and histopathology for tumors larger than 1 cm based on T2-weighted imaging. Using DCE-MR imaging, Lemaitre and colleagues[104] underestimated tumor volume in 7% to 40% of cases depending on the tumor size, with the best correlation obtained for intermediate-sized tumors and worse correlation for smaller and larger tumors. Mazaheri and colleagues[105] reported that combined T2-weighted imaging and DWI can significantly improve the accuracy of prostate peripheral zone tumor volume measurement compared with T2 alone.

## Assessing Aggressiveness

Multiparametric MR imaging may have the potential of providing information about the biologic aggressiveness of prostate cancer. Numerous studies have shown a significant association between the ADC value and the Gleason score.[39,106–110] Rastinehad and colleagues[111] showed statistically significant correlation between the suspicion of lesions on MR imaging and the D'Amico risk stratification of the lesion after targeted biopsy. A negative correlation between the ADC value and the Gleason score as well as the D'Amico clinical risk score was also reported by Turkbey and colleagues.[112] In some of these studies the ADC was shown to be a good discriminator of low-risk, intermediate-risk, and high-risk cancer.[109,112] Although the ADC value is the most reported parameter to have strong association with the Gleason score, other parameters have also been reported. In one study, $K^{trans}$ was reported to be moderately correlated with the Gleason score,[80] whereas in another the washout gradient was the only parameter that correlated with the Gleason score.[45] Multiple other studies have showed a correlation between the MR spectroscopy parameters and the Gleason score.[110,113]

The data on assessing tumor aggressiveness are strong and promising, but the correlation between MR parameters and Gleason score are not strong enough to allow immediate clinical implementation. Further research is needed to improve the ability of MR imaging in identification of aggressive prostate cancer, which is the principal goal of prostate cancer management.

## Role of MR imaging in Active Surveillance

As an increasing percentage of patients are diagnosed at early stage with expected slow progression of the disease, there is a growing adoption of active surveillance protocols. In active surveillance, patients with favorable-risk prostate cancer are monitored using annual serum PSA, digital rectal examination, and TRUS GB with appropriate treatment provided to patients who show evidence of disease progression. The exact definition of favorable-risk prostate cancer varied between studies but generally included some combination of Gleason 6 or less, no Gleason pattern of 4 or 5, PSA 10 ng/mL or less, PSA density of less than 0.2 ng/mL per cm$^3$, clinical local stage of T2 or lower, no more than 3 positive core biopsies, and no core greater than 50% involved.[114,115] The limitations of this approach arise because of a high possibility of underestimating the disease on the initial biopsy with subsequent upgrade in up to one-third of the patients.[116,117] In particular, patients with anterior tumor represented a notable component of those failing active surveillance[118] because the anterior gland is often undersampled.[13,14] The emerging role of active surveillance combined with the limitations of the current paradigm call for more accurate ways in selecting the appropriate patients for active surveillance as well as a less invasive method for following them. MR imaging is well suited to play a potential role in active surveillance given its established and potential usefulness in tumor detection, volume estimation, and assessment of aggressiveness as well as biopsy guidance. MR imaging can potentially play 2 roles in surveillance protocols. First, it can play a role in patient selection for active surveillance. Abnormal prostate MR imaging results suggesting cancer were reported to be associated with increased risk with Gleason score upgrade on subsequent biopsy.[119,120] The ADC value was also reported to be an independent predictor of adverse repeat biopsy findings and shorter time to radical treatment.[121] Second, MR imaging can be used to monitor patients who are on active surveillance. In a study by Giles and colleagues,[122] ADC values at repeat biopsy were significantly lower in patients in whom the Gleason increased as opposed to those with stable Gleason score. The tumor volume and the ADC values were independent predictors of histologic progression. Similar correlation between low ADC values and adverse histology on repeat biopsy and shorter time to deferred radical treatment were reported by van As and colleagues.[123]

Similar to other indications for MR imaging, large-scale studies may be needed before there is a widespread integration of MR imaging into active surveillance protocols; however, the initial results are promising for an emerging role.[124]

### Image-guided Interventions

MR imaging of the prostate has created the opportunity for targeted biopsies and intervention in the prostate. Targeted biopsies of suspicious lesions on MR imaging promise to significantly improve the accuracy of prostate biopsy and ameliorate the limitations of the current biopsy paradigm. MR can aid prostate biopsy in 3 ways. In MR imaging–directed TRUS GB (also referred to as cognitive registration), the sectors that contained suspicious lesions on MR imaging are sampled using TRUS GB. Information from MR imaging is conveyed to the urologist performing the TRUS GB either verbally or via mutually designed prostate diagrams. Targeted core biopsies are most often obtained in addition to the standard systematic cores. Multiple studies have reported improved yield of biopsies when directed by MR imaging results.[125–132] These studies have reported on the accuracy of various combinations of T2-weighted, DCE MR imaging, ADC, and MRSI in directing the biopsies, with a general trend toward improved targeting using multiparametric techniques. In a systematic review, Moore and colleagues[133] compared the outcomes for MR imaging–directed biopsy alone with systematic biopsy and reported that both techniques detected cancer in an equivalent number of men. However, in MR imaging–directed biopsy, this was achieved using fewer biopsies, with a reduction in the diagnosis of clinically insignificant cancer. A limitation of MR imaging–directed TRUS biopsy is that the suspicious lesion is often not directly visualized on TRUS and thus there is a degree of subjectivity in targeting the lesion. An emerging technique that promises to mitigate this limitation is the MR-TRUS fusion–guided biopsy. Preprocedural MR imaging data are fused with real-time TRUS to direct the needle under real-time TRUS guidance into the tumor-suspicious regions identified previously on MR imaging. Studies have reported improved detection with MR-TRUS fusion–guided biopsy compared with systemic biopsy.[132,134,135] In a study by Portalez and colleagues[136] designed to validate the European Society of Urogenital Radiology scoring system of prostate cancer, MR imaging/3D TRUS fusion technology was used to guide biopsies to suspicious lesions

identified on MR imaging. Fusion-targeted biopsies were 11-fold more likely to show cancer than random cores. The suspicion score correlated with the probability of positive biopsies, whereas 83% of the most suspicious lesions had positive biopsies compared with 3% of the least suspicious lesions. Using MR imaging/ultrasonography fusion, Pinto and colleagues[134] likewise reported a higher detection rate for more suspicion lesions than for the less suspicious lesions. In addition, MR imaging can be used to directly guide the biopsy in real-time (in-bore MR-guided biopsies). A T2-weighted fast spin echo sequence is typically used to localize the region of interest, an MR imaging–compatible needle and guide are directed toward the lesion, and a T2-weighted sequence is used to confirm the position of the needle in the tumor-suspicious region.[137] A transrectal approach in a closed-bore magnet is the most commonly used approach in the recent literature.[137] The prostate cancer detection rates at MR imaging–guided biopsy in most of these studies ranged from 38% to 59% following negative TRUS GB.[12,138–145] This rate compares favorably with a detection rate of 10% to 17% on repeat TRUS-guided biopsy.[143,146]

Based on these results and others, Ahmed and colleagues[147] proposed a new strategy of performing the MR imaging before the biopsy, thereby eliminating the biopsy-related artifacts, improving the biopsy yield, and potentially avoiding some biopsies. Furthermore, Rosenkrantz and colleagues[148] reported 100% sensitivity for MR imaging in predicting the presence of tumor on subsequent biopsy, making MR imaging an attractive potential alternative in the prebiopsy work-up of patients. Although a few centers are already performing MR imaging before biopsy, a widespread acceptance of this shift in work-up strategy would require larger studies validating its diagnostic accuracy as well as discussing its cost-effectiveness. Guidelines on which patients would be best served by this strategy may also be needed.

In addition to directing biopsy, localization of prostate cancer by MR imaging is enabling focal therapy for tumors under MR imaging guidance. The goal of focal therapy is to eradicate known cancer foci and to minimize damage to surrounding prostate tissue with the intention of preserving normal urinary and sexual function.[149] Some ablative techniques are in the early stages of investigation, including laser ablation, cryoablation, photodynamic ablation, electroporation, and HIFU ablation. In addition to localizing the targeted tumor, MR imaging can direct the ablation device, thermally monitor the ablation, and depict the ablated tissue. A phase 1 trial of focal laser ablation has recently shown feasibility and safety in clinically low-risk prostate cancer.[150] MR imaging–guided focal cryoablation of the prostate in patients with local recurrence after radiation therapy was also recently shown to be feasible and safe.[151] The oncologic efficacy and impact of these focal therapy methods on patient outcomes need to be further evaluated with phase II and III studies.

### Posttreatment Evaluation

Increasing PSA after treatment of prostate cancer indicates local recurrence, metastatic disease, or both. MR imaging can detect local recurrences after radical prostatectomy or radiation therapy and can also be used as an imaging tool for the whole body for detection of metastatic disease. Local recurrence after prostatectomy is a frequent occurrence[152,153] and it is often diagnosed based on increase in PSA (>0.2 ng/mL). The clinical dilemma becomes distinguishing local recurrence from metastasis. Multiparametric MR is useful in evaluating the prostatic fossa after prostatectomy in patients with biochemical recurrence. The accuracy of MR imaging for detecting recurrence depends on the size of the recurrence and on the PSA value. The reported sensitivities varied from 85% to 97% and the reported specificities from 90% to 100%.[154–156] It is increasingly common that patients present with suspected local recurrence based on mild increase in the PSA (<1 ng/mL) with no clinically palpable disease. The data on the diagnostic performance of MR imaging in these patients are sparse. Liauw and colleagues[157] reported their experience with 88 patients after radical prostatectomy referred to salvage radiotherapy evaluation with no clinically palpable recurrence and with a median PSA of 0.3 (interquartile range, 0.19–0.71) who were further evaluated by endorectal MR imaging. The likelihood of radiologists identifying local

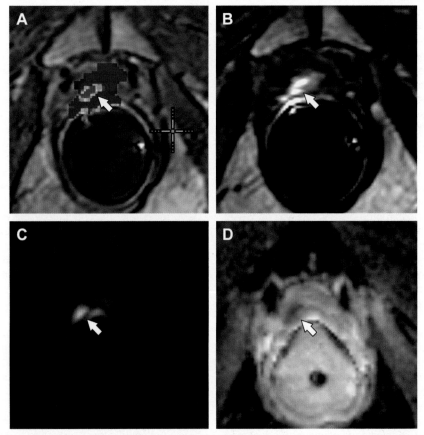

**Fig. 14.** Local recurrence after prostatectomy. A 64-year-old patient with increasing PSA after prostatectomy and radiation. Color map from DCE-MR imaging (A) analysis shows a focal area of suspicious kinetics depicted in red in the prostate bed, consistent with local recurrence (*arrow*). A corresponding image from the DCE data set (B) shows the hyperenhancement of the focus of recurrence (*arrow*). DWI b-800 image (C) and ADC map (D) show corresponding restricted diffusion (*arrow*). This focus of recurrence was difficult to see on the T2 sequence.

recurrence on MR imaging related to the PSA level. The incidence of radiologic local recurrence by PSA was 8% for PSA less than or equal to 0.19 ng/mL, 18% for PSA 0.19 to less than or equal to 0.30 ng/mL, 35% for PSA 0.30 to less than or equal to 0.72 ng/mL, and 38% for PSA greater than 0.72 ng/mL ($P = .04$). In evaluating patients after prostatectomy, we recommend that particular attention be paid to DCE-MR imaging (**Fig. 14**). Unlike in evaluating the prostate gland, for which DCE-MR imaging lacks specificity, in the prostatectomy bed it is a more useful sequence and can be quite specific. Multiple studies agree that DCE-MR imaging is the most useful sequence in detecting local recurrence[154–156]; however, more recently Panebianco and colleagues[156] reported that DWI showed an accuracy that approached that of DCE-MR imaging. The most common site of recurrence is at the vesicourethral anastomosis (67%–76%) followed by the retrovesical region around the seminal vesicle bed and the resection site of the vas deferens (22%–33%).[157,158]

Likewise, in the evaluation of patients for biochemical recurrence after external beam radiation therapy, the multiparametric approach is essential, particularly because the T2-weighted sequences are not as sensitive after radiation therapy because of radiation-induced changes to the signal of the peripheral zone. DCE-MR imaging is reported to be accurate with high interobserver agreement[159] and with small reports of reasonable sensitivity and specificity of 72% to 93% and 85% to 100%, respectively.[160,161] Tamada and colleagues[162] investigated the use of DCE-MR imaging and DWI after brachytherapy in 16 patients with biochemical recurrence and reported sensitivity and specificity of 50% and 98% for DCE-MR imaging and 68% and 95% for DWI. Donati and colleagues[163] reported that the combination of T2-weighted images and DWI resulted in significantly better diagnostic accuracy compared with T2-weighted alone and that the addition of DCE-MR imaging did not further improve the accuracy.

## SUMMARY

MR imaging of the prostate is playing an increasing role in the management of prostate cancer. T2-weighted imaging and DWI are the most promising components of the well-accepted multiparametric prostate MR imaging. In addition to more conventional indications such as preoperative staging, emerging and promising indications for prostate MR imaging include cancer localization before biopsies using MR-ultrasonography fusion and focal therapies,

triage and follow-up of patients for active surveillance, and posttreatment follow-up. There is a need for standardization of image acquisition and interpretation techniques and validating the role of MR imaging in large, multicenter trials in these emerging clinical indications.

## REFERENCES

1. Siegel R, Naishadham D, Jemal A. Cancer statistics, 2013. CA Cancer J Clin 2013;63(1):11–30.
2. Siegel R, Naishadham D, Jemal A. Cancer statistics, 2012. CA Cancer J Clin 2012;62(1):10–29.
3. Albertsen PC. The unintended burden of increased prostate cancer detection associated with prostate cancer screening and diagnosis. Urology 2010; 75(2):399–405.
4. Moyer VA. Screening for prostate cancer: U.S. Preventive Services Task Force recommendation statement. Ann Intern Med 2012;157(2):120–34.
5. Hodge KK, McNeal JE, Terris MK, et al. Random systematic versus directed ultrasound guided transrectal core biopsies of the prostate. J Urol 1989;142(1):71–4 [discussion: 74–5].
6. Raja J, Ramachandran N, Munneke G, et al. Current status of transrectal ultrasound-guided prostate biopsy in the diagnosis of prostate cancer. Clin Radiol 2006;61(2):142–53.
7. Durkan GC, Sheikh N, Johnson P, et al. Improving prostate cancer detection with an extended-core transrectal ultrasonography-guided prostate biopsy protocol. BJU Int 2002;89(1):33–9.
8. Presti JC Jr, Chang JJ, Bhargava V, et al. The optimal systematic prostate biopsy scheme should include 8 rather than 6 biopsies: results of a prospective clinical trial. J Urol 2000;163(1):163–6 [discussion: 166–7].
9. Thompson IM, Pauler DK, Goodman PJ, et al. Prevalence of prostate cancer among men with a prostate-specific antigen level < or =4.0 ng per milliliter. N Engl J Med 2004;350(22):2239–46.
10. Yakar D, Hambrock T, Hoeks C, et al. Magnetic resonance-guided biopsy of the prostate: feasibility, technique, and clinical applications. Topics in magnetic resonance imaging. Top Magn Reson Imaging 2008;19(6):291–5.
11. Chun FK, Steuber T, Erbersdobler A, et al. Development and internal validation of a nomogram predicting the probability of prostate cancer Gleason sum upgrading between biopsy and radical prostatectomy pathology. Eur Urol 2006;49(5):820–6.
12. Franiel T, Stephan C, Erbersdobler A, et al. Areas suspicious for prostate cancer: MR-guided biopsy in patients with at least one transrectal US-guided biopsy with a negative finding–multiparametric MR imaging for detection and biopsy planning. Radiology 2011;259:162–72.

13. Lawrentschuk N, Haider MA, Daljeet N, et al. 'Prostatic evasive anterior tumours': the role of magnetic resonance imaging. BJU Int 2010;105(9):1231–6.

14. Bott SR, Young MP, Kellett MJ, et al, Contributors to the UCLHTRPD. Anterior prostate cancer: is it more difficult to diagnose? BJU Int 2002;89(9):886–9.

15. Partin AW, Mangold LA, Lamm DM, et al. Contemporary update of prostate cancer staging nomograms (Partin tables) for the new millennium. Urology 2001;58(6):843–8.

16. Akin O, Sala E, Moskowitz CS, et al. Transition zone prostate cancers: features, detection, localization, and staging at endorectal MR imaging. Radiology 2006;239(3):784–92.

17. Bonekamp D, Jacobs MA, El-Khouli R, et al. Advancements in MR imaging of the prostate: from diagnosis to interventions. Radiographics 2011; 31(3):677–703.

18. McNeal JE, Redwine EA, Freiha FS, et al. Zonal distribution of prostatic adenocarcinoma. Correlation with histologic pattern and direction of spread. Am J Surg Pathol 1988;12(12):897–906.

19. Vargas HA, Akin O, Franiel T, et al. Normal central zone of the prostate and central zone involvement by prostate cancer: clinical and MR imaging implications. Radiology 2012;262(3):894–902.

20. Cohen RJ, Shannon BA, Phillips M, et al. Central zone carcinoma of the prostate gland: a distinct tumor type with poor prognostic features. J Urol 2008;179(5):1762–7.

21. Ayala AG, Ro JY, Babaian R, et al. The prostatic capsule: does it exist? Its importance in the staging and treatment of prostatic carcinoma. Am J Surg Pathol 1989;13(1):21–7.

22. White S, Hricak H, Forstner R, et al. Prostate cancer: effect of postbiopsy hemorrhage on interpretation of MR images. Radiology 1995;195(2):385–90.

23. Barrett T, Vargas HA, Akin O, et al. Value of the hemorrhage exclusion sign on T1-weighted prostate MR images for the detection of prostate cancer. Radiology 2012;263(3):751–7.

24. Qayyum A, Coakley FV, Lu Y, et al. Organ-confined prostate cancer: effect of prior transrectal biopsy on endorectal MRI and MR spectroscopic imaging. Am J Roentgenol 2004;183(4):1079–83.

25. Barentsz JO, Richenberg J, Clements R, et al. ESUR prostate MR guidelines 2012. Eur Radiol 2012;22(4):746–57.

26. Heijmink SW, Fütterer JJ, Hambrock T, et al. Prostate cancer: body-array versus endorectal coil MR Imaging at 3 T—comparison of image quality, localization, and staging performance. Radiology 2007;244(1):184–95.

27. Engelbrecht MR, Jager GJ, Laheij RJ, et al. Local staging of prostate cancer using magnetic resonance imaging: a meta-analysis. Eur Radiol 2002; 12(9):2294–302.

28. Sosna J, Pedrosa I, Dewolf WC, et al. MR imaging of the prostate at 3 tesla: comparison of an external phased-array coil to imaging with an endorectal coil at 1.5 tesla. Acad Radiol 2004;11(8): 857–62.

29. Beyersdorff D, Taupitz M, Winkelmann B, et al. Patients with a history of elevated prostate-specific antigen levels and negative transrectal US-guided quadrant or sextant biopsy results: value of MR imaging. Radiology 2002;224(3):701–6.

30. Turkbey B, Merino MJ, Gallardo EC, et al. Comparison of endorectal coil and nonendorectal coil T2W and diffusion-weighted MRI at 3 Tesla for localizing prostate cancer: correlation with whole-mount histopathology. J Magn Reson Imaging 2013. http://dx.doi.org/10.1002/jmri.24317.

31. Dickinson L, Ahmed HU, Allen C, et al. Magnetic resonance imaging for the detection, localisation, and characterisation of prostate cancer: recommendations from a European Consensus Meeting. Eur Urol 2011;59(4):477–94.

32. Rosenkrantz AB, Neil J, Kong X, et al. Prostate cancer: comparison of 3D T2-weighted with conventional 2D T2-weighted imaging for image quality and tumor detection. Am J Roentgenol 2010; 194(2):446–52.

33. Cornud F, Rouanne M, Beuvon F, et al. Endorectal 3D T2-weighted 1 mm-slice thickness MRI for prostate cancer staging at 1.5 Tesla: should we reconsider the indirects signs of extracapsular extension according to the D'Amico tumor risk criteria? Eur J Radiol 2012;81(4):e591–7.

34. Metens T, Miranda D, Absil J, et al. What is the optimal b value in diffusion-weighted MR imaging to depict prostate cancer at 3T? Eur Radiol 2012; 22(3):703–9.

35. Rosenkrantz AB, Hindman N, Lim RP, et al. Diffusion-weighted imaging of the prostate: comparison of b1000 and b2000 image sets for index lesion detection. J Magn Reson Imaging 2013;38(3): 694–700.

36. Kitajima K, Takahashi S, Ueno Y, et al. Clinical utility of apparent diffusion coefficient values obtained using high b-value when diagnosing prostate cancer using 3 tesla MRI: comparison between ultra-high b-value (2000 s/mm$^2$) and standard high b-value (1000 s/mm$^2$). J Magn Reson Imaging 2012;36(1):198–205.

37. Katahira K, Takahara T, Kwee T, et al. Ultra-high-b-value diffusion-weighted MR imaging for the detection of prostate cancer: evaluation in 201 cases with histopathological correlation. Eur Radiol 2011;21(1):188–96.

38. Ueno Y, Kitajima K, Sugimura K, et al. Ultra-high b-value diffusion-weighted MRI for the detection of prostate cancer with 3-T MRI. J Magn Reson Imaging 2013;38(1):154–60.

39. Vargas HA, Akin O, Franiel T, et al. Diffusion-weighted endorectal MR imaging at 3 T for prostate cancer: tumor detection and assessment of aggressiveness. Radiology 2011;259(3):775–84.

40. Verma S, Turkbey B, Muradyan N, et al. Overview of dynamic contrast-enhanced MRI in prostate cancer diagnosis and management. Am J Roentgenol 2012;198(6):1277–88.

41. Bonekamp D, Macura KJ. Dynamic contrast-enhanced magnetic resonance imaging in the evaluation of the prostate. Top Magn Reson Imaging 2008;19(6):273–84.

42. Isebaert S, De Keyzer F, Haustermans K, et al. Evaluation of semi-quantitative dynamic contrast-enhanced MRI parameters for prostate cancer in correlation to whole-mount histopathology. Eur J Radiol 2012;81(3):e217–22.

43. Kim JK, Hong SS, Choi YJ, et al. Wash-in rate on the basis of dynamic contrast-enhanced MRI: usefulness for prostate cancer detection and localization. J Magn Reson Imaging 2005;22(5):639–46.

44. Valentini AL, Gui B, Cina A, et al. T2-weighted hypointense lesions within prostate gland: differential diagnosis using wash-in rate parameter on the basis of dynamic contrast-enhanced magnetic resonance imaging–hystopatology correlations. Eur J Radiol 2012;81(11):3090–5.

45. Chen Y-J, Chu W-C, Pu Y-S, et al. Washout gradient in dynamic contrast-enhanced MRI is associated with tumor aggressiveness of prostate cancer. J Magn Reson Imaging 2012;36(4):912–9.

46. Verma S, Rajesh A, Futterer JJ, et al. Prostate MRI and 3D MR spectroscopy: how we do it. AJR Am J Roentgenol 2010;194(6):1414–26.

47. Weinreb JC, Blume JD, Coakley FV, et al. Prostate cancer: sextant localization at MR imaging and MR spectroscopic imaging before prostatectomy—results of ACRIN Prospective Multi-institutional Clinicopathologic Study. Radiology 2009;251(1):122–33.

48. Villeirs GM, De Meerleer GO, De Visschere PJ, et al. Combined magnetic resonance imaging and spectroscopy in the assessment of high grade prostate carcinoma in patients with elevated PSA: a single-institution experience of 356 patients. Eur J Radiol 2011;77(2):340–5.

49. Casciani E, Polettini E, Bertini L, et al. Contribution of the MR spectroscopic imaging in the diagnosis of prostate cancer in the peripheral zone. Abdom Imaging 2007;32(6):796–802.

50. Fütterer JJ, Engelbrecht MR, Huisman HJ, et al. Staging prostate cancer with dynamic contrast-enhanced endorectal MR Imaging prior to radical prostatectomy: experienced versus less experienced readers. Radiology 2005;237(2):541–9.

51. Wassberg C, Akin O, Vargas HA, et al. The incremental value of contrast-enhanced MRI in the detection of biopsy-proven local recurrence of prostate cancer after radical prostatectomy: effect of reader experience. Am J Roentgenol 2012;199(2):360–6.

52. Mullerad M, Hricak H, Wang L, et al. Prostate cancer: detection of extracapsular extension by genitourinary and general body radiologists at MR imaging. Radiology 2004;232(1):140–6.

53. Rosenkrantz AB, Kim S, Lim RP, et al. Prostate cancer localization using multiparametric MR imaging: comparison of Prostate Imaging Reporting and Data System (PI-RADS) and Likert Scales. Radiology 2013;269(2):482–92.

54. Roethke MC, Kuru TH, Schultze S, et al. Evaluation of the ESUR PI-RADS scoring system for multiparametric MRI of the prostate with targeted MR/TRUS fusion-guided biopsy at 3.0 Tesla. Eur Radiol 2013; 24(2):344–52.

55. Tamada T, Sone T, Jo Y, et al. Prostate cancer: relationships between postbiopsy hemorrhage and tumor detectability at MR diagnosis. Radiology 2008;248(2):531–9.

56. Turkbey B, Choyke PL. Multiparametric MRI and prostate cancer diagnosis and risk stratification. Curr Opin Urol 2012;22(4):310–5. http://dx.doi.org/10.1097/MOU.0b013e32835481c2.

57. Wang L, Mazaheri Y, Zhang J, et al. Assessment of biologic aggressiveness of prostate cancer: correlation of MR signal intensity with Gleason grade after radical prostatectomy. Radiology 2008;246(1):168–76.

58. Langer DL, van der Kwast TH, Evans AJ, et al. Intermixed normal tissue within prostate cancer: effect on MR imaging measurements of apparent diffusion coefficient and T2—sparse versus dense cancers. Radiology 2008;249(3):900–8.

59. Delongchamps NB, Rouanne M, Flam T, et al. Multiparametric magnetic resonance imaging for the detection and localization of prostate cancer: combination of T2-weighted, dynamic contrast-enhanced and diffusion-weighted imaging. BJU Int 2011;107(9):1411–8.

60. Langer DL, van der Kwast TH, Evans AJ, et al. Prostate cancer detection with multi-parametric MRI: logistic regression analysis of quantitative T2, diffusion-weighted imaging, and dynamic contrast-enhanced MRI. J Magn Reson Imaging 2009;30(2):327–34.

61. Isebaert S, Van den Bergh L, Haustermans K, et al. Multiparametric MRI for prostate cancer localization in correlation to whole-mount histopathology. J Magn Reson Imaging 2012;37(6): 1392–401.

62. Turkbey B, Pinto PA, Mani H, et al. Prostate cancer: value of multiparametric MR imaging at 3 T for detection—histopathologic correlation. Radiology 2010;255(1):89–99.

63. Rosenkrantz AB, Kopec M, Kong X, et al. Prostate cancer vs. post-biopsy hemorrhage: diagnosis with T2- and diffusion-weighted imaging. J Magn Reson Imaging 2010;31(6):1387–94.

64. Ogura K, Maekawa S, Okubo K, et al. Dynamic endorectal magnetic resonance imaging for local staging and detection of neurovascular bundle involvement of prostate cancer: correlation with histopathologic results. Urology 2001;57(4):721–6.

65. Rosenkrantz AB, Chandarana H, Gilet A, et al. Prostate cancer: utility of diffusion-weighted imaging as a marker of side-specific risk of extracapsular extension. J Magn Reson Imaging 2012;38(2): 312–9.

66. Outwater EK, Petersen RO, Siegelman ES, et al. Prostate carcinoma: assessment of diagnostic criteria for capsular penetration on endorectal coil MR images. Radiology 1994;193(2):333–9.

67. Cornud F, Flam T, Chauveinc L, et al. Extraprostatic spread of clinically localized prostate cancer: factors predictive of pT3 tumor and of positive endorectal MR imaging examination results. Radiology 2002;224(1):203–10.

68. Pierorazio PM, Ross AE, Schaeffer EM, et al. A contemporary analysis of outcomes of adenocarcinoma of the prostate with seminal vesicle invasion (pT3b) after radical prostatectomy. J Urol 2011;185(5):1691–7.

69. Sapre N, Pedersen J, Hong MK, et al. Re-evaluating the biological significance of seminal vesicle invasion (SVI) in locally advanced prostate cancer. BJU Int 2012;110:58–63.

70. Eberhardt SC, Carter S, Casalino DD, et al. ACR Appropriateness Criteria Prostate Cancer—pretreatment detection, staging, and surveillance. J Am Coll Radiol 2013;10(2):83–92.

71. Soylu FN, Peng Y, Jiang Y, et al. Seminal Vesicle invasion in prostate cancer: evaluation by using multiparametric endorectal MR imaging. Radiology 2013;267(3):797–806.

72. Sala E, Akin O, Moskowitz CS, et al. Endorectal MR imaging in the evaluation of seminal vesicle invasion: diagnostic accuracy and multivariate feature analysis. Radiology 2006;238(3):929–37.

73. Noguchi M, Stamey TA, Neal JE, et al. An analysis of 148 consecutive transition zone cancers: clinical and histological characteristics. J Urol 2000; 163(6):1751–5.

74. Li H, Sugimura K, Kaji Y, et al. Conventional MRI capabilities in the diagnosis of prostate cancer in the transition zone. Am J Roentgenol 2006;186(3): 729–42.

75. Oto A, Kayhan A, Jiang Y, et al. Prostate cancer: differentiation of central gland cancer from benign prostatic hyperplasia by using diffusion-weighted and dynamic contrast-enhanced MR imaging. Radiology 2010;257(3):715–23.

76. Hoeks CM, Hambrock T, Yakar D, et al. Transition Zone prostate cancer: detection and localization with 3-T multiparametric MR imaging. Radiology 2013;266(1):207–17.

77. Turkbey B, Mani H, Shah V, et al. Multiparametric 3T prostate magnetic resonance imaging to detect cancer: histopathological correlation using prostatectomy specimens processed in customized magnetic resonance imaging based molds. J Urol 2011;186(5):1818–24.

78. Jung SI, Donati OF, Vargas HA, et al. Transition zone prostate cancer: incremental value of diffusion-weighted endorectal MR imaging in tumor detection and assessment of aggressiveness. Radiology 2013;269(2):493–503.

79. Haider MA, van der Kwast TH, Tanguay J, et al. Combined T2-weighted and diffusion-weighted MRI for localization of prostate cancer. Am J Roentgenol 2007;189(2):323–8.

80. Peng Y, Jiang Y, Yang C, et al. Quantitative analysis of multiparametric prostate MR images: differentiation between prostate cancer and normal tissue and correlation with Gleason score—a computer-aided diagnosis development study. Radiology 2013;267(3):787–96.

81. Sung YS, Kwon HJ, Park BW, et al. Prostate cancer detection on dynamic contrast-enhanced MRI: computer-aided diagnosis versus single perfusion parameter maps. AJR Am J Roentgenol 2011; 197(5):1122–9.

82. Bostwick DG. Staging prostate cancer–1997: current methods and limitations. Eur Urol 1997; 32(Suppl 3):2–14.

83. Bloch BN, Furman-Haran E, Helbich TH, et al. Prostate cancer: accurate determination of extracapsular extension with high-spatial-resolution dynamic contrast-enhanced and T2-weighted MR imaging—initial results. Radiology 2007;245(1):176–85.

84. Bloch BN, Genega E, Costa D, et al. Prediction of prostate cancer extracapsular extension with high spatial resolution dynamic contrast-enhanced 3-T MRI. Eur Radiol 2012;22(10):2201–10.

85. Greene KL, Albertsen PC, Babaian RJ, et al. Prostate specific antigen best practice statement: 2009 update. J Urol 2009;182(5):2232–41.

86. Mohler J, Bahnson RR, Boston B, et al. Prostate cancer. J Natl Compr Canc Netw 2010;8(2): 162–200.

87. Roehl KA, Antenor JA, Catalona WJ. Serial biopsy results in prostate cancer screening study. J Urol 2002;167(6):2435–9.

88. Djavan B, Ravery V, Zlotta A, et al. Prospective evaluation of prostate cancer detected on biopsies 1, 2, 3 and 4: when should we stop? J Urol 2001; 166(5):1679–83.

89. Mian BM, Naya Y, Okihara K, et al. Predictors of cancer in repeat extended multisite prostate

biopsy in men with previous negative extended multisite biopsy. Urology 2002;60(5):836–40.

90. Cookson MS, Fleshner NE, Soloway SM, et al. Correlation between Gleason score of needle biopsy and radical prostatectomy specimen: accuracy and clinical implications. J Urol 1997; 157(2):559–62.

91. Steinberg DM, Sauvageot J, Piantadosi S, et al. Correlation of prostate needle biopsy and radical prostatectomy Gleason grade in academic and community settings. Am J Surg Pathol 1997; 21(5):566–76.

92. Heidenreich A, Bellmunt J, Bolla M, et al. EAU guidelines on prostate cancer. Part 1: screening, diagnosis, and treatment of clinically localised disease. Eur Urol 2011;59(1):61–71.

93. Nix JW, Turkbey B, Hoang A, et al. Very distal apical prostate tumours: identification on multiparametric MRI at 3 Tesla. BJU Int 2012;110(11 Pt B): E694–700.

94. Tamada T, Sone T, Higashi H, et al. Prostate cancer detection in patients with total serum prostate-specific antigen levels of 4-10 ng/mL: diagnostic efficacy of diffusion-weighted imaging, dynamic contrast-enhanced MRI, and T2-weighted imaging. AJR Am J Roentgenol 2011; 197(3):664–70.

95. Langer DL, van der Kwast TH, Evans AJ, et al. Prostate tissue composition and MR measurements: investigating the relationships between ADC, T2, K(trans), v(e), and corresponding histologic features. Radiology 2010;255(2):485–94.

96. Rosenkrantz AB, Mendrinos S, Babb JS, et al. Prostate cancer foci detected on multiparametric magnetic resonance imaging are histologically distinct from those not detected. J Urol 2012; 187(6):2032–8.

97. Kirkham AP, Emberton M, Allen C. How good is MRI at detecting and characterising cancer within the prostate? Eur Urol 2006;50(6):1163–75.

98. Vargas HA, Wassberg C, Akin O, et al. MR imaging of treated prostate cancer. Radiology 2012;262(1): 26–42.

99. Doo K, Sung D, Park B, et al. Detectability of low and intermediate or high risk prostate cancer with combined T2-weighted and diffusion-weighted MRI. Eur Radiol 2012;22(8):1812–9.

100. Scheidler J, Hricak H, Vigneron DB, et al. Prostate cancer: localization with three-dimensional proton MR spectroscopic imaging – clinicopathologic study. Radiology 1999;213(2):473–80.

101. Fütterer JJ, Heijmink SW, Scheenen TW, et al. Prostate cancer localization with dynamic contrast-enhanced MR imaging and proton MR spectroscopic imaging. Radiology 2006;241(2):449–58.

102. Hoeks CM, Barentsz JO, Hambrock T, et al. Prostate cancer: multiparametric MR imaging for detection, localization, and staging. Radiology 2011;261(1):46–66.

103. Nakashima J, Tanimoto A, Imai Y, et al. Endorectal MRI for prediction of tumor site, tumor size, and local extension of prostate cancer. Urology 2004; 64(1):101–5.

104. Lemaitre L, Puech P, Poncelet E, et al. Dynamic contrast-enhanced MRI of anterior prostate cancer: morphometric assessment and correlation with radical prostatectomy findings. Eur Radiol 2009; 19(2):470–80.

105. Mazaheri Y, Hricak H, Fine SW, et al. Prostate tumor volume measurement with combined T2-weighted imaging and diffusion-weighted MR: correlation with pathologic tumor volume. Radiology 2009; 252(2):449–57.

106. Yoshimitsu K, Kiyoshima K, Irie H, et al. Usefulness of apparent diffusion coefficient map in diagnosing prostate carcinoma: correlation with stepwise histopathology. J Magn Reson Imaging 2008;27(1):132–9.

107. Tamada T, Sone T, Jo Y, et al. Apparent diffusion coefficient values in peripheral and transition zones of the prostate: comparison between normal and malignant prostatic tissues and correlation with histologic grade. J Magn Reson Imaging 2008;28(3): 720–6.

108. Verma S, Rajesh A, Morales H, et al. Assessment of aggressiveness of prostate cancer: correlation of apparent diffusion coefficient with histologic grade after radical prostatectomy. AJR Am J Roentgenol 2011;196(2):374–81.

109. Hambrock T, Somford DM, Huisman HJ, et al. Relationship between apparent diffusion coefficients at 3.0-T MR imaging and Gleason grade in peripheral zone prostate cancer. Radiology 2011;259(2):453–61.

110. Kobus T, Vos PC, Hambrock T, et al. Prostate cancer aggressiveness: in vivo assessment of MR spectroscopy and diffusion-weighted imaging at 3 T. Radiology 2012;265(2):457–67.

111. Rastinehad AR, Baccala AA Jr, Chung PH, et al. D'Amico risk stratification correlates with degree of suspicion of prostate cancer on multiparametric magnetic resonance imaging. J Urol 2011;185(3): 815–20.

112. Turkbey B, Shah VP, Pang Y, et al. Is apparent diffusion coefficient associated with clinical risk scores for prostate cancers that are visible on 3-T MR images? Radiology 2011;258(2):488–95.

113. Zakian KL, Sircar K, Hricak H, et al. Correlation of proton MR spectroscopic imaging with Gleason score based on step-section pathologic analysis after radical prostatectomy. Radiology 2005; 234(3):804–14.

114. Klotz L, Zhang L, Lam A, et al. Clinical results of long-term follow-up of a large, active surveillance

cohort with localized prostate cancer. J Clin Oncol 2010;28(1):126–31.

115. Stattin P, Holmberg E, Johansson JE, et al. Outcomes in localized prostate cancer: National Prostate Cancer Register of Sweden follow-up study. J Natl Cancer Inst 2010;102(13):950–8.

116. Ouzzane A, Puech P, Villers A. MRI and surveillance. Curr Opin Urol 2012;22(3):231–6.

117. Porten SP, Whitson JM, Cowan JE, et al. Changes in prostate cancer grade on serial biopsy in men undergoing active surveillance. J Clin Oncol 2011;29(20):2795–800.

118. Duffield AS, Lee TK, Miyamoto H, et al. Radical prostatectomy findings in patients in whom active surveillance of prostate cancer fails. J Urol 2009; 182(5):2274–9.

119. Fradet V, Kurhanewicz J, Cowan JE, et al. Prostate cancer managed with active surveillance: role of anatomic MR imaging and MR spectroscopic imaging. Radiology 2010;256(1):176–83.

120. Vargas HA, Akin O, Afaq A, et al. Magnetic resonance imaging for predicting prostate biopsy findings in patients considered for active surveillance of clinically low risk prostate cancer. J Urol 2012; 188(5):1732–8.

121. deSouza NM, Riches SF, VanAs NJ, et al. Diffusion-weighted magnetic resonance imaging: a potential non-invasive marker of tumour aggressiveness in localized prostate cancer. Clin Radiol 2008;63(7): 774–82.

122. Giles SL, Morgan VA, Riches SF, et al. Apparent diffusion coefficient as a predictive biomarker of prostate cancer progression: value of fast and slow diffusion components. AJR Am J Roentgenol 2011;196(3):586–91.

123. van As NJ, de Souza NM, Riches SF, et al. A study of diffusion-weighted magnetic resonance imaging in men with untreated localised prostate cancer on active surveillance. Eur Urol 2009;56(6):981–8.

124. Turkbey B, Mani H, Aras O, et al. Prostate cancer: can multiparametric MR imaging help identify patients who are candidates for active surveillance? Radiology 2013;268(1):144–52.

125. Lawrentschuk N, Fleshner N. The role of magnetic resonance imaging in targeting prostate cancer in patients with previous negative biopsies and elevated prostate-specific antigen levels. BJU Int 2009;103(6):730–3.

126. Kumar V, Jagannathan NR, Kumar R, et al. Transrectal ultrasound-guided biopsy of prostate voxels identified as suspicious of malignancy on three-dimensional (1)H MR spectroscopic imaging in patients with abnormal digital rectal examination or raised prostate specific antigen level of 4-10 ng/ml. NMR Biomed 2007;20(1):11–20.

127. Sciarra A, Panebianco V, Ciccariello M, et al. Value of magnetic resonance spectroscopy imaging and dynamic contrast-enhanced imaging for detecting prostate cancer foci in men with prior negative biopsy. Clin Cancer Res 2010;16(6):1875–83.

128. Cheikh AB, Girouin N, Colombel M, et al. Evaluation of T2-weighted and dynamic contrast-enhanced MRI in localizing prostate cancer before repeat biopsy. Eur Radiol 2009;19(3):770–8.

129. Watanabe Y, Nagayama M, Araki T, et al. Targeted biopsy based on ADC map in the detection and localization of prostate cancer: a feasibility study. J Magn Reson Imaging 2013;37(5):1168–77.

130. Watanabe Y, Terai A, Araki T, et al. Detection and localization of prostate cancer with the targeted biopsy strategy based on ADC Map: a prospective large-scale cohort study. J Magn Reson Imaging 2012;35(6):1414–21.

131. Haffner J, Lemaitre L, Puech P, et al. Role of magnetic resonance imaging before initial biopsy: comparison of magnetic resonance imaging-targeted and systematic biopsy for significant prostate cancer detection. BJU Int 2011;108(8 Pt 2):E171–8.

132. Puech P, Rouvière O, Renard-Penna R, et al. Prostate cancer diagnosis: multiparametric MR-targeted biopsy with cognitive and transrectal US–MR fusion guidance versus systematic biopsy—prospective multicenter study. Radiology 2013;268(2):461–9.

133. Moore CM, Robertson NL, Arsanious N, et al. Image-guided prostate biopsy using magnetic resonance imaging–derived targets: a systematic review. Eur Urol 2013;63(1):125–40.

134. Pinto PA, Chung PH, Rastinehad AR, et al. Magnetic resonance imaging/ultrasound fusion guided prostate biopsy improves cancer detection following transrectal ultrasound biopsy and correlates with multiparametric magnetic resonance imaging. J Urol 2011;186(4):1281–5.

135. Natarajan S, Marks LS, Margolis DJ, et al. Clinical application of a 3D ultrasound-guided prostate biopsy system. Urol Oncol 2011;29(3):334–42.

136. Portalez D, Mozer P, Cornud F, et al. Validation of the European Society of Urogenital radiology scoring system for prostate cancer diagnosis on multiparametric magnetic resonance imaging in a cohort of repeat biopsy patients. Eur Urol 2012; 62(6):986–96.

137. Yacoub JH, Verma S, Moulton JS, et al. Imaging-guided prostate biopsy: conventional and emerging techniques. Radiographics 2012;32(3): 819–37.

138. Zangos S, Eichler K, Engelmann K, et al. MR-guided transgluteal biopsies with an open low-field system in patients with clinically suspected prostate cancer: technique and preliminary results. Eur Radiol 2005;15(1):174–82.

139. Engelhard K, Hollenbach H, Kiefer B, et al. Prostate biopsy in the supine position in a standard 1.5-T

scanner under real time MR-imaging control using a MR-compatible endorectal biopsy device. Eur Radiol 2006;16(6):1237–43.

140. Hambrock T, Futterer JJ, Huisman HJ, et al. Thirty-two-channel coil 3T magnetic resonance-guided biopsies of prostate tumor suspicious regions identified on multimodality 3T magnetic resonance imaging: technique and feasibility. Invest Radiol 2008;43(10):686–94.

141. Anastasiadis AG, Lichy MP, Nagele U, et al. MRI-guided biopsy of the prostate increases diagnostic performance in men with elevated or increasing PSA levels after previous negative TRUS biopsies. Eur Urol 2006;50(4):738–48 [discussion: 748–9].

142. Beyersdorff D, Winkel A, Hamm B, et al. MR imaging-guided prostate biopsy with a closed MR unit at 1.5 T: initial results. Radiology 2005;234(2):576–81.

143. Hambrock T, Somford DM, Hoeks C, et al. Magnetic resonance imaging guided prostate biopsy in men with repeat negative biopsies and increased prostate specific antigen. J Urol 2010;183(2):520–7.

144. Roethke M, Anastasiadis AG, Lichy M, et al. MRI-guided prostate biopsy detects clinically significant cancer: analysis of a cohort of 100 patients after previous negative TRUS biopsy. World J Urol 2012;30(2):213–8.

145. Hoeks CM, Schouten MG, Bomers JG, et al. Three-Tesla magnetic resonance–guided prostate biopsy in men with increased prostate-specific antigen and repeated, negative, random, systematic, transrectal ultrasound biopsies: detection of clinically significant prostate cancers. Eur Urol 2012;62(5):902–9.

146. Pondman KM, Futterer JJ, ten Haken B, et al. MR-guided biopsy of the prostate: an overview of techniques and a systematic review. Eur Urol 2008; 54(3):517–27.

147. Ahmed HU, Kirkham A, Arya M, et al. Is it time to consider a role for MRI before prostate biopsy? Nat Rev Clin Oncol 2009;6(4):197–206.

148. Rosenkrantz AB, Mussi TC, Borofsky MS, et al. 3.0 T multiparametric prostate MRI using pelvic phased-array coil: utility for tumor detection prior to biopsy. Urol Oncol 2013;31(8):1430–5.

149. Bomers JG, Sedelaar JP, Barentsz JO, et al. MRI-guided interventions for the treatment of prostate cancer. AJR Am J Roentgenol 2012;199(4):714–20.

150. Oto A, Sethi I, Karczmar G, et al. MR imaging–guided focal laser ablation for prostate cancer: phase I trial. Radiology 2013;267(3):932–40.

151. Bomers JG, Yakar D, Overduin CG, et al. MR imaging–guided focal cryoablation in patients with recurrent prostate cancer. Radiology 2013;268(2):451–60.

152. Han M, Partin AW, Zahurak M, et al. Biochemical (prostate specific antigen) recurrence probability following radical prostatectomy for clinically localized prostate cancer. J Urol 2003;169(2):517–23.

153. Freedland SJ, Presti JC Jr, Amling CL, et al. Time trends in biochemical recurrence after radical prostatectomy: results of the SEARCH database. Urology 2003;61(4):736–41.

154. Cirillo S, Petracchini M, Scotti L, et al. Endorectal magnetic resonance imaging at 1.5 Tesla to assess local recurrence following radical prostatectomy using T2-weighted and contrast-enhanced imaging. Eur Radiol 2009;19(3):761–9.

155. Sciarra A, Panebianco V, Salciccia S, et al. Role of dynamic contrast-enhanced magnetic resonance (MR) imaging and proton MR spectroscopic imaging in the detection of local recurrence after radical prostatectomy for prostate cancer. Eur Urol 2008; 54(3):589–600.

156. Panebianco V, Barchetti F, Sciarra A, et al. Prostate cancer recurrence after radical prostatectomy: the role of 3-T diffusion imaging in multi-parametric magnetic resonance imaging. Eur Radiol 2013; 23(6):1745–52.

157. Liauw SL, Pitroda SP, Eggener SE, et al. Evaluation of the prostate bed for local recurrence after radical prostatectomy using endorectal magnetic resonance imaging. Int J Radiat Oncol Biol Phys 2013;85(2):378–84.

158. Nguyen DP, Giannarini G, Seiler R, et al. Local recurrence after retropubic radical prostatectomy for prostate cancer does not exclusively occur at the anastomotic site. BJU Int 2013;112(4):E243–9.

159. Rouvière O, Valette O, Grivolat S, et al. Recurrent prostate cancer after external beam radiotherapy: value of contrast-enhanced dynamic MRI in localizing intraprostatic tumor—correlation with biopsy findings. Urology 2004;63(5):922–7.

160. Haider MA, Chung P, Sweet J, et al. Dynamic contrast-enhanced magnetic resonance imaging for localization of recurrent prostate cancer after external beam radiotherapy. Int J Radiat Oncol Biol Phys 2008;70(2):425–30.

161. Kara T, Akata D, Akyol F, et al. The value of dynamic contrast-enhanced MRI in the detection of recurrent prostate cancer after external beam radiotherapy: correlation with transrectal ultrasound and pathological findings. Diagn Interv Radiol 2011;17(1):38–43.

162. Tamada T, Sone T, Jo Y, et al. Locally recurrent prostate cancer after high-dose-rate brachytherapy: the value of diffusion-weighted imaging, dynamic contrast-enhanced MRI, and T2-weighted imaging in localizing tumors. AJR Am J Roentgenol 2011;197(2):408–14.

163. Donati OF, Jung SI, Vargas HA, et al. Multiparametric prostate MR imaging with T2-weighted, diffusion-weighted, and dynamic contrast-enhanced sequences: are all pulse sequences necessary to detect locally recurrent prostate cancer after radiation therapy? Radiology 2013;268(2):440–50.

# MR Angiography of the Abdomen and Pelvis

Jad Bou Ayache, MD[a], Jeremy D. Collins, MD[b],*

## KEYWORDS

- MR angiography • Abdominal vascular imaging • Pelvic vascular imaging • MR venography
- Transplant vascular imaging

## KEY POINTS

- Magnetic resonance (MR) angiography relies on spoiled gradient-echo imaging with the administration of gadolinium-based contrast media. Mask subtraction is used to increase the conspicuity of the vasculature.
- MR angiography can be performed well at either 1.5 or 3 T. Imaging at 3 T offers the advantage of longer T1 relaxivity, which further suppresses signal from background nonvascular tissue.
- Noncontrast MR angiographic techniques are available from all manufacturers. Sequences can be optimized for evaluation of the arteries and veins in the abdomen and pelvis. Many of these techniques rely on balanced, steady-state free precession pulse sequences.
- MR angiography enables assessment of the mesenteric arteries, renal arteries, and pelvic arteries. The dynamic nature of the acquisition permits simultaneous evaluation of the arterial and venous vasculature.
- Congenital venous anomalies and abdominopelvic venous thrombosis are assessed well with MR angiography. Although all gadolinium-based contrast media are able to evaluate the venous vasculature with late-phase acquisitions, blood pool contrast agents with steady-state imaging are ideal for this application.
- MR angiography is an important complementary diagnostic modality in the vascular evaluation of solid organ transplants by Doppler ultrasonography. Noncontrast techniques have extended its availability to patients with renal dysfunction.
- Representative standard clinical protocols for contrast-enhanced MR angiography, noncontrast MR angiography, and MR venography are listed in **Boxes 1–3**, respectively.

## INTRODUCTION

Magnetic resonance (MR) angiography is a robust technique that complements other diagnostic imaging modalities for imaging the vasculature. Although lacking the spatial resolution of computed tomography (CT), the lack of ionizing radiation, improved contrast resolution, and ability to image in multiple phases of contrast enhancement are several of the advantages of MR angiography for assessment of the vasculature. MR angiography has traditionally relied on contrast-enhanced spoiled gradient-echo techniques to evaluate the vasculature of the abdomen and pelvis.[1] Mask

Funding Sources: None.

Conflicts of Interest: Northwestern University Department of Radiology has a research agreement with Siemens Medical Systems.

[a] Department of Radiology, Northwestern University, 737 North Michigan Avenue, Suite 1600, Chicago, IL 60611, USA; [b] Divisions of Cardiovascular Imaging and Interventional Radiology, Department of Radiology, Northwestern University, 737 North Michigan Avenue, Suite 1600, Chicago, IL 60611, USA

* Corresponding author. Department of Radiology, Northwestern University Feinberg School of Medicine, 737 North Michigan Avenue, Suite 1600, Chicago, IL 60611.

E-mail address: collins@fsm.northwestern.edu

Radiol Clin N Am 52 (2014) 839–859
http://dx.doi.org/10.1016/j.rcl.2014.02.017

subtraction is commonly used to reduce signal from background tissues, and generate postprocessed maximum-intensity projection and volume-rendered images of the vasculature.

Multiple contrast agents are available for contrast-enhanced MR angiography. Most are considered extracellular contrast agents, which freely distribute out of the vasculature into the interstitium. Imaging with these contrast agents relies primarily on careful timing of the contrast arrival with the acquisition of the central lines of k-space in the vessel of interest to optimize vascular conspicuity. Gadolinium-based blood pool contrast agents are also available, which bind reversibly to albumin. These agents achieve a prolonged vascular dwell time and enable steady-state venous and arterial imaging. Although both types of gadolinium-based contrast agents generate robust first-pass MR angiographic images, imaging protocols need to be optimized to take full advantage of steady-state imaging with blood pool contrast agents.

Although patients with stage 3 renal insufficiency are commonly imaged with gadolinium-based contrast media, these agents are not routinely administered to patients with stage 4 or 5 renal insufficiency, owing to concerns regarding the risk for nephrogenic systemic fibrosis (NSF). A systemic disease associated with exposure to gadolinium-based contrast media, the risk of NSF is greatest in patients with stage 4 or 5 renal insufficiency and those on chronic dialysis. Noncontrast MR angiographic techniques offer safe diagnostic imaging options for these patients.

Noncontrast MR imaging techniques have shown promise for vascular imaging of the abdomen and pelvis. Noncontrast techniques optimized for both arterial and venous assessment are available from most MR scanner manufacturers. Familiarity with the pulse sequences is necessary to appropriately apply these in the abdomen and pelvis, optimizing for arterial and/or venous evaluation. When optimized for the vascular region of interest, noncontrast techniques can clearly depict the vasculature often with image quality similar to that of subtracted contrast-enhanced techniques.

## MR ANGIOGRAPHIC TECHNIQUES
### Contrast-Enhanced MR Angiography

First-pass gadolinium-enhanced MR angiography is the mainstay of MR vascular imaging protocols (**Box 1**). This technique relies on an infusion of gadolinium contrast, timed carefully to initiate the acquisition coinciding with contrast arrival in the vasculature of interest. The length of the contrast

---

**Box 1**
**MR angiography protocol for abdomen and pelvis**

*Contrast*

Normal glomerular filtration rate (GFR): double-dose extravascular contrast agent, or gadofosveset trisodium 0.12 mL/kg

Decreased GFR (30–59 mL/min/1.73 m$^2$): gadofosveset trisodium 0.12 mL/kg, or single dose extravascular contrast agent

*Acquisition*

Scout

Axial half-Fourier acquisition single-shot turbo spin echo (HASTE)

Coronal HASTE

Axial pregadolinium 3D gradient echo[a]

Coronal pregadolinium 3D gradient echo[a]

Timing bolus

3D MR angiography[a]

   Slab thickness depending on area of interest

   Partition thickness 1–1.5 mm

Axial postgadolinium 3D gradient echo

Coronal postgadolinium 3D gradient echo

*Postprocessing*

MIP reconstructions as needed

   [a] Breath-hold.

---

bolus must be carefully optimized with the duration of the acquisition to minimize signal contamination from venous structures. For first-pass MR angiography, tricks of k-space sampling are used to build in a buffer between the length of the contrast bolus and the acquisition time. The central lines of k-space are filled initially, contributing to image contrast, while the peripheral lines are filled afterwards, contributing to image sharpness. This action mitigates the influence of slight differences in arterial transit on image quality of MR angiography. Mask subtraction is applied to further improve the conspicuity of the arteries.

Abdominal and pelvic MR angiography is often performed with multiple phases of imaging. Each phase is acquired sequentially, separated by breath-holds. This approach enables visualization of the pelvic, portal, and systemic veins (**Fig. 1**). The same mask acquisition is applied across all angiographic phases.

Time-resolved MR angiography (TR-MRA) is another contrast-enhanced technique applied in abdominal and pelvic MR imaging. Important

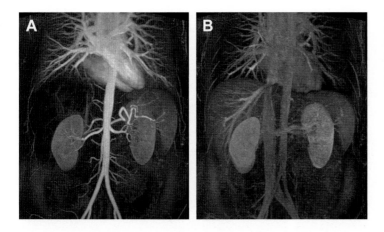

**Fig. 1.** Contrast-enhanced magnetic resonance (MR) angiography of the abdomen and pelvis. Arterial (*A*) and venous (*B*) phase acquisitions are displayed using a maximum-intensity projection (MIP) technique.

trade-offs are made to achieve a very short effective temporal resolution or frame update time. Similar to first-pass MR angiography, a mask acquisition is acquired and used to subtract from subsequent contrast-enhanced phases. A short, effective temporal resolution is achieved by sharing k-space data between adjacent phases (viewsharing) and varying the update rates of the central and peripheral lines of k-space. By varying the number of slices and phase-encoding steps, a range of effective temporal resolutions can be achieved. This technique is commonly used to query retrograde flow in the gonadal veins in patients with chronic pelvic pain. TR-MRA can also be used to demonstrate collateral arterial and venous pathways.

## Noncontrast Techniques for Abdomen and Pelvis

All scanner manufacturers have embraced noncontrast MR angiographic solutions for vascular imaging (**Box 2**). Noncontrast techniques should be considered to augment contrast-enhanced approaches or avoid the need for contrast media. Approaches for noncontrast arterial and venous imaging have been optimized. The principal limitations to the application of noncontrast angiographic techniques in the abdomen and pelvis are (1) nonvascular, nonrespiratory motion, (2) acquisition times beyond a comfortable breath-hold necessitating respiratory gating, and (3) a limited field of view. A comprehensive review of noncontrast MR angiographic techniques is outside the scope of this article. However, 3 techniques are particularly useful for vascular assessment in the abdomen and pelvis.

3-Dimensional (3D) MR angiography with balanced steady-state free precession (bSSFP) takes advantage of the native bright blood signal

of this technique, depending on the T2/T1 ratio.[2] A volume of tissue is imaged, with suppression of the stationary tissue and a dedicated venous suppression volume, to depict the arterial vasculature in a region of interest. Signal intensity depends on vascular inflow with a user-specified inflow time. Although signal loss can occur in regions of flow acceleration, as the technique depends on inflow the visualization of distal branches excludes critical arterial stenoses and increases reader confidence (**Fig. 2**).

Quiescent interval single-shot (QISS) MR angiography is an emerging technique for arterial and venous imaging in the abdomen and pelvis.[3] This technique is based on a 2-dimensional (2D) bSSFP pulse sequence. To improve arterial conspicuity, QISS MR angiography combines

---

**Box 2**
**Noncontrast MR angiography**

*Contrast*

None

*Acquisition*

Scout

Axial and coronal HASTE

Axial and coronal bSSFP

3D MR angiography precontrast mask

Quiescent interval single-shot (ECG gated, 3 average)[a]

For optimal imaging the images should be orthogonal to blood flow

3D bSSFP (ECG gated)[b]

± Coronal 3D short-tau inversion recovery[b]

[a] Breath-hold.
[b] Free breathing.

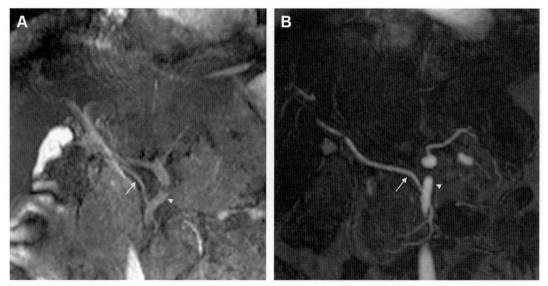

**Fig. 2.** 3-Dimensional (3D) balanced steady-state free precession (bSSFP) noncontrast MR angiography (*A*) and contrast-enhanced MR angiography (*B*), demonstrating a replaced right hepatic artery (*arrow*) arising from the proximal superior mesenteric artery (*arrowhead*).

stationary tissue suppression, a dedicated fat-saturation pulse, and a venous inflow suppression pulse with electrocardiographic (ECG) gating for diastolic acquisition. Applications in the abdomen integrate concatenated breath-holds, dividing a slab of 70 3-mm slices into 5 breath-holds. This technique is well suited for imaging the abdominal aorta and aortic branches orthogonal to the imaging slices (**Fig. 3**). When optimized, noncontrast techniques can approach the diagnostic utility

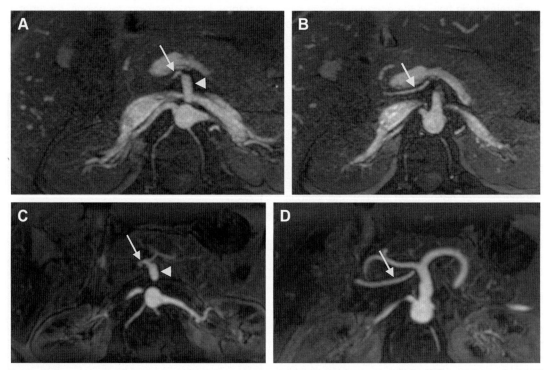

**Fig. 3.** Quiescent interval single-shot (QISS) MR angiography (*A, B*) and contrast-enhanced MR angiography (*C, D*) demonstrate a replaced right hepatic artery (*arrow*) arising from the proximal superior mesenteric artery (*arrowhead*), coursing into the right upper quadrant.

of contrast-enhanced MR angiography (see **Fig. 10B–D**).

3D T2-weighted short-tau inversion recovery (STIR) is a useful technique for evaluating the arteries and veins in the abdomen and pelvis. As this technique is not based on bSSFP pulse sequences, it is complementary to the previously discussed techniques for abdominal and pelvic vascular assessment. Although this technique has primarily been evaluated for MR neurography,[4] the authors have found it useful for evaluating the vasculature of the abdomen and pelvis. The veins in particular are well depicted with 3D T2 STIR (**Fig. 4**). Although a respiratory navigator can be applied, in the authors' experience it is not necessary in patients with a regular breathing pattern.

### Field-Strength Considerations

MR angiography performs well at 1.5 T because of the strong T1-shortening effect of the paramagnetic rare earth element gadolinium. At higher field strengths, the T1 relaxation of tissues is prolonged. Although the relaxivity of gadolinium-based contrast media is similar at 1.5 and 3 T, the longer T1 of background tissues at 3 T increases the conspicuity of vascular enhancement. This process translates into improved vascular contrast to noise for contrast-enhanced spoiled gradient-echo MR angiography, and potentially enables MR angiography with lower doses of contrast. Finally, higher fields generate superior signal-to-noise ratios and enable higher-resolution imaging while providing improved

flexibility, with choice of flip angle to reduce the specific absorption ratio and shorten the acquisition time.

### Contrast Agents

Contrast-enhanced MR angiography is performed clinically using either extracellular or blood pool contrast agents. Extracellular contrast agents freely distribute into the perivascular interstitium. MR angiographic protocols with these agents rely primarily on optimizing TR-MRA or first-pass MR angiographic techniques during the first pass of the contrast agent. Timing the MR angiography acquisition with peak enhancement of the vascular structure of interest is critical to achieving superior image quality with extracellular contrast agents.

Blood pool contrast agents enable flexible protocols that take advantage of both the first-pass acquisition and angiographic imaging in the steady state of vascular enhancement. The only blood pool contrast agent approved for use by the Food and Drug Administration is gadofosveset trisodium, which binds reversibly to albumin, achieving 79.8% and 87.4% albumin protein binding at 3 minutes and 4 hours, respectively.[5] Binding to albumin enables this agent to maintain 56% of the peak early plasma concentration at 1 hour. Steady-state imaging can be performed with high-resolution 3D T1-weighted gradient-echo sequences with submillimeter isotropic voxels in the pelvis, whereby breath-holding is not necessary (**Fig. 5**). Respiratory navigator-based sequences may be necessary in the abdomen to achieve a desired spatial resolution in the steady

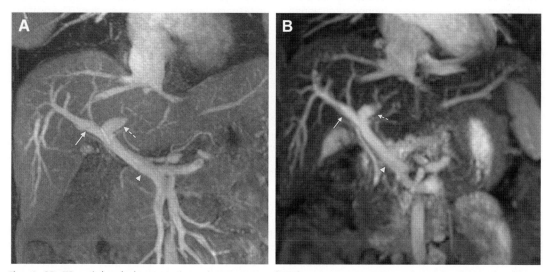

**Fig. 4.** 3D T2-weighted short-tau inversion recovery (STIR) noncontrast MR angiography (*A*) and contrast-enhanced MR angiography (*B*) demonstrate wide patency of the main (*arrowhead*), left (*dashed arrow*), and right (*solid arrow*) portal veins.

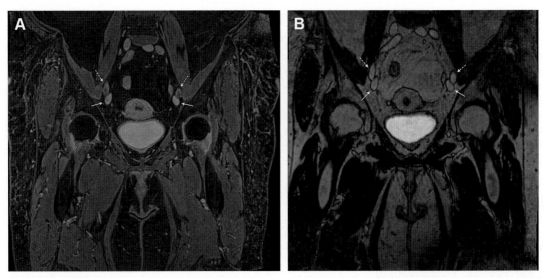

**Fig. 5.** Steady-state imaging with a blood pool contrast agent. (*A*) 3D T1-weighted gradient-echo image and (*B*) 3D bSSFP acquisition with a respiratory navigator clearly demonstrate patency in the pelvic arteries (*dashed arrow*) and veins (*solid arrow*).

state (see **Fig. 5**). Blood pool contrast agents are most useful for venous imaging or to extend the volume of MR angiographic coverage to several regions of the body in a single examination.

## CLINICAL APPLICATIONS: ARTERIAL IMAGING
### Renal Artery Stenosis

Hypertension is a common condition affecting 1 in 5 adults. The majority (90%) of hypertension is idiopathic or essential, with secondary hypertension accounting for the remainder. Renovascular hypertension is the most common type of secondary hypertension, and has higher prevalence among patients with severe hypertension and end-stage renal disease. There are numerous causes of reduced renal perfusion with resultant renovascular hypertension, the most common being renal artery stenosis secondary to either atherosclerotic disease (90%) or fibromuscular dysplasia (FMD) (10%). Other less common causes include vasculitis, atheroembolic disease, dissection, posttraumatic occlusion, and extrinsic compression of a renal artery or the kidney itself.

MR angiography leads the American College of Radiology guidelines appropriateness criteria to evaluate patients with high index of suspicion of renovascular hypertension with normal slightly diminished renal function, sharing the classification with CT in the normal renal function group and Doppler ultrasonography in the diminished renal function group.[6,7]

Extrarenal structures must be evaluated in every MR angiogram of the renal arteries. Adrenal masses such as pheochromocytoma and functioning adenomas may be the cause of secondary hypertension. The para-aortic sympathetic chains, including the organ of Zuckerkandl, may harbor extra-adrenal pheochromocytoma, and this can and should be ruled out on every MR angiography examination.

Identification of the anatomy of the renal arteries should be the first step in analyzing renal MR angiography. The number of vessels should be identified, because accessory renal arteries are common variants and may contribute to renovascular hypertension. This aspect is also important in planning interventions and surgery. The distribution of disease can suggest the underlying etiology. Atherosclerosis often involves the ostium or proximal vessel with coexistent aortic atherosclerotic disease, whereas FMD classically involves the mid to distal portions of the renal arteries. Assessment of the renal parenchyma is essential, including cortical thickness, organ size, and symmetry, as renal infarcts can sometimes point to the symptomatic organ. This evaluation is easily performed using a T2-weighted sequence such as half-Fourier acquisition single-shot turbo spin echo or postcontrast T1-weighted 2D and 3D gradient-echo images.

FMD is more common in young women (<40 years), and affects the distal two-thirds of the artery. Several pathologic classifications are present: intimal fibroplasia (10%), medial FMD (75%–80%), perimedial fibroplasia (10%–15%), medial hyperplasia (1%–2%), and adventitial fibroplasia (<1%). Medial FMD is the most common subtype, presenting as discrete web-like stenoses and small saccular aneurysms resembling a string of beads angiographically (**Fig. 6**). Involvement may be focal (**Fig. 7**), segmental, or diffuse. Perimedial fibroplasia also displays a string-of-beads appearance but usually forms fewer and smaller aneurysms. The narrowing in this subtype may be substantial. Intimal fibroplasia, on the other hand, presents as a smooth tubular or concentric focal narrowing (**Fig. 8**).[8] The remaining two subtypes are rare and are not discussed further. The finding of FMD should prompt a search for involvement of other vessels including the carotid and intracerebral vessels, mesenteric arteries, and iliac arteries.[8]

Atherosclerotic disease is the most common cause of renovascular hypertension. The distribution usually spans the proximal third of the renal artery, predominantly the ostium (**Fig. 9**). The plaque is usually an extension of contiguous abdominal aortic atherosclerotic plaque. Although atherosclerotic disease is more common in elderly patients, with a slight male predominance, it may coexist with FMD (see **Fig. 6**). The distinction between FMD and atherosclerosis is essential because management differs greatly. Percutaneous transluminal angioplasty is the primary therapy for FMD,[9] although large, multicenter, randomized controlled studies have proven that medical therapy and renal artery stenting have similar outcomes in management of hemodynamically significant atherosclerotic disease.[10,11]

Dissections can be a cause of renovascular hypertension, and are more common in patients with atherosclerosis, FMD, or vasculitis, and patients with previous endovascular or surgical aortic manipulation. The appearance of dissection is usually an abrupt cutoff or decrease in caliber of the artery, usually accompanied by poststenotic dilatation.

## Mesenteric Artery Stenosis and Flow-Related Aneurysms

Isolated mesenteric artery stenosis is often unrecognized clinically, owing to the abundance of collateral pathways in the mesentery. As flow is diverted through collateral pathways to bypass a hemodynamically significant proximal mesenteric stenosis, flow-related aneurysms may develop. This section discusses challenges in evaluating the significance of celiac axis stenosis and potential complications from flow-related aneurysms.

### Median arcuate ligament syndrome

Compression of the median arcuate ligament is a common variant present in 12% to 49% of the population. It is important to differentiate isolated imaging findings of compression-associated celiac stenosis from median arcuate ligament syndrome (MALS) with the clinical presentation of abdominal pain. The cause of abdominal pain in MALS may be related to mesenteric ischemia caused by celiac axis stenosis or compression of the celiac plexus by the median arcuate ligament.[12] Celiac artery compression manifests as downward displacement of the vessel with narrowing (**Fig. 10**). This ligament is formed by muscle fibers attaching the right and left diaphragmatic crura defining the anterior aortic hiatus. The abnormality has been implicated in mesenteric ischemia; however, the clinical significance of the extent of celiac artery narrowing is controversial. Celiac narrowing resulting from associated compression of the median arcuate ligament is accentuated at end-expiration, with the least amount of dynamic compression occurring at end-inspiration. Therefore, when assessing for the potential hemodynamic implications of compression of the median arcuate ligament, it is advised to acquire images in end-inspiration.[13] Poststenotic dilatation (see **Fig. 10**A) and the presence of prominent pancreaticoduodenal collaterals are secondary signs of hemodynamically significant celiac axis stenosis. The definitive diagnosis is performed with an angiogram in both inspiration and expiration showing persistent narrowing. Management of symptomatic cases may

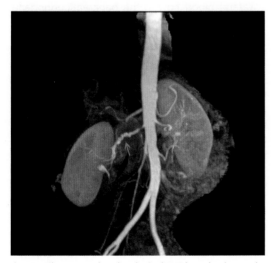

**Fig. 6.** Fibromuscular dysplasia (FMD) and atherosclerosis. Coronal MIP image of the abdominal aorta in a 51-year-old woman with renovascular hypertension. The mid and distal portion of the right renal artery demonstrates a beads-on-a-string appearance (*thick red arrow*) typical of medial subtype fibromuscular dysplasia. Severe narrowing just distal to the ostium (*thin red arrow*) is also present, typical of atherosclerotic disease.

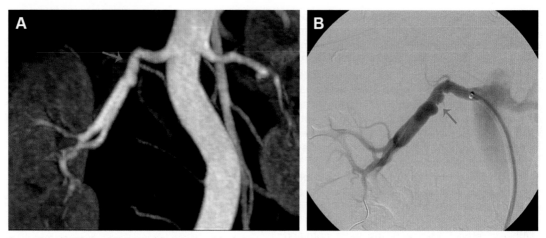

Fig. 7. Focal FMD in a 53-year-old woman with short-segment involvement of the mid right renal artery, showing a beads-on-a-string appearance (*arrow*) both on contrast-enhanced MR angiography (*A*) and digital subtraction angiography (*B*).

require surgical release of the ligament. Both open and laparoscopic techniques have been described.[14,15] Endovascular stenting is reserved for high-risk surgical patients or patients with

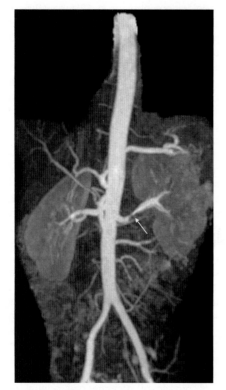

Fig. 8. Intimal fibroplasia. Contrast-enhanced MR angiography in a 26-year-old woman with renovascular hypertension demonstrates focal severe stenosis in the distal left main renal artery extending to involve the trifurcation (*solid arrow*). The tapered smooth narrowing is typical of intimal fibroplasia.

recurrence due to repetitive stress on the stent increasing the risk of fracture.[16]

## Flow-related aneurysms

Inferior pancreaticoduodenal artery aneurysms are associated with proximal celiac artery or superior mesenteric artery stenosis. Celiac stenosis may be due to median arcuate ligament impingement or atherosclerosis, and, less likely, FMD. Superior mesenteric artery stenosis is most commonly secondary to atherosclerotic disease. The increase in collateral blood flow in the pancreaticoduodenal vascular bed is hypothesized as the cause for inferior pancreaticoduodenal artery aneurysms.[17] Aneurysms in the arc of Buhler, a rare arterial communication between the proximal superior mesenteric artery and celiac artery, and dorsal pancreatic artery are also associated with pancreaticoduodenal aneurysms. These collateral pathway aneurysms rupture more often than other splanchnic aneurysms, and may have dramatic presentation with hemorrhagic shock. There is no clear association with size of the aneurysm and risk of rupture.[18] Catheter embolization is the treatment of choice.[19] Simultaneous treatment of the causative narrowing of mesenteric artery is often performed at the same time.

Close follow-up of these aneurysms has recently been advocated in small retrospective studies.[20] These aneurysms are now more frequently diagnosed with MR angiography of the abdomen (**Fig. 11**). Narrowing of the celiac artery and superior mesenteric artery should always prompt a search for pancreaticoduodenal aneurysms. MR angiography is a valuable tool in following up this subgroup of patients to assess for recanalization.[21]

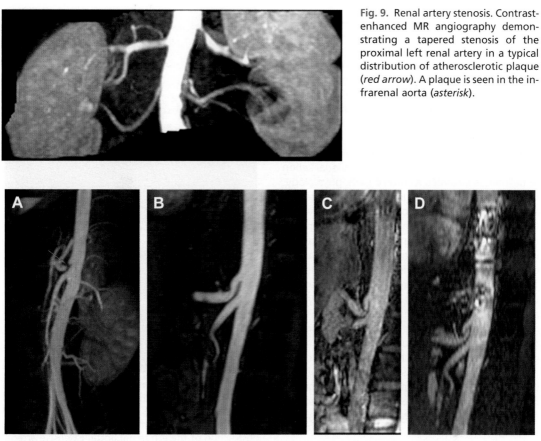

**Fig. 9.** Renal artery stenosis. Contrast-enhanced MR angiography demonstrating a tapered stenosis of the proximal left renal artery in a typical distribution of atherosclerotic plaque (*red arrow*). A plaque is seen in the infrarenal aorta (*asterisk*).

**Fig. 10.** A 31-year-old man with abdominal pain and dynamic stenosis of the proximal celiac axis. (*A*) Sagittal end-expiration maximum intensity projection (MIP) image demonstrating apparent severe stenosis of the celiac axis with a downward course, post-stenotic dilation. Sagittal end-inspiration MIP from MRA illustrates the dynamic nature of the lesion with only mild residual stenosis at end-inspiration. 3D bSSFP non-contrast MRA at end-expiration demonstrates a similar appearance to (*A*) and QISS non-contrast MRA at end-inspiration demonstrates a similar appearance to (*B*). Finding are consistent with median arcuate ligament syndrome.

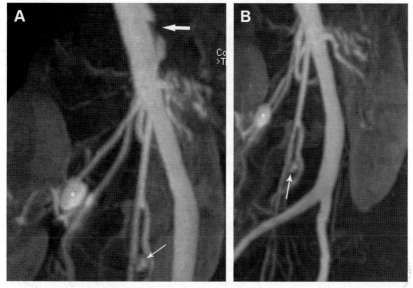

**Fig. 11.** Compression of celiac axis with flow-related aneurysm. Parasagittal (*A*) and coronal (*B*) contrast-enhanced MR angiography MIP images demonstrate celiac stenosis (*thick arrow*), with a flow-related aneurysm along the inferior pancreaticoduodenal arcade (*thin arrow*). A renal artery aneurysm is noted incidentally (*asterisk*).

## Leriche Syndrome

Leriche syndrome is described as the clinical triad of impotence, buttock claudication, and absent femoral pulses.[22] Impotence is a classic presentation in males. This syndrome is associated with infrarenal occlusion of the abdominal aorta. The common femoral arterial pulses are nonpalpable on physical examination. Treatment is indicated for symptomatic claudication.

MR angiography of the abdomen and pelvis readily depicts infrarenal occlusion. Visualization of collaterals indicates a chronic pathophysiology. Collateral pathways include systemic-systemic, systemic-visceral, and visceral-visceral pathways. Of special clinical significance are the superior epigastric (branch of the internal thoracic artery)–inferior epigastric pathway and gonadal artery collaterals, when arising from the renal arteries. The former may be compromised in coronary artery bypass using internal thoracic artery bypass and transverse laparotomies, whereas the latter may be compromised in renal artery manipulation/surgery and scrotal surgery.[23] More common collateral pathways include the intercostal-lumbar-iliolumbar arteries (**Fig. 12**). Surgical bypass is the mainstay of treatment for chronic presentations with endovascular approaches, namely, combination catheter thrombolysis and stenting in select patients.

An important imaging differential diagnosis for infrarenal aortic occlusion is acute thromboembolism. Patients present with acute onset of ischemia with a lack of lower extremity pulses without developed collaterals on MR angiography. An expeditious evaluation for a proximal vascular cause such as dissection, plaque, or aneurysm, or an intracardiac source of thromboembolism can be performed at the same time. Treatment involves endovascular approaches with catheter thrombolysis and stenting or surgical thrombectomy.

## Iliac Artery Aneurysms

Iliac artery aneurysms are coexistent in 10% to 20% of patients with abdominal aortic aneurysms, with isolated aneurysms accounting for 2% of patients with aortoiliac aneurysms.[24] Isolated internal iliac artery aneurysms are much less common, with an incidence of 0.03% to 0.04% in large autopsy series.[25] Atherosclerosis is the underlying cause in 80% of cases. Internal iliac artery aneurysms often present late, and because of their location deep in the pelvis, rupture at presentation carries a 58% mortality rate.[26]

Internal iliac artery aneurysms are now often discovered incidentally on surveillance imaging performed for other indications. An internal iliac

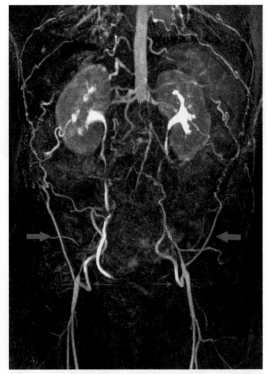

**Fig. 12.** Leriche syndrome in a 60-year-old man with impotence, buttock and thigh claudication, and reduced femoral pulses. Coronal contrast-enhanced MR angiography MIP image demonstrates complete obstruction of the infrarenal aorta. Extensive arterial collateralization involving the intercostal (*interposed between dark red lines*), deep circumflex iliac (*thick red arrows*), and inferior epigastric (*thin red arrows*) arteries reconstitutes the common femoral arteries.

artery measuring more than 1.5 cm is considered aneurysmal, similar to the definition of a common iliac artery aneurysm (**Fig. 13**). Although there are few data regarding the natural history of internal iliac artery aneurysms, clinical management mirrors that of common iliac artery aneurysms. Common iliac artery aneurysms measuring less than 3.0 cm demonstrate a slow rate of progression (1.1 mm/y) compared with those larger than 3 cm, which enlarge at a faster rate (2.6 mm/y). Clouding this assessment, others have demonstrated stability over 4 years for aneurysms 2.0 to 2.5 cm in size as well as progressive enlargement at 2.9 mm/y regardless of size. Nevertheless, rupture of common iliac artery aneurysms smaller than 3.5 cm is exceedingly rare.

MR angiography is well equipped to identify and characterize iliac artery aneurysms. Measurements should be performed on a dedicated workstation using doubly oblique multiplanar reformatted images. Other complications include thrombosis and thromboembolization. Repair is considered

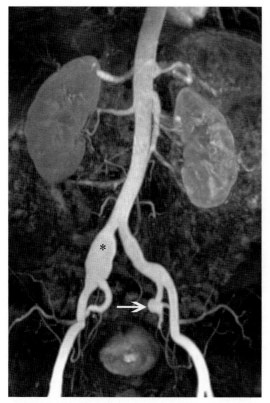

**Table 1**
Usefulness of MR angiography in vasculitis decreases with size of vessel involved

| | MR Angiography Usefulness |
| --- | --- |
| **Large vessel** | |
| Giant-cell arteritis | +++ |
| Takayasu arteritis | +++ |
| Idiopathic aortitis | +++ |
| **Medium vessel** | |
| Polyarteritis nodosa | ++ |
| Kawasaki disease | ++ |
| **Small vessel** | |
| Henoch-Schönlein purpura | − |
| Microscopic polyangitis | − |
| Churg-Strauss syndrome | − |
| Other small-vessel vasculitides | − |

**Fig. 13.** Internal and common iliac artery aneurysms. Contrast-enhanced MR angiography MIP image in a 50-year-old man demonstrates a fusiform right common iliac artery aneurysm (*asterisk*) coexistent with a left internal iliac artery aneurysm (*arrow*).

for iliac artery aneurysms 3.0 to 3.5 cm in size. Endovascular repair is the preferred therapy, with a reported success rate of 71%.[27]

## Vasculitis

MR imaging with MR angiography is very useful in the assessment and follow-up of vasculitis involving medium- to large-sized abdominal vessels. MR angiography is not useful in evaluation of the small vessel vasculitides because of resolution limitations (**Table 1**). MR imaging enables an accurate assessment of wall thickening, edema, and enhancement of vessel walls using black blood prepared T1-weighted and T2-weighted sequences.

One of the more common vasculitides to affect medium-sized abdominal arteries is polyarteritis nodosa (PAN) with involvement of both renal and mesenteric vessels. PAN usually is more common in adults and has a subacute presentation. Large vessel vasculitis such as Takayasu arteritis, giant-cell arteritis, and idiopathic aortitis can all involve the abdominal aorta. MR angiography

findings of vasculitis are nonspecific include aneurysms and strictures usually involving more than 1 segment. When combined with vessel-wall thickening, perivascular inflammation, and mural enhancement, MR angiography becomes more specific in comparison with other cross-sectional imaging (**Fig. 14**). However, the spatial resolution of MR imaging essentially limits assessment of small vessel vasculitis to conventional angiography alone. Assessment of the entire vascular tree in the absence of ionizing radiation is perhaps the greatest advantage of MR imaging in assessing multifocal vasculitis.[28] Differentiating acute medium- and large-vessel vasculitis from an infectious aortitis with aneurysm is difficult, and relies on clinical assessment and blood work to demonstrate elevated inflammatory markers without signs of systemic infection.

## CLINICAL APPLICATIONS: VENOUS IMAGING
### Congenital Variants of the Inferior Vena Cava and Renal Veins

Numerous variants of the inferior vena cava (IVC) and renal veins have been described. Although rarely a cause of patient symptoms, these become important in the evaluation of lower extremity deep venous thrombosis, infertility, planning urologic procedures, and organ transplantation. Rarer variants include solitary left-sided IVC (0.2%–0.5%), duplicated IVC (0.2%–3%), infrahepatic caval interruption with azygous continuation of the IVC (0.6%).[29] Circumaortic (8.7%) and retroaortic

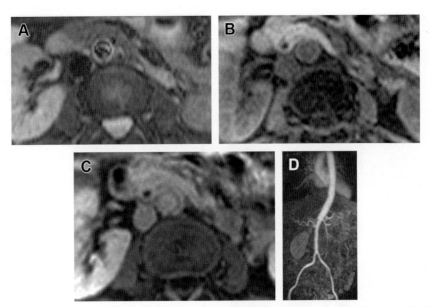

Fig. 14. Idiopathic aortitis. Axial MR 2-dimensional (2D) STIR (*A*) image through the mid abdominal aorta demonstrates high signal within the aortic wall. Precontrast (*B*) and postcontrast (*C*) T1-weighted gradient-echo images through the mid abdominal aorta demonstrate wall thickening with diffuse enhancement. There is segmental mild stenosis of the infrarenal abdominal aorta on contrast-enhanced MR angiography (*D*).

courses of the left renal vein (2.1%) are more common variants.[29]

A solitary left-sided IVC or duplicated IVC should be acknowledged before IVC filter placement. Circumaortic and retroaortic renal veins require surgical planning in patients planned for nephrectomy or organ donation. Moreover, the circumaortic renal veins drain different structures, with the cranial vein draining the adrenal vein and the inferior vein draining the gonadal vein. This drainage is important in planning intravenous interventions such as adrenal vein sampling and varicose vein embolization.

Contrast-enhanced MR angiography and noncontrast MR venography are techniques well suited for the evaluation of congenital venous variants (**Box 3**). Contrast-enhanced MR angiography using blood pool contrast agents enables steady-state venography, clearly depicting various venous drainage pathways in the retroperitoneum without limitation based on the intravenous location or contrast injection rate.

## May-Thurner Syndrome

Deep venous thrombosis is more common in the left lower extremity than in the right. This fact has long been attributed to left common iliac vein compression by the right common iliac artery. Although there is often a mild degree of

---

**Box 3**
**MR venography protocol for abdomen and pelvis**

*Contrast*

GFR (>30 mL/min/1.73 m²): gadofosveset trisodium 0.12 mL/kg, or single dose extravascular contrast agent

*Acquisition*

Scout

Axial and coronal HASTE

Axial and coronal bSSFP

Axial and coronal pregadolinium T1 3D gradient echo[a]

3D MR angiography precontrast mask

Automatic bolus detection

3D MR angiography arterial/venous/delayed

Axial and coronal postgadolinium 3D gradient echo[a]

   Maximum-intensity projection arterial and venous phase

   Steady-state imaging

High-resolution steady-state multiplanar reformatted coronal and axial 3D gradient echo

[a] Breath-hold.

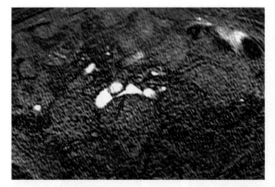

**Fig. 15.** May-Thurner syndrome in a 49-year-old woman with swollen left leg. Unenhanced axial QISS MR angiography image demonstrates left common iliac vein compression (*thick blue arrow*) by the right common iliac artery (*thick red arrow*). Right common iliac vein (*thin blue arrow*) and left common iliac artery (*thin red arrow*) are denoted for anatomic reference.

compression of the more posterior left common iliac vein by the crossing right common iliac artery, it is when the compression is significant (~70%) that the risk of deep venous thrombosis increases. Of note, compression of the left common iliac vein more than 70% or to a diameter of less than 4 mm is associated with lower incidence of pulmonary emboli.[30,31]

May-Thurner syndrome is due to chronic injury to the left common iliac vein by the crossing right common iliac artery. Angiographically it is characterized by the formation of intraluminal spurs and webs leading to obstruction to blood flow, and can present with acute deep venous thrombosis (**Fig. 15**). There is contralateral presentation of symptoms in the presence of a left-sided IVC with associated right common iliac vein stenosis (**Fig. 16**). Although rare, fatal venous hemorrhages associated with May-Thurner syndrome have been reported.[32]

MR angiography is an excellent technique to delineate the extent of venous thrombosis in the pelvic veins, enabling clear depiction of any associated IVC or renal venous anomalies that would affect the treatment plan. Doppler ultrasonography is the most appropriate imaging modality to make a diagnosis of lower extremity deep venous thrombosis; however, the extent of pelvic deep venous thrombosis can only be inferred indirectly with this technique. CT venography is limited because of the need for ipsilateral venous access, adequate outflow to opacify collateral channels during the first pass of venous injected contrast media, and poor contrast resolution during late-phase venous imaging when contrast is administered via the uninvolved extremity. MR angiography in the steady state using blood pool contrast agents or late-phase MR angiography using extracellular contrast agents can optimally delineate the extent of deep venous thrombosis in the pelvis. Patients who experience iliofemoral deep venous thrombosis are at risk of developing post-thrombotic syndrome, an important etiology leading to patient disability and reduced quality of life.

## CLINICAL APPLICATIONS: VASCULAR COMPLICATIONS OF TRANSPLANTATION

MR imaging, and MR angiography in particular, play an important role in investigating potential transplant complications in clinical practice. Although not the first-line imaging modality for evaluation of graft dysfunction, MR is an important tool for further investigation of abnormalities detected on screening examinations. In practice, noncontrast MR angiographic techniques are preferred in patients with transplants. Gadolinium-based contrast agents can be administered to patients with stable moderate or better renal insufficiency (glomerular filtration rate >30 mL/min/m²).

### Pancreas Transplant Complications

Pancreatic transplantation is performed for the treatment of type 1 diabetes. Owing to the

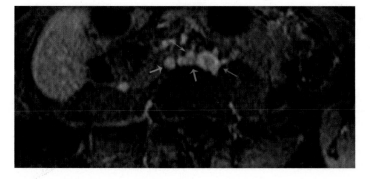

**Fig. 16.** Right common iliac vein stenosis with a left-sided inferior vena cava (IVC). Variant anatomy with a left-sided IVC changes the relationship of the crossing arteries and veins at the pelvic brim. There is compression of the right common iliac vein (*thick blue arrow*) by the left common iliac artery (*thin red arrow*) in this patient with a left-sided IVC. The central left common iliac vein is denoted by a thin blue arrow and the right common iliac artery by a thick red arrow.

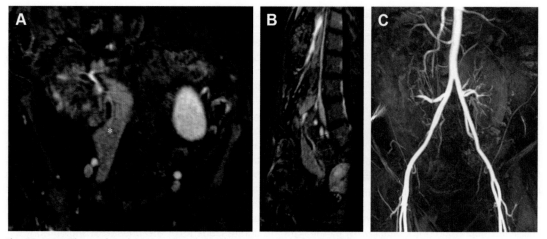

**Fig. 17.** Transplant-related pancreatic venous thrombosis. Subtracted oblique (*A*) and sagittal (*B*) oriented venous phase-contrast enhanced MR angiography in a 49-year-old woman with pancreas and kidney transplant presenting with hyperglycemia. Large thrombi (*blue arrows*) are present in both the donor splenic and superior mesenteric veins (*A*, *B*). Coronal arterial phase MIP contrast-enhanced MR angiography (*C*) demonstrates patency of both the transplant pancreatic (*small red arrow*) and renal (*large red arrow*) arteries. Pancreatic parenchyma is demarcated with an asterisk.

prevalence of renal disease in this population, concomitant kidney transplantation is common. Knowledge of the postsurgical anatomy is essential to identifying complications and mapping the graft vascular anatomy. Vascular thrombosis (**Fig. 17**) and anastomotic stenosis are second only to graft rejection as causes of graft dysfunction. Understanding the specific pancreatic transplant procedure is essential to interpreting the vascular evaluation. Two surgical procedures have been described for pancreatic transplantation: systemic bladder drainage and portal enteric drainage.

The systemic bladder drainage procedure involves placement of the pancreas in the lower pelvis. The venous drainage is into the systemic vasculature (iliac veins) and exocrine drainage to the urinary bladder. The donor splenic and superior mesenteric arteries are anastomosed to the recipient's iliac arteries via a Y graft formed from the donor's iliac arteries. The venous drainage with this type of graft is into the recipient's iliac veins. The pancreas is anastomosed to the bladder by an interposition duodenal graft (**Fig. 18**). Complications arose using this technique, which was associated with higher risk of graft failure. In addition there were high rates of hyperinsulinemia, leading to insulin resistance caused by systemic venous drainage. Urinary infections and pancreatitis are more common with this procedure.

These complications decreased through use of the portal enteric technique, whereby the pancreas is placed in the mid aspect of the

abdomen and oriented cranially. The exocrine drainage is into the recipient's small bowel using the interposition duodenal graft. The transplanted superior mesenteric artery and splenic artery are connected to a donor Y graft, again formed from the donor's iliac arteries. A long synthetic graft is

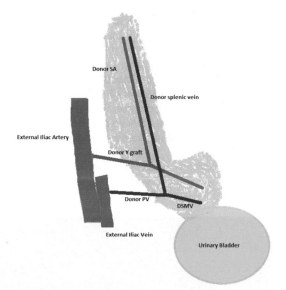

**Fig. 18.** The bladder systemic drainage pancreatic transplant procedure. Exocrine secretion is via the urinary bladder. Venous drainage is via the common iliac vein. The donor superior mesenteric and splenic arteries are anastomosed to the common iliac artery using the donor Y graft. DSMV, donor superior mesenteric vein; PV, pancreatic vein; SA, splenic artery.

then used to connect the Y graft and the common iliac artery. The venous drainage of the donor's superior mesenteric vein, splenic vein, and portal vein is into the superior mesenteric vein (**Fig. 19**).

Vascular thrombosis and arterial stenosis are easily diagnosed at MR angiography as filling defects or narrowing at anastomotic sites, highlighting the importance of familiarization with the surgical technique. Although vascular complications are often suspected at [99m]Tc radionuclide perfusion imaging, the underlying etiology is unknown. MR angiography combined with MR imaging allows assessment of both the graft and the vasculature in a single examination. Transplant rejection manifests as inhomogeneous enhancement of the pancreas with normal vasculature, although biopsy is necessary to enable differentiation from other entities on imaging, especially pancreatitis.[33–35]

### Kidney Transplant Complications

There were 77,520 active candidates for kidney transplantation as of December 1, 2013; annual transplants to date only amount to 19,262.[36] This discrepancy between supply and demand of these

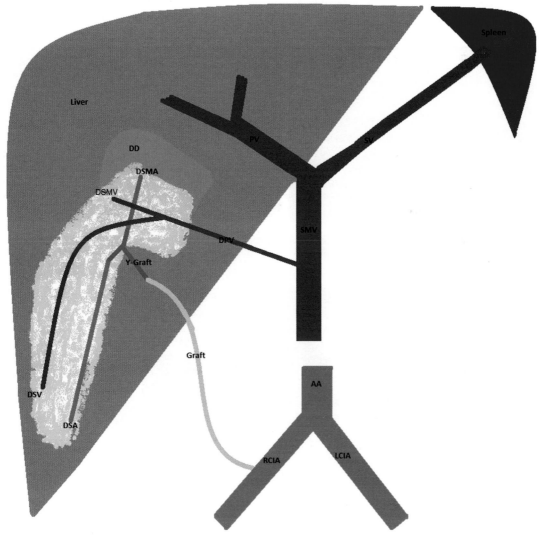

**Fig. 19.** Enteric-portal drainage pancreatic transplant. Donor venous drainage is via the superior mesenteric vein. The donor superior mesenteric artery and donor splenic artery are anastomosed to the donor Y graft, which in turn is anastomosed to a long graft connecting the Y graft to the right common iliac artery. Exocrine secretions are drained into the small bowel using a duodenal interposition graft. AA, abdominal aorta; DD, donor duodenum; DPV, donor portal vein; DSMV, donor superior mesenteric vein; DSV, donor splenic vein; LCIA, left common iliac artery; PV, portal vein; RCIA, right common iliac artery; SMV, superior mesenteric vein; SV, splenic vein.

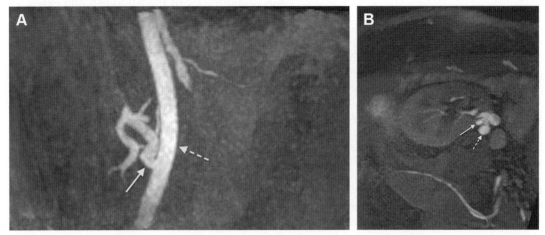

**Fig. 20.** Noncontrast assessment of renal transplant artery: Oblique multiplanar reformatted images of 3D bSSFP MR angiography (*A*) and QISS MR angiography (*B*) demonstrate a widely patent renal transplant artery (*solid arrow*) arising from the right external iliac artery (*dashed arrow*).

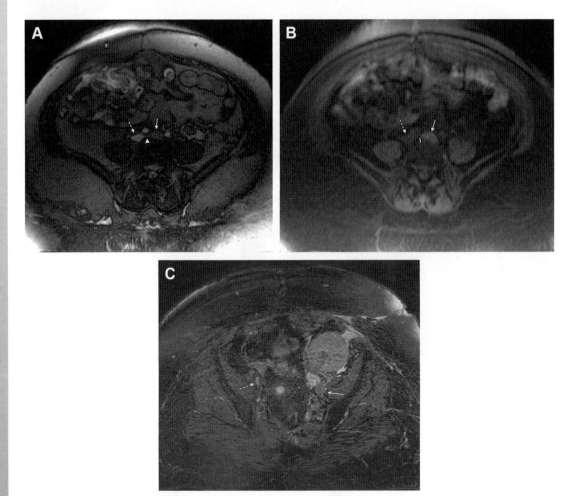

**Fig. 21.** Transplant-related renal vein thrombosis: Axial single-shot bSSFP image (*A*) through the common iliac vein confluence demonstrates an expanded, low-signal left common iliac vein (*solid arrow*), with narrowing centrally (*arrowhead*), and normal signal in the right common iliac vein (*dashed arrow*). Axial T1-weighted fat-suppressed 2D image (*B*) demonstrates high T1 signal within the left common iliac vein (*solid arrow*) with low signal in the contralateral right common iliac vein (*dashed arrow*). QISS noncontrast MR angiography (*C*) demonstrates an expanded left external iliac vein (*solid arrow*) with low signal compared with the contralateral right external iliac vein (*dashed arrow*), consistent with venous thrombosis underlying a May-Thurner vein lesion.

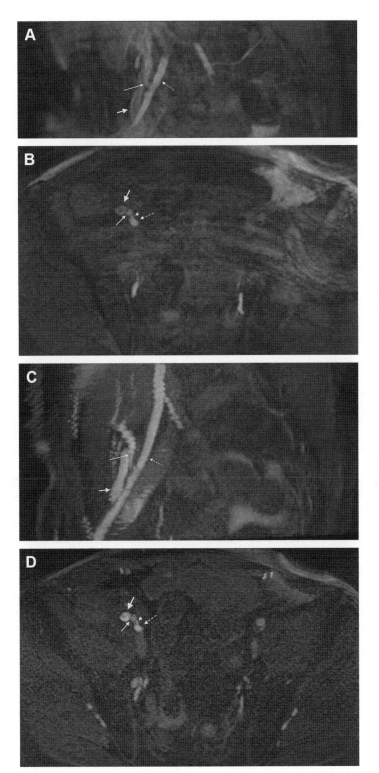

**Fig. 22.** Transplant-related renal artery stenosis. Oblique multiplanar reformatted images from 3D bSSFP MR angiography (*A*, *B*) and QISS noncontrast MR angiography (*C*, *D*) demonstrate moderate transplant arterial anastomotic stenosis (*arrowhead*) confirmed at catheter angiography (*E*). Dashed arrows demarcate the external iliac artery, solid arrows denote the proximal transplant renal artery, and thick arrows indicate the transplant vein.

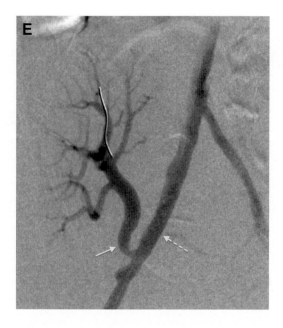

**Fig. 22.** (*continued*)

organs makes the perioperative and postoperative follow-up essential in ensuring good outcomes. The kidney is usually placed in the intraperitoneal pelvis with anastomosis of the grafted artery and vein to the ipsilateral external iliac artery and vein, respectively.

Renal transplant vascular complications are an important yet infrequent cause of graft dysfunction, accounting for less than 10% of complications in the early perioperative period.[37] MR imaging has become the study of choice for evaluation of renal grafts with suspected vascular complications detected on surveillance Doppler ultrasonography. Noncontrast MR angiography coupled with MR imaging enables the interrogation of vascular, parenchymal, and perirenal abnormalities in a noninvasive fashion, without exposure to gadolinium-based contrast media (**Fig. 20**). Renal arterial stenosis, arterial thrombosis, and venous thrombosis account for most vascular complications. Complete visualization of the arterial and venous vasculature deep in the pelvis can more definitively delineate the underlying cause of renal allograft compromise (**Figs. 21** and **22**). Accurate and timely diagnosis, especially in vascular complications, is essential in guiding prompt medical and surgical treatment.[38]

## Liver Transplant Complications

Liver transplant vascular complications are relatively uncommon, occurring in 9% of orthotopic liver transplants in a single-center series.[39] Findings of heterogeneous parenchymal enhancement, infarcts, ascites, and biliary dilatation should prompt a search for vascular complications. Hepatic artery stenosis, portal venous thrombosis, hepatic artery thrombosis, and hepatic artery rupture are the most common vascular complications. Prompt diagnosis is vital to preserve the graft and reduce recipient morbidity and mortality.

Hepatic artery thrombosis is the most feared complication in the early postoperative period, and frequently requires retransplantation. It is usually detected by ultrasonography in the immediate postoperative period and is confirmed at diagnostic catheter angiography. Hepatic artery thrombosis has been reported to occur in 3% to 12% of liver transplant recipients. Hepatic artery stenosis is usually at the anastomosis and usually develops within 3 months of liver transplantation, and has been reported to occur in 5% to 11% of transplant recipients.[40,41] MR angiography is often requested to confirm the clinical suspicion of hepatic artery stenosis detected at Doppler ultrasonography and to guide therapeutic management (**Fig. 23**). Imaging follow-up is elected in patients with noncritical stenoses of the hepatic artery.

Portal vein thrombosis is a rare vascular complication, occurring in 1% to 2% of transplant recipients. Doppler ultrasonography demonstrates no flow within the portal venous system. MR angiography is often requested to better delineate the extent of portal and mesenteric venous thrombosis. At MR angiography, deep venous thrombosis appears as a filling defect, which demonstrates varied degrees of T1 hyperintensity.

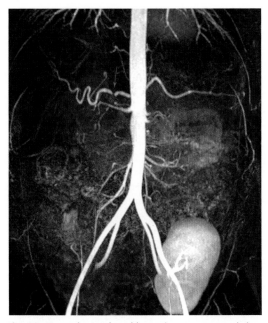

**Fig. 23.** Transplant-related hepatic artery stenosis in a 43-year-old woman with liver and kidney transplants. Coronal MIP image shows severe narrowing of the hepatic artery anastomosis (*arrow*). The transplanted kidney is seen in the left pelvis.

Anastomotic portal vein stenosis is usually at the level of the anastomosis, but can also occur at clamp locations (**Fig. 24**).

Hepatic vein stenosis is an uncommon complication with varied incidence based on the surgical approach, being reported to occur in 1% to 11% of orthotopic liver transplants. There are 4 common surgical approaches for hepatic venous anastomoses in orthotopic liver transplants. The piggyback technique is associated in some series with higher degrees of hepatic venous stenosis, and involves anastomosing the cranial end of the donor IVC to a common ostium created from either all 3 recipient hepatic venous ostia or the common middle and left venous ostium. The side-to-side technique involves creating longitudinal incisions in the recipient and donor IVC, anastomosing these primarily. The end-to-side approach involves anastomosing the cranial end of the donor IVC to the side of the recipient's IVC. The cavoplasty technique has a low incidence of hepatic venous stenosis and involves fashioning a triangular orifice from all 3 recipient hepatic venous ostia, extending the orifice with a longitudinal incision on the IVC; this is matched with a similarly configured incision along the posterior wall of the donor's IVC. Knowledge of the hepatic venous anastomotic surgical technique is valuable in assessing for abnormalities of the graft hepatic veins. Delayed hepatic vein stenosis is caused by intimal hyperplasia and fibrosis.[42] Hepatic vein stenosis can be isolated, but as a consequence of the surgical approaches outlined herein is usually associated with IVC stenosis (**Fig. 25**).

Other associated complications such as biliary stricture and intrahepatic fluid collections are usually secondary to ischemia, and are strongly associated with hepatic artery abnormalities. Biliary

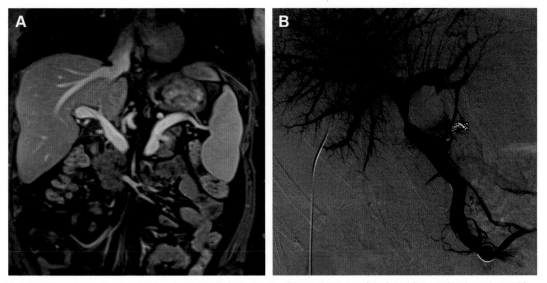

**Fig. 24.** Liver transplant portal vein stenosis. Contrast-enhanced T1-weighted gradient-echo imaging with a blood pool contrast agent in the steady state (*A*) demonstrates moderate narrowing of the portal vein at the anastomosis (*arrow*). Moderate stenosis was confirmed at catheter portography (*B*) before balloon angioplasty.

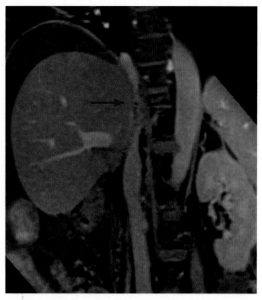

**Fig. 25.** IVC stenosis in a 61-year-old man with history of liver transplantation, ascites, and lower abdomen and extremity edema. Coronal contrast-enhanced 3D T1-weighted gradient-echo image shows long-segment IVC stenosis (*arrow*).

strictures are easily evaluated at the same time with MR cholangiopancreatography.

## SUMMARY

State-of-the-art MR angiography enables evaluation of vascular structures in the abdomen and pelvis. Evolution of noncontrast techniques has now enabled robust solutions for vascular imaging in patients for whom gadolinium-based contrast media are contraindicated. In addition, the availability of blood pool contrast agents has improved the diagnostic armamentarium for venous assessment while the widespread dissemination of 3-T clinical scanners has improved the image quality of spoiled gradient-echo MR angiography. MR angiography continues to be an important diagnostic tool for abdomen and pelvis applications.

## REFERENCES

1. Prince MR. Gadolinium-enhanced MR aortography. Radiology 1994;191(1):155–64.
2. Scheffler K, Lehnhardt S. Principles and applications of balanced SSFP techniques. Eur Radiol 2003;13(11):2409–18.
3. Edelman RR, Sheehan JJ, Dunkle E, et al. Quiescent interval single shot unenhanced magnetic resonance angiography of peripheral vascular disease: technical considerations and clinical feasibility. Magn Reson Med 2010;63(4):951–8.
4. Jarvik JG, Yuen E, Haynor DR, et al. MR nerve imaging in a prospective cohort of patients with suspected carpal tunnel syndrome. Neurology 2002; 58(11):1597–602.
5. Gadofosveset trisodium (Ablavar) [package insert]. North Billerica, MA: Lantheus Medical Imaging.
6. Amis ES Jr, Bigongiari LR, Bluth EI, et al. Radiologic investigation of patients with renovascular hypertension. American College of Radiology. ACR Appropriateness Criteria. Radiology 2000;215(Suppl):663–70.
7. Harvin HJ, Casalino DD, Remer EM, et al. Expert Panel on Urologic Imaging. ACR Appropriateness Criteria; Reno-vascular Hypertension. 2012. Available at: http://www.acr.org/~/media/ACR/Documents/AppCriteria/Diagnostic/RenovascularHypertension. pdf. Accessed April 11, 2014.
8. Begelman SM, Olin JW. Fibromuscular dysplasia. Curr Opin Rheumatol 2000;12(1):41–7.
9. Meuse MA, Turba UC, Sabri SS, et al. Treatment of renal artery fibromuscular dysplasia. Tech Vasc Interv Radiol 2010;13(2):126–33.
10. Cooper CJ, Murphy TP, Cutlip DE, et al. Stenting and medical therapy for atherosclerotic renal-artery stenosis. N Engl J Med 2014;370(1):13–22.
11. ASTRAL Investigators, Wheatley K, Ives N, et al. Revascularization versus medical therapy for renal-artery stenosis. N Engl J Med 2009;361(20): 1953–62.
12. Skeik N, Cooper LT, Duncan AA, et al. Median arcuate ligament syndrome: a nonvascular, vascular diagnosis. Vasc Endovascular Surg 2011;45(5): 433–7.
13. Lee VS, Morgan JN, Tan AG, et al. Celiac artery compression by the median arcuate ligament: a pitfall of end-expiratory MR imaging. Radiology 2003;228(2):437–42.
14. Jimenez JC, Harlander-Locke M, Dutson EP. Open and laparoscopic treatment of median arcuate ligament syndrome. J Vasc Surg 2012; 56(3):869–73.
15. Grotemeyer D, Duran M, Iskandar F, et al. Median arcuate ligament syndrome: vascular surgical therapy and follow-up of 18 patients. Langenbecks Arch Surg 2009;394(6):1085–92.
16. Duffy AJ, Panait L, Eisenberg D, et al. Management of median arcuate ligament syndrome: a new paradigm. Ann Vasc Surg 2009;23(6):778–84.
17. Kadir S, Athanasoulis CA, Yune HY, et al. Aneurysms of the pancreaticoduodenal arteries in association with celiac axis occlusion. Cardiovasc Radiol 1978; 1(3):173–7.
18. Kallamadi R, Demoya MA, Kalva SP. Inferior pancreaticoduodenal artery aneurysms in association with celiac stenosis/occlusion. Semin Intervent Radiol 2009;26(3):215–23.
19. Murata S, Tajima H, Fukunaga T, et al. Management of pancreaticoduodenal artery aneurysms: results of

superselective transcatheter embolization. AJR Am J Roentgenol 2006;187(3):W290–8.

20. Takao H, Doi I, Watanabe T, et al. Natural history of true pancreaticoduodenal artery aneurysms. Br J Radiol 2010;83(993):744–6.

21. Kurosaka K, Kawai T, Shimohira M, et al. Time-resolved magnetic resonance angiography for assessment of recanalization after coil embolization of visceral artery aneurysms. Pol J Radiol 2013; 78(1):64–8.

22. Leriche R, Morel A. The syndrome of thrombotic obliteration of the aortic bifurcation. Ann Surg 1948;127(2):193–206.

23. Hardman RL, Lopera JE, Cardan RA, et al. Common and rare collateral pathways in aortoiliac occlusive disease: a pictorial essay. AJR Am J Roentgenol 2011;197(3):W519–24.

24. Sakamoto I, Sueyoshi E, Hazama S, et al. Endovascular treatment of iliac artery aneurysms. Radiographics 2005;25(Suppl 1):S213–27.

25. Brunkwall J, Hauksson H, Bengtsson H, et al. Solitary aneurysms of the iliac arterial system: an estimate of their frequency of occurrence. J Vasc Surg 1989;10(4):381–4.

26. Brin BJ, Busuttil RW. Isolated hypogastric artery aneurysms. Arch Surg 1982;117(10):1329–33.

27. Antoniou GA, Nassef AH, Antoniou SA, et al. Endovascular treatment of isolated internal iliac artery aneurysms. Vascular 2011;19(6):291–300.

28. Raman SV, Aneja A, Jarjour WN. CMR in inflammatory vasculitis. J Cardiovasc Magn Reson 2012;14:82.

29. Bass JE, Redwine MD, Kramer LA, et al. Spectrum of congenital anomalies of the inferior vena cava: cross-sectional imaging findings. Radiographics 2000;20(3):639–52.

30. Narayan A, Eng J, Carmi L, et al. Iliac vein compression as risk factor for left- versus right-sided deep venous thrombosis: case-control study. Radiology 2012;265(3):949–57.

31. Chan KT, Popat RA, Sze DY, et al. Common iliac vein stenosis and risk of symptomatic pulmonary embolism: an inverse correlation. J Vasc Interv Radiol 2011;22(2):133–41.

32. Hughes RL, Collins KA, Sullivan KE. A case of fatal iliac vein rupture associated with May-Thurner syndrome. Am J Forensic Med Pathol 2013;34(3): 222–4.

33. Hagspiel KD, Nandalur K, Burkholder B, et al. Contrast-enhanced MR angiography after pancreas transplantation: normal appearance and vascular complications. AJR Am J Roentgenol 2005;184(2): 465–73.

34. Hagspiel KD, Nandalur K, Pruett TL, et al. Evaluation of vascular complications of pancreas transplantation with high-spatial-resolution contrast-enhanced MR angiography. Radiology 2007;242(2):590–9.

35. Vandermeer FQ, Manning MA, Frazier AA, et al. Imaging of whole-organ pancreas transplants. Radiographics 2012;32(2):411–35.

36. Heimbach JK. Infrastructure, logistics and regulation of transplantation: UNOS. Anesthesiol Clin 2013;31(4):659–66.

37. Salehipour M, Salahi H, Jalaeian H, et al. Vascular complications following 1500 consecutive living and cadaveric donor renal transplantations: a single center study. Saudi J Kidney Dis Transpl 2009;20(4): 570–2.

38. Onniboni M, De Filippo M, Averna R, et al. Magnetic resonance imaging in the complications of kidney transplantation. Radiol Med 2013;118(5):837–50.

39. Langnas AN, Marujo W, Stratta RJ, et al. Vascular complications after orthotopic liver transplantation. Am J Surg 1991;161(1):76–82 [discussion: 82–3].

40. Glockner JF, Forauer AR. Vascular or ischemic complications after liver transplantation. AJR Am J Roentgenol 1999;173(4):1055–9.

41. Bhargava P, Vaidya S, Dick AA, et al. Imaging of orthotopic liver transplantation: review. AJR Am J Roentgenol 2011;196(Suppl 3):WS15–25 [quiz: S35–8].

42. Strovski E, Liu D, Scudamore C, et al. Magnetic resonance venography and liver transplant complications. World J Gastroenterol 2013;19(36):6110–3.

# Dealing with Vascular Conundrums with MR Imaging

Wirana Angthong, MD[a,b], Richard C. Semelka, MD[a,*]

## KEYWORDS

- Vascular imaging • Body imaging • Magnetic resonance imaging • Abdominal vascular imaging

## KEY POINTS

- The use of thin-section three-dimensional (3D) gradient-echo tissue-imaging sequences provides comprehensive information on vessel lumen, vessel wall, and surrounding organs. These techniques can adequately answer almost all clinical questions related to vascular diseases.
- The use of high T1-relaxivity gadolinium-based contrast agent, which persists in the vascular space for a longer duration than other standard gadolinium agents, is suitable to improve the performance of body vascular imaging, particularly in studies that combined multiple territories (eg, abdominal and pelvic vascular imaging).
- Implementation of the motion-resistant magnetic resonance (MR) sequences, including radial acquisition 3D gradient-echo and two-dimensional water excitation-magnetization-prepared rapid-acquisition gradient-echo has permitted acceptable image quality in noncooperative patients for the diagnosis of vascular abnormalities.
- A non–contrast-enhanced MR angiography technique is the preferred examination for the diagnosis of vascular disease in the setting of pregnancy and severely impaired renal function.
- The combination of parallel imaging and 3 T is beneficial in increasing image quality and minimizing specific absorption rate.

## INTRODUCTION

Body magnetic resonance (MR) imaging using thin-section tissue-imaging sequences has evolved into a versatile imaging approach for use in a variety of vascular applications. MR imaging using an MR angiography technique has replaced many diagnostic angiographic procedures, thus decreasing the cost and morbidity of diagnosis.[1–3] The advantage of tissue-imaging MR imaging is that it can serve as a 1-stop-shop modality, replacing the classic combination of cross-sectional imaging and conventional angiography in the evaluation of organ/tissues and vascular diseases, such as in settings of preoperative diagnostic workup of abdominal tumors or posttreatment follow-up.[4–7] MR imaging has surpassed computed tomography (CT) in several important aspects. First, because of the lack of ionizing radiation, MR imaging can be performed repeatedly for the follow-up of patients without the concern of radiation exposure. Therefore, MR imaging can be used as a modality in patients in whom radiation effects are especially undesirable. Second, gadolinium-based contrast agents (GBCA) are considerably safer than iodine-based contrast

Funding Source: None.
Conflict of Interest: None.
[a] Department of Radiology, University of North Carolina Hospitals, UNC at Chapel Hill, CB 7510, 2001 Old Clinic Building, Chapel Hill, NC 27599-7510, USA; [b] Department of Radiology, HRH Princess Maha Chakri Sirindhorn Medical Center, Srinakharinwirot University, 62 Moo 7, Khlong Sip, Ongkharak, Nakhon Nayok, Thailand
* Corresponding author.
*E-mail address:* richsem@med.unc.edu

Radiol Clin N Am 52 (2014) 861–882
http://dx.doi.org/10.1016/j.rcl.2014.02.002

agents used in contrast-enhanced CT.[8] There is a lesser association with nephrotoxicity and allergic reactions with MR contrast agents.[9]

Technical advances in the introduction of 3-T MR imaging is especially beneficial in vascular imaging combined with tissue imaging. This factor reflects that 3-T MR generates higher-quality images because of higher in-plane and through-plane spatial and temporal resolution compared with 1.5 T. The higher signal at 3 T also has more pronounced contrast enhancement effect of vascular structures.[10,11] Application of parallel imaging provides reduced acquisition time, facilitating imaging coverage of multiple territories (eg, chest, abdomen, and pelvis), with high image quality maintained. In this article, the usefulness of tissue-sequence MR imaging for the evaluation of vascular abnormalities is reviewed and characteristic MR imaging features are illustrated. Comprehensive MR imaging protocols in cooperative and noncooperative patients are also discussed.

## IMAGING TECHNIQUES
### Non–Contrast-Enhanced MR Angiography

Non–contrast-enhanced MR angiography has achieved recent increased interest as a result of concern over the safety of GBCAs. These techniques are particularly important for vascular assessments in patients with chronic kidney disease. Fast imaging acquisition sequences such as flow-independent balanced steady-state free-precession sequences (b-SSFP) have been used in a wide range of applications. These applications have various acronyms for the different vendors, such as TrueFISP (true fast imaging with steady-state precession) (Siemens, Germany), FIESTA (GE Medical Systems, Milwaukee, WI, USA), and b-TFE (Philips, The Netherlands). The b-SSFP technique is a free-precession gradient-echo (GE) sequence, with balanced gradients in all directions.[12] It possesses T2-weighted and T1-weighted information, uses short repetition time (TR)/echo time (TE) (approximately 2–3/1–1.5 milliseconds), and renders high signal for fluid. This flow-independent technique allows bright blood to be shown in all directions (**Fig. 1**). b-SSFP is commonly used in coronary, thoracic, and renal angiography.[13,14] Abdominal vascular imaging can be used with breath hold, or with a respiratory-triggered or navigator-gated free-breathing acquisition.[12,15] The major advantages of b-SSFP are the short acquisition time and high signal-to-noise ratio (SNR). A major drawback of the b-SSFP sequence is vulnerability to susceptibility artifacts because of field inhomogeneity, tissue interface, and metallic implants.[12]

Traditional noncontrast time-of-flight (TOF) and phase-contrast (PC) MR angiography do not achieve reproducible image quality in body imaging because of longer acquisition times and susceptibility to motion artifact. The shortcomings of both techniques include overestimation of the severity of the stenosis from turbulent flow caused by intravoxel dephasing phenomena. Consequently, both techniques are not generally used in vascular application in body MR imaging.[16]

### Contrast-Enhanced MR Angiography and Postprocessing Techniques

Contrast-enhanced MR angiography has emerged as a major technique for the evaluation of vascular disease. Ultrashort TR and TE are performed to achieve the fastest possible imaging speed (TR <4 milliseconds, TE <3 milliseconds). The total scan times range from 10 to 30 seconds.[16] The application of higher flip angles (range from 25° to 50°) improves background suppression and enhances intravascular contrast (**Fig. 2**).[16,17] The center of k-space contains the bulk signal and contrast information, and the periphery of k-space contains fine spatial resolution information. For optimal contrast enhancement, the center of k-space should be acquired when the contrast agent arrives into the vessel of interest. The timing of sequence acquisition can be determined by test bolus, automatic triggering on contrast agent arrival, or fluoroscopic real-time monitoring.[13,17]

Artifacts related to turbulent flow encountered with TOF or PC MR angiography are minimal with contrast-enhanced MR angiography. Although flow is important, this technique does not generate high signal based primarily on flow, but rather on T1 shortening effect of circulating GBCA. Further approaches to improve the performance of contrast-enhanced MR angiography are the use of high T1-relaxivity GBCA. For example, gadobenate dimeglumine (Multihance, Bracco, Milan, Italy) has shown a weak protein binding property, and therefore, it provides greater and longer-lasting vascular enhancement at standard doses compared with other standard GBCAs.[8,18] Kroencke and colleagues[19] reported that gadobenate dimeglumine is an effective and safe agent for contrast-enhanced MR angiography of abdominal aorta and renal arteries at a dose of 0.1 mmol/kg.

Imaging at 3 T provides an approximately 1.4 × SNR compared with 1.5 T, an improved background suppression as a result of the prolonged T1 relaxation time of most tissues, and increased contrast agent enhancement effect.[20] Therefore, 3-T MR imaging is an excellent modality for MR angiography in conjunction with parallel imaging, which

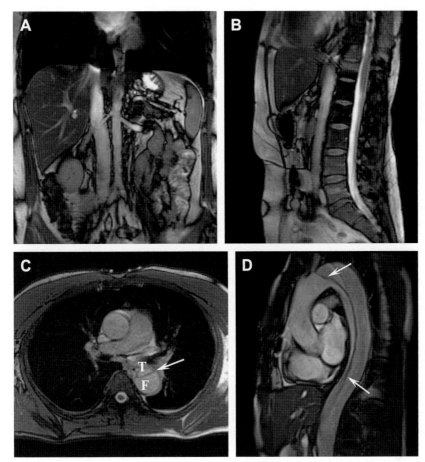

Fig. 1. b-SSFP of the abdominal aorta (*A, B*). (*A*) Coronal and (*B*) sagittal images show normal appearance of abdominal aorta with bright blood signal. b-SSFP in a 47-year-old man with Stanford type B aortic dissection (*C, D*). (*C*) Transverse image obtained at the level of the right pulmonary artery shows the intimal flap (*arrow*) between the true lumen (T) and false lumen (F). (*D*) Sagittal image shows the intimal flap originating distal to the origin of the left subclavian artery extending into the abdominal aorta (*arrows*).

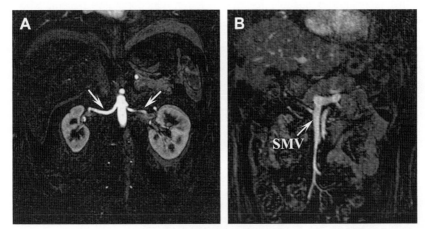

Fig. 2. Source images of subtraction contrast-enhanced MR angiography obtained at 3.0 T with gadobenate di-meglumine at a dose of 0.05 mmol/kg. (*A*) Coronal arterial phase contrast-enhanced MR angiography of the abdominal aorta shows adequate visualization of the renal arteries (*arrows*). (*B*) Coronal venous phase contrast-enhanced MR angiography shows a normal. SMV, superior mesenteric vein (*arrow*).

facilitates increased spatial resolution, shortens scan time and decreases specific absorption rate.[21]

The MR angiography data acquired can be post-processed either by maximum intensity projection (MIP), multiplanar construction (MPR) (**Fig. 3**), or volumetric display, with MIP being the most common means of showing data. MIP technique shows the voxel with the highest signal intensity within each projection ray through a volume of data, in which the background signal is low and arterial contrast is high.[17] It provides a good overview and is useful in tracking tortuous vessels. Consequently, MIP images achieve high acceptance by clinicians. However, accurate diagnosis is usually based on the source images; evaluation should not rely solely on the MIP images. MPR is often used to reconstruct images in planar orientation, such as orthogonal, oblique, or curved planes. The combination of postprocessed image data sets with source images in MR angiography provides maximal diagnostic accuracy of assessing vascular diseases.[4,22]

## Contrast-Enhanced Fat-Suppressed T1-Weighted Three-Dimensional–GE Sequences

Three-dimensional (3D)-GE sequences can be obtained with large volume coverage, very thin sections, and high spatial resolution in a single breath-holding time. On newer MR systems, especially 3 T, slice thickness may be 2 mm or thinner, achieving near isotropic resolution, and as a result, these 3D data sets can be reconstructed in multiple planes, with minimal loss in image resolution. When compared with contrast-enhanced MR angiography, the lower flip angle used with 3D-GE sequences (reduced to 12°–15°), results in increased signal of the background soft tissue structures.[23] This technique is suitable for dynamic contrast-enhanced studies, because of its excellent sensitivity for enhancement in tissues and organs. A minimum of 2 postcontrast sequences are needed: one acquired in the hepatic arterial dominant phase (HADP) and the second in the hepatic venous or interstitial phase. HADP is characterized by the presence of contrast in the hepatic arteries, portal veins, renal veins, splenic vein, and superior mesenteric vein; the absence of contrast in the hepatic veins (HVs). Various enhancement patterns of liver lesions and other organs are also distinctive on HADP. Appropriate timing can be reliably judged by vessel enhancement. In our institution, to achieve timing for the contrast-enhanced HADP, we use a bolus-tracking technique with the following approach. The contrast agent is monitored by the technologist as it travels through the vascular system. With the perception of contrast in the descending aorta, patients are instructed to suspend breathing using an 8-second instruction command, and the sequence is initiated thereafter. 3D-GE sequences are used routinely on newer MR systems in the evaluation of the chest, abdomen, and pelvis and are used in evaluating solid organs. If section thickness is 3.5 mm or less, acceptable vascular information is also presented on these images (**Fig. 4**).[17] In general, 3D-GE can adequately answer almost all clinical questions related to vascular diseases.

## Motion-Resistant Protocol in Noncooperative Patients

Separate protocols are necessary for noncooperative patients that use sequences that are fundamentally motion resistant. The acquisition time of routinely used MR imaging sequences is generally too long for high diagnostic quality of vascular imaging in noncooperative patients who are unable to suspend respiration for more than 10 seconds.

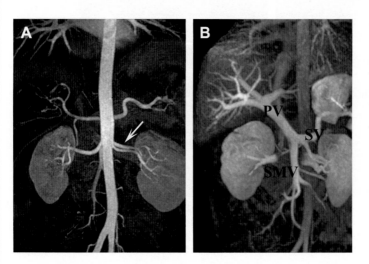

Fig. 3. MIP reconstruction of coronal source images MR angiography. (A) MIP image of the abdominal aorta at 3.0 T shows early bifurcation of the left renal artery (*arrow*). (B) MIP image of the portal venous system at 1.5 T shows well-delineated superior mesenteric vein (SMV), splenic vein (SV), and main portal vein (PV).

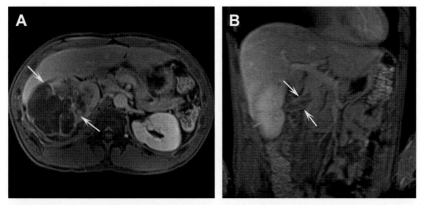

**Fig. 4.** A 37-year-old man with undifferentiated sarcoma of the right kidney. (*A*) Transverse T1-weighted interstitial phase postgadolinium 3D-GE image shows heterogeneous enhancing renal mass involving the renal cortex and medulla (*arrows*), with central area of necrosis. (*B*) Coronal interstitial phase postgadolinium 3D-GE image shows enhancing tumor thrombus within the right renal vein (*arrows*).

Contrast-enhanced two-dimensional (2D) water excitation-magnetization-prepared rapid-acquisition GE (WE-MPRAGE) and 3D radial GE sequences achieve good image quality in a free-breathing manner.[24,25]

MPRAGE sequences, including turbo fast low-angle shot (turboFLASH), are generally performed as a single shot, with image acquisition time of 1 to 2 seconds.[24] In patients who cannot cooperate, the use of an MPRAGE sequence may generate adequate quality without the need for breath holding.

A free-breathing T1-weighted fat-suppressed 3D radial GE sequence acquires radial k-space filling with the use of a multishot radial acquisition technique. MR imaging datasets are acquired in multiple overlapping radial lines, each of which includes data sampled from the center to the periphery of k-space. This sequence acquisition is performed in a free-breathing manner without trigger or navigation techniques. It provides motion insensitivity in noncooperative patients.[25] Both MR-RAGE and a free-breathing radial 3D-GE sequence are feasible for vascular imaging and may be indicated in patients who are unable to suspend respiration (**Figs. 5** and **6**).

## ABDOMINAL VASCULAR IMAGING

The major problem in abdominal MR imaging is motion artifacts. The shorter scan time of 3D-GE sequences facilitates breath-hold imaging to minimizing motion artifact. In the studies that combined multiple territories (eg, abdominal and pelvic vascular imaging), it is more imperative to use high T1-relaxivity GBCA such as gadobenate dimeglumine, which persists in the vascular space for a longer duration than other standard gadolinium agents.[8] Imaging on a 3-T system is preferred

for evaluation of fine anatomic details of visceral vessels (eg, hepatic or superior mesenteric arteries), which provides further reduction in slice thickness (1.5–2 mm), with less partial volume effect. This advantage also renders reconstruction of images in any plane.[10,11]

### Problem Solving

#### Flow artifact versus thrombosis
To distinguish flow artifact from venous thrombosis, it is useful to acquire images directly in planes; generally, transverse and coronal planes are sufficient. Multiplanar data should be obtained as separate acquisitions. Comparing transverse with coronal images, real thrombosis should have the same configuration and distribution as would be anticipated comparing 1 plane with the next (**Fig. 7**). In addition, thrombosis should appear identical on early hepatic venous (or portal venous) and interstitial phase images. We routinely perform this procedure with a coronal acquisition as the fourth data set after 3 transverse acquisitions. Another critical point to emphasize is that caution should be taken to generally avoid interpretation of venous thrombosis based on arterial phase images alone, because admixing of contrast media can simulate thrombosis.

#### Bland thrombosis versus tumor thrombosis
MR imaging usually enables the distinction between bland thrombosis and tumor thrombosis. Bland thrombosis is generally low signal intensity on T2-weighted images and does not enhance after contrast administration. Tumor thrombosis is higher signal intensity or soft tissue signal on T2-weighted images, frequently expands the luminal diameter, and may show appreciable enhancement after contrast administration. Tumor

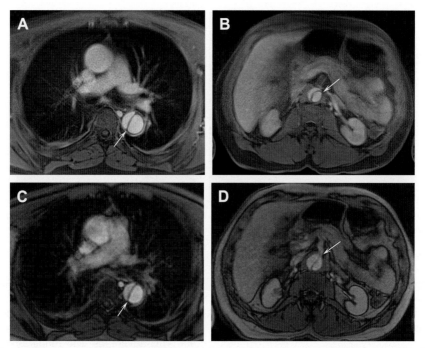

**Fig. 5.** Motion-resistant protocol in 59-year-old man with Stanford type B aortic dissection using 2 difference techniques: free-breathing T1-weighted 3D radial GE sequences (*A, B*) and contrast-enhanced 2D MPRAGE (*C, D*). Both techniques clearly show an intimal flap in the thoracoabdominal aorta (*arrows*).

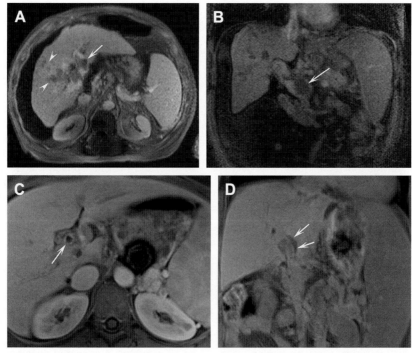

**Fig. 6.** Motion-resistant protocol in 2 different noncooperative patients. A 62-year-old man with hepatitis C viral cirrhosis (*A, B*). (*A*) Transverse and (*B*) coronal interstitial phase WE-MPRAGE images show diffuse-type HCC (*arrowheads*) with malignant portal venous thrombosis in right, left, and main portal veins (*arrows, A, B*). A 32-year-old woman with primary sclerosing cholangitis after liver transplantation (*C, D*). (*C*) Transverse and (*D*) coronal interstitial phase free-breathing T1-weighted 3D radial GE sequences show main portal vein thrombosis (*arrows, C, D*). Although the images are acquired without breath holding, there is no motion artifact.

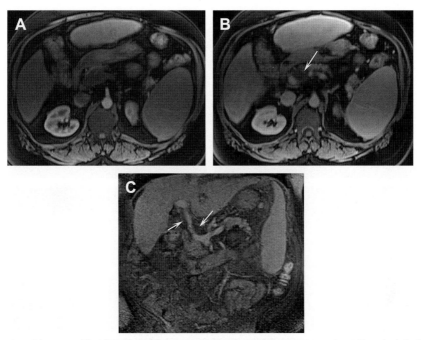

Fig. 7. A 51-year-old man with bland portal venous thrombosis. (*A*) Transverse hepatic arterial phase and (*B*) venous phase postgadolinium 3D-GE images show bland thrombus in the main portal vein extending into the SMV. Thrombus is best visualized on the late phase image as a nonenhanced signal-void structure (*arrow, B*). (*C*) Coronal interstitial phase postgadolinium image shows thrombus having the same configuration and distribution as shown on the transverse image (*arrows, C*).

thrombosis is most often observed in the setting of diffuse hepatocellular carcinoma, in which it is contiguous with the tumor. Bland thrombosis may be observed in the setting of cirrhosis and various inflammatory or infectious processes involving organs in the portal circulation (**Fig. 8**).[26]

*Vessel versus mass*
A vessel may be distinguished from a mass by the observation that the signal intensity of vessels follows the course of enhancement characteristics of comparable vessels and vascular structures (artery, portal vein, and HV). In addition, vessels usually retain contrast, especially when using an agent with a longer intravascular dwell time. Focal hepatic masses follow their own enhancement course, which usually seem to either fade quickly (such as hepatic adenoma, focal nodular hyperplasia [FNH]) or wash out on delayed interstitial phase images (such as hepatocellular carcinoma, carcinoid metastasis) (**Fig. 9**). Hemangiomas tend to retain contrast.

*Type of vessel*
Distinguishing vessel type may be established based on time of appearance of enhancement. Arterial entities follow the enhancement course of arteries (such as vascular aneurysms), whereas venous entities follow the enhancement course of veins (such as venous varices). Portal and HVs can also be differentiated by the temporal opacification of these structures.

Some focal hepatic lesions are difficult to distinguish from vascular aneurysm, for example, small fast-enhancing hemangioma may mimic the appearance of vascular aneurysm on early phase postgadolinium images. Small hemangioma may show intense uniform enhancement on early phase and tend to maintain the signal intensity or fade toward background intensity. However, small hemangiomas are distinctively bright signal intensity on T2-weighted images, whereas vascular aneurysms may or may not be bright and often are not. Comparison of signal is critical to the surrounding vessels, in which vascular aneurysm should show the same signal intensity as surrounding vessels on the image. The routine combination of T2-weighted information with serial dynamic contrast-enhanced study is useful to establish the correct diagnosis of these entities.

*Clinical Considerations*

*Abdominal aortic aneurysm*
Aneurysm is defined as enlargement of arterial diameter by 50% or more from its normal caliber, which for an abdominal aortic aneurysm (AAA) is greater than or equal to 3 cm.[16] Most AAAs are

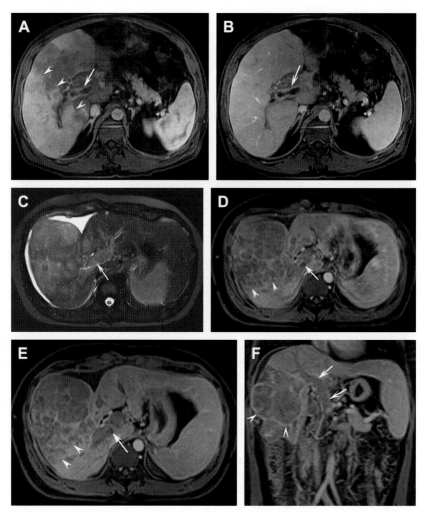

**Fig. 8.** Bland thrombosis versus tumor thrombosis. A 77-year-old man with infected bland portal venous thrombosis in the setting of liver abscess (*A, B*). (*A*) Transverse hepatic arterial phase postgadolinium 3D-GE image shows transient increased enhancement of the right lobe of the liver (*arrowheads*), which reflects increased hepatic arterial supply caused by an autoregulatory mechanism as a result of portal venous thrombosis (*arrow*). (*B*) Transverse interstitial phase image shows bland thrombus in the right portal vein with enhancing vessel wall (*arrow*). Note the intense mural enhancement of the portal vein wall on the delayed image. A 30-year-old man with malignant portal venous thrombosis (*C–F*). There are multiple irregular, ill-defined foci of diffuse hepatocellular carcinoma (HCC) scattered throughout the right hepatic lobe, which show moderately hyperintense signal intensity on T2-weighted fat-suppressed single-shot echo train spin-echo image (*C*). The right and main portal veins are expanded with tumor thrombus (*arrow*). (*D*) Transverse hepatic arterial phase image shows early heterogeneous enhancement of the tumor thrombus (*arrow*) with comparable imaging feature to diffuse HCC (*arrowheads*). (*E*) Transverse and (*F*) coronal interstitial phase images show washout of tumor thrombus (*arrows*) and diffuse HCC (*arrowheads*).

atherosclerotic. Atherosclerotic aneurysm is typically fusiform, although focal eccentric aneurysm is occasionally encountered. Aneurysms are frequently infrarenal (84%) (**Fig. 10**) but can also involve the entire abdominal aorta (4%) or be limited to the pararenal region (12%).[16] Important evaluations in imaging aortic aneurysms include the maximum diameter, the length, the characteristic of mural thrombi, and involvement of visceral vessels. All these findings can be characterized precisely with contrast-enhanced MR angiography.[22] Assessment of the aortic wall, intraluminal thrombus, periaortic tissue, and abdominal viscera are accomplished on postgadolinium 3D-GE.

Infected aortic aneurysm or mycotic aneurysm caused by bacterial infection results in fragility of the vessel wall, causing saccular outpouching, which typically involves the suprarenal portion of

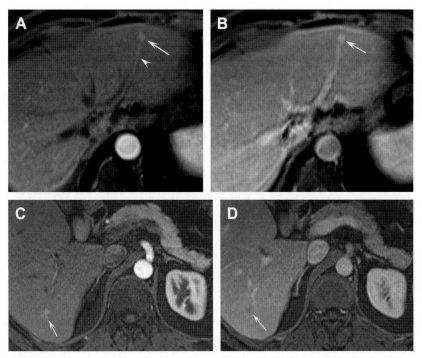

Fig. 9. Vessel versus mass. A 63-year-old woman with small portal vein varix (*A, B*). (*A*) Transverse hepatic arterial phase image and (*B*) interstitial phase image show a 9-mm moderately hyperenhancing lesion in segment 2 (*arrow*), which follows the course of enhancement of the portal vein and is consistent with small portal vein varix. Notice the early filling of the left HV (*arrowhead, A*) consistent with rapid transit. A 54-year-old man with small hepatocellular carcinoma (*C, D*). (*C*) Transverse hepatic arterial phase image shows hyperenhancing nodule in segment 5/6 (*arrow*) and washout with capsular enhancement on delayed interstitial phase image (*D*). Notice how the solid mass and the varix both show early enhancement, but the mass shows washout (*arrow, D*), and the varix shows persistent enhancement comparable with venous structures.

the abdominal aorta.[16] MR imaging can show the aneurysm itself and also show wall thickening and periaortic abscess. Inflammatory aortic aneurysm is a variant of atherosclerotic aneurysm in which an inflammatory reaction or fibrotic changes develop in the periaortic region of the retroperitoneum.[1] The mural and extramural changes are probably the result of a local autoallergic reaction to certain components of atherosclerotic plaque. Inflammatory aneurysm may affect the abdominal or thoracic aorta. The mural and extramural findings may be best shown on

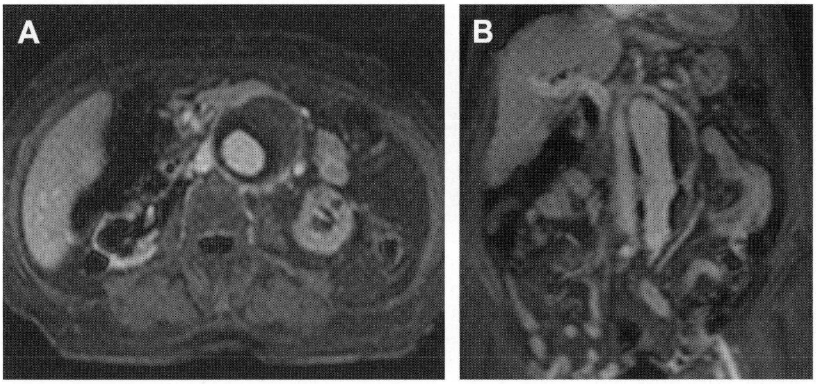

Fig. 10. Contrast-enhanced 2D WE-MPRAGE in a 79-year-old woman with atherosclerotic aneurysm of the abdominal aorta. (*A*) Transverse and (*B*) coronal interstitial phase WE-MPRAGE images show a large fusiform infrarenal aortic aneurysm. An aortic aneurysm containing high signal intensity intraluminal gadolinium and low signal intensity mural thrombus is evident.

interstitial phase postgadolinium 3D-GE as marked enhancement of the vessel wall and ill-defined infiltrative enhancing surrounding tissue, which is most prominent around the anterior and lateral walls of aneurysm.[1]

### Aortic dissection

Aortic dissection occurs when blood leaks from the aortic lumen through an intimal tear into the tunica media, separating media from intima. Aortic dissection usually originates in the thoracic aorta. Contrast-enhanced MR angiography techniques permit determining the type of aortic dissection by ascertaining involvement of the ascending thoracic aorta, and clearly delineate the true and false lumen, location of the intimal flap, entry site, the full extent of dissection, and the relation to the visceral vessels.[27] These data are crucial for the planning of surgical or endovascular therapy. Postgadolinium 3D-GE sequences are advantageous for showing the intimal flap and the extent of dissection. The intimal flap appears as a hypointense line with a linear, arc, or S shape in transverse plane. The true and false lumens can be distinguished by temporal appearance of contrast in the particular vascular compartment (faster in the true lumen) signal intensity, morphologic features, the relationship between the lumina, and the presence of thrombosis (**Box 1**, **Fig. 11**). Contrast-enhanced MR angiography during the venous phase reliably distinguishes slow flow and intraluminal thrombosis, both of which may be observed in the false lumen. Slow flow

shows high signal intensity, whereas thrombus shows low signal intensity.[16,27] There are limitations to the use of MR imaging. First, it cannot be performed readily in unstable patients. Second, it cannot detect small volume calcification of the arterial wall or intimal flap. Third, some endovascular stents produce substantial susceptibility artifacts related to the metallic composition of the stent.[27]

### Visceral artery aneurysm

Most aneurysms of the visceral arteries are detected incidentally. The distribution and frequency of aneurysms among visceral vessels are as follows: splenic (60%), hepatic (20%), superior mesenteric (5.5%), and celiac (4%) arteries.[28] Splenic artery aneurysms are usually asymptomatic. The risk of rupture is approximately 2% to 10%, with mortality of 36%.[29] Splenic artery aneurysms are usually small, saccular, and occur frequently in the distal portion of splenic artery. Most hepatic artery aneurysms involve the extrahepatic portion (78%) in the proper hepatic artery or common hepatic artery (**Fig. 12**).[3,28] Although aneurysms of hepatic arteries are typically caused by trauma or iatrogenic procedures, aneurysms of the splenic artery occur secondary to atherosclerosis, portal hypertension, or pancreatitis.[3] Imaging assessment of arterial anatomy and variations is crucial to determine the appropriate treatment. MR imaging is a fast, accurate, and noninvasive technique for showing visceral artery aneurysms. Contrast-enhanced MR angiography can replace diagnostic invasive angiography in most cases.[28] As mentioned earlier, attention must be paid to the temporal appearance of high signal in the suspected aneurysm, which should be comparable with other arteries.

### Mesenteric arterial ischemia

Acute mesenteric arterial ischemia is an acute interruption of mesenteric blood supply, which is caused by embolism, thrombosis, nonocclusive ischemia, or aortic dissection. Acute emboli in the superior mesenteric artery (SMA) is the most common cause and is responsible for 40% to 50% of cases of acute mesenteric ischemia.[30] These patients typically have a clinical history of cardiovascular disease. Most emboli in the SMA lodge just beyond the origin of the middle colic artery. Contrast-enhanced MR angiography can show abrupt termination of the vessel (cutoff sign) or filling defects in the vessel lumen (**Table 1**).

Acute thrombotic occlusion is responsible for 20% to 30% of all cases of acute mesenteric ischemia. It is typically associated with preexisting atherosclerosis. In contrast to acute SMA

---

**Box 1**
**Differentiation of the true lumen and the false lumen in aortic dissection**

- Signal intensity: the true lumen is higher signal intensity (enhances early) than the false lumen on arterial phase images

- Size: the true lumen is usually smaller than the false lumen

- Shape: the true lumen is frequently thin or flat, appearing elliptical on transverse plane images; the false lumen is usually expanded, appearing crescentic or winding around the true lumen on transverse plane images

- The presence of thrombosis: mural thrombus is usually observed in the false lumen, which appears as low signal intensity on postgadolinium 3D-GE

- The presence of slow flow: slow flow is usually observed in the false lumen, which appears as high signal intensity in the lumen on postgadolinium 3D-GE

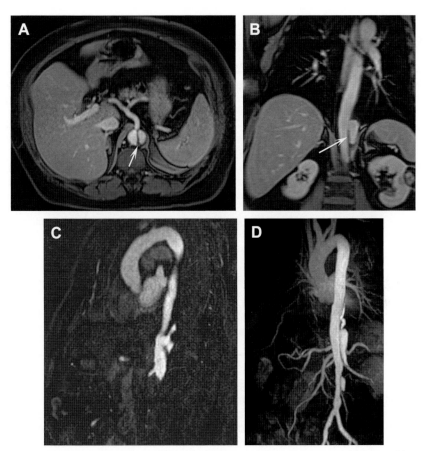

**Fig. 11.** A 61-year-old woman with abdominal aortic dissection. (*A*) Transverse and (*B*) coronal interstitial phase postgadolinium 3D-GE images show low signal intensity linear structure of the intimal flap (*arrow*), which separates the true and false lumen. (*C*) Oblique sagittal contrast-enhanced MR angiography source image and (*D*) MIP reconstruction obtained in a coronal plane clearly show the extent and relationship of aortic dissection with major aortic branches. No involvement of major aortic branches is shown.

embolism, the abdominal symptoms associated with acute SMA thrombosis may be more insidious, because of the development of collateral circulation. Occlusion by SMA thrombosis is characteristically within the first 2 cm of its origin, in contrast to acute embolic occlusion, which is generally observed more distally.[31] Contrast-enhanced MR angiography can show collateral vessels.

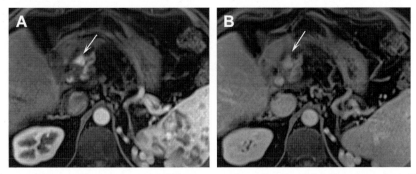

**Fig. 12.** A 54-year-old man with an aneurysm of the common hepatic artery after liver transplantation. (*A*) Transverse hepatic arterial phase image shows an early hyperenhancing lesion of the common hepatic artery anastomosis (*arrow*), which retains contrast on delayed interstitial phase image (*arrow*) (*B*). The enhancement features are identical to surrounding arteries.

**Table 1**
**Main clinical characteristics and radiographic findings of mesenteric arterial ischemia**

| | Main Clinical Characteristics | Radiographic Findings |
|---|---|---|
| Acute mesenteric embolism | Typical history of cardiovascular disease (emboli usually originate from left atrial or ventricular thrombi)<br>Abrupt catastrophic onset of abdominal symptom | Emboli in SMA frequently lodge just beyond the origin of middle colic artery<br>Cutoff sign or intraluminal filling defect on contrast-enhanced MR angiography |
| Acute mesenteric thrombosis | Typically associated with preexisting atherosclerotic disease<br>Abdominal symptoms may be more insidious<br>≤50% of cases have previously experienced symptoms of chronic mesenteric ischemia before the acute event | SMA thrombosis usually develops within the first 2 cm of its origin<br>Usually no defined intraluminal filling defect<br>Development of collateral circulation can be observed |
| Chronic mesenteric ischemia | Almost always caused by severe atherosclerosis<br>Characterized by a classic clinical triad of postprandial abdominal pain, weight loss, and food avoidance | Stenosis or occlusion in affected mesenteric vessel with collateral circulation |

Chronic mesenteric ischemia is invariably caused by severe atherosclerosis and is characterized by a classic clinical triad of postprandial abdominal pain, weight loss, and the patient's avoidance of food.[30] It is generally considered that at least 2 of the 3 main vessels should be affected either by occlusive or stenotic disease to produce clinical symptoms, although stenosis or occlusion in only 1 affected vessel may result in this.[30] Although atherosclerosis of mesenteric branches is frequent in advanced age, chronic mesenteric ischemia is uncommon, because of the rich arterial supply of mesenteric collateral circulation.[5] The marginal artery of Drummond is situated along the mesenteric border of the colon, which connects between right, middle, and left colic arteries. The arc of Riolan is situated more centrally. It is classically described as connecting the middle colic branch of the SMA with the left colic branch of the inferior mesenteric artery. It forms a short loop that runs close to the root of the mesentery (**Fig. 13**). 3D-GE tissue-imaging sequences provide additional information of bowel changes, such as wall thickening and abnormal enhancement. Contrast-enhanced MR angiography is accepted as a noninvasive screening modality for patients suspected of having mesenteric ischemia.[31] The use of MIP images can visualize the entire vascular anatomy at different phases of contrast enhancement.

*Portal venous thrombosis*

Thrombosis of the portal vein can develop at the intrahepatic or extrahepatic level. Portal venous thrombosis is most often observed in the setting of hepatic cirrhosis, but may be associated with a variety of different disease processes, such as severe intra-abdominal infection, malignancy, or hypercoagulable stage.[2,3] On MR imaging, thrombosis of the intrahepatic portion of the portal vein may produce segmental or lobar wedge-shaped areas of increased enhancement on hepatic arterial phase secondary to compensatory increased hepatic arterial supply to the thrombosed hepatic segment. On later phase images, differential enhancement quickly fades. Homogeneous hepatic enhancement is observed, reflecting that the concentration of gadolinium in the hepatic arteries and portal veins equilibrates and that the liver parenchyma receives GBCA from both vessel types. Distinction between acute and chronic portal venous thrombosis is important for clinical management. In the acute setting, portal vein thrombus may resolve with anticoagulation therapy. However, once the thrombosis has become a long-standing process, the likelihood of therapeutic recanalization is greatly reduced. Acute thrombus may show mild hyperintensity on T2-weighted images compared with low signal in the chronic setting.[3] Chronic portal venous occlusion leads to development of cavernous transformation in the porta hepatis. If

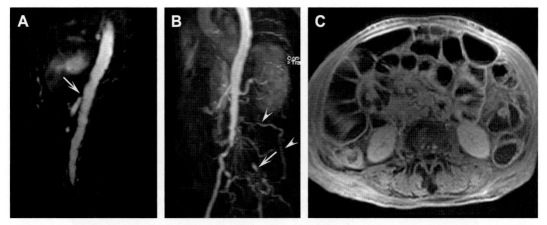

Fig. 13. A 71-year-old woman with a history of peripheral vascular disease who presents with abdominal pain and weight loss. (*A*) Contrast-enhanced MR angiography source image shows severe atherosclerosis of the abdominal aorta, complete occlusion of the celiac axis, and high-grade stenosis of the SMA ostium (*arrow*). (*B*) MIP reconstruction obtained in an oblique coronal plane shows occlusion of the left common iliac artery with distal reconstitution (*arrow*). The inferior mesentery artery was reconstituted via the Riolan arch (*arrowheads*). (*C*) Transverse T1-weighted interstitial phase postgadolinium 3D-GE image shows dilation and abnormal wall enhancement and thickening of the entire small bowel.

thrombus also involves the superior mesenteric vein, this may preclude future transplantation.[3] Postgadolinium 3D-GE sequence performs well in distinguishing tumor from bland portal venous thrombosis.[32] MR imaging is generally considered superior to CT in determining the presence and extent of tumor thrombosis (**Fig. 14**).[26,30] MR imaging is unmatched in its ability to diagnose thrombophlebitis secondary to infected venous clot. At MR imaging, thrombophlebitis may be diagnosed when periportal edema, thickening, and enhancing portal venous wall are observed in the setting of portal vein thrombosis and fever or sepsis.[33]

### Budd-Chiari syndrome

Budd-Chiari syndrome (BCS) is an uncommon obstruction of hepatic venous outflow secondary to a variety of causes. Most cases of BCS are idiopathic; specific causes of BCS are hematologic disorders, pregnancy, intravascular web/membrane, or tumor thrombus. Hepatic venous outflow obstruction leads to increase of sinusoidal pressure and diminished portal venous flow, which develop centrilobular congestion followed by necrosis and atrophy.[34] MR imaging features include HV occlusion or narrowing, and inferior vena cava (IVC) or HV thrombosis.[3]

In acute BCS, the peripheral hepatic parenchyma is hypointense on T1-weighted images and hyperintense on T2-weighted images. This appearance reflects the presence of hepatic edema. After contrast administration, the peripheral liver enhances less than the central region, reflecting diminished blood supply from both hepatic arterial and portal venous systems in the peripheral liver caused by increased tissue pressure. The caudate lobe shows early increased enhancement, which persists on late phase images, reflecting a separate blood supply, and as a result, lesser tissue pressure than peripheral liver (**Table 2**).

In the subacute syndrome, the enhancement of the caudate lobe is less prominent than the heterogeneously increased enhancement in peripheral liver on hepatic arterial phase images (**Fig. 15**). The pattern of enhancement in subacute BCS reflects the development of capsular-based collaterals. Caudate lobe hypertrophy is mild, and intrahepatic collateral vessels are not pronounced in the subacute setting.

In the chronic stage, there is development of portal hypertension and cirrhosis. Hepatic edema is not a prominent feature, and fibrosis develops. Fibrosis of peripheral liver can be observed that appears mildly hypointense on T1-weighted and T2-weighted images. The enhancement differences between peripheral and central region on dynamic postgadolinium MR images become more subtle. The caudate lobe often undergoes compensatory massive hypertrophy. Characteristic curvilinear intrahepatic collaterals and capsular-based collaterals can be identified on postgadolinium 3D-GE.[32] The development of benign large regenerative nodules may be observed in chronic BCS, termed adenomatous hyperplastic nodules, and resulting from increased regenerative activity in response to continuous

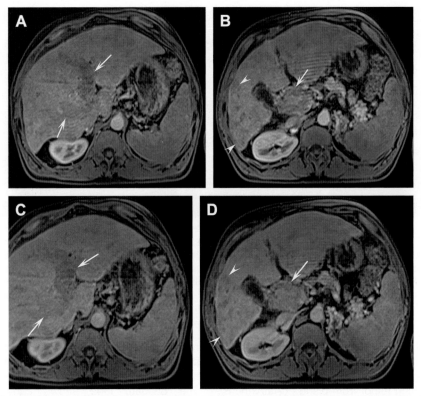

**Fig. 14.** A 50-year-old man with malignant portal venous thrombosis. (*A, B*) Transverse hepatic arterial phase images show mild heterogeneous enhancing tumor thrombus causing expansion of the right, left, and main portal veins (*arrows*). There are multiple irregular, ill-defined foci of diffuse HCC scattered throughout the right hepatic lobe (*arrowheads*). (*C, D*) Transverse venous phase images show washout of tumor thrombus (*arrows*) and of portions of diffuse HCC (*arrowheads*).

congestive changes in liver parenchyma. There is no evidence that these nodules degenerate to malignancy. These benign nodules are usually multiple, with a typical diameter of 0.5 to 4.0 cm, and show homogeneous mildly and moderately intense enhancement on hepatic arterial phase images (**Fig. 16**). They show high signal intensity on T1-weighted images and intermediate to low signal intensity on T2-weighted images.[32,35]

### Hereditary hemorrhagic telangiectasia (Osler-Weber-Rendu syndrome)

Hereditary hemorrhagic telangiectasia (HHT) is an autosomal-dominant multiorgan disorder that presents with a wide range of symptoms, including recurrent epistaxis, mucocutaneous telangiectasia, and visceral involvement. HHT is caused by a genetic defect of fibroelastic fibers and affects tissue in the vicinity of the vessel walls, with multiple telangiectasias accompanied by arteriovenous malformations (AVM).[34] Hepatic involvement occurs in 30% to 73% of patients with HHT, and most often, they are asymptomatic from the liver disease. Three different and concurrent types of

vascular shunts are responsible for parenchymal and biliary abnormalities, namely hepatic artery to HV, hepatic artery to portal vein, and portal vein to HV.[36] These patients can be divided into 3 clinical patterns: (1) high-output cardiac failure as a result of the presence of arteriovenous shunts, (2) portal hypertension as a result of arterioportal shunt, and (3) ischemic biliary disease related to arteriovenous shunt.[37] MR imaging findings of HHT are characterized by the presence of telangiectasia (round hyperenhancing lesion <10 mm), large confluent vascular mass (similar lesion >10 mm), hepatic AVM (shunts between major hepatic vessels), transient perfusion disorders, and enlargement of the hepatic artery (**Fig. 17**).[36,37] Liver in patients with HHT may show hepatocellular regenerative activity, leading to the development of FNH. The prevalence of FNH in patients with HHT is 100-fold greater than in the general population.[36] MR imaging permits delineating parenchyma and vascular and biliary abnormalities in HHT and can be used to assess the outcome of an interventional procedure in symptomatic patients.[38]

| Table 2 Classic imaging findings of BCS | |
| --- | --- |
| **Classic Imaging Findings** | |
| Acute BCS | Presence of hepatic edema in peripheral liver: hypointense on T1-weighted and hyperintense on T2-weighted images, and diminished enhancement on postgadolinium images <br> Early increased enhancement of the caudate lobe and central liver |
| Subacute BCS | Development of capsular-based collaterals: increased enhancement of peripheral region and less enhancement of the caudate lobe <br> Caudate lobe hypertrophy is mild |
| Chronic BCS | Development of fibrosis: hypointense on T1-weighted and T2-weighted images <br> Massive caudate lobe hypertrophy <br> Characteristic development of curvilinear intrahepatic collateral vessels and benign enhancing large regenerative nodules |

## IVC disease

In general, an abdominal protocol using pregadolinium and postgadolinium 3D-GE images provides sufficient evaluation of the IVC for patient management. At least 1 sequence should be performed in the sagittal or coronal plane, because this permits direct visualization of the longitudinal extent of the IVC. Tumor-related invasion of the IVC can be well shown on MR imaging, in the setting of extension of tumor from primary tumors in adjacent organs or more rarely, as primary malignancy of the IVC. Primary leiomyosarcoma may rarely arise from the wall of the IVC. Slow growth allows for the formation of retroperitoneal collateral vessels, and these tumors are usually large at presentation. 3D-GE shows the relationship of the tumor and the extent of involvement (**Fig. 18**).[29] Malignancies that commonly extend directly into the IVC include renal cell carcinoma, hepatocellular carcinoma, adrenal cortical carcinoma, neuroblastoma, Wilms tumor, and extraadrenal paraganglioma (**Fig. 19**).[39] MR imaging features that distinguish malignant from bland thrombus include the presence of a contiguous adjacent mass, thrombus that enlarges the vessel lumen, and enhancement of the thrombus. However, bland downstream thrombus may coexist with malignant thrombus more superiorly in the IVC.[39] Determination of the extent of malignant

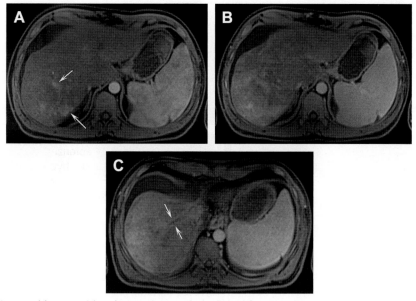

**Fig. 15.** A 39-year-old man with subacute BCS and myeloproliferative disease. (*A*) Transverse hepatic arterial phase image shows mildly heterogeneous enhancement of the peripheral region (*arrows*). (*B*) Transverse venous phase image shows mildly diminished enhancement of the caudate lobe, which enhances less than peripheral liver. This appearance is consistent with subacute syndrome. (*C*) Transverse venous phase image at the level of hepatic dome shows right HV thrombosis (*arrows*).

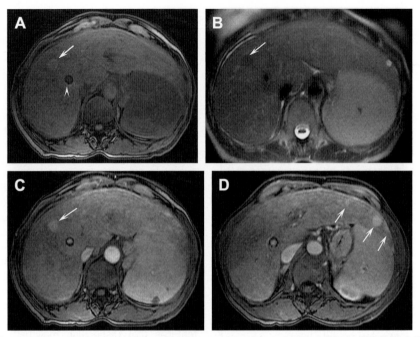

**Fig. 16.** A 60-year-old woman with multiple adenomatous hyperplasia in the setting of chronic BCS. Transverse (*A*) pregadolinium T1-weighted and (*B*) T2-weighed fat-suppressed single-shot echo train spin-echo images show hepatic nodules with mild hyperintensity on T1-weighted and slight hypointensity on T2-weighed images (*arrow*). Transjugular intrahepatic portosystemic shunt is also shown (*arrowhead*). (*C, D*) Transverse hepatic arterial phase postgadolinium images show numerous hyperenhancing nodules scattered in both hepatic lobes (*arrows*), which fade to isointensity on late phase images (*not shown*).

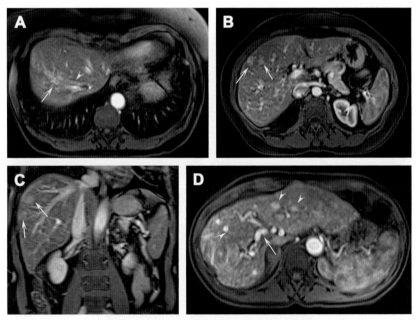

**Fig. 17.** A 63-year-old woman with HHT. (*A, B*) Transverse hepatic arterial phase images show multifocal small hyperenhancing lesions that parallel the enhancement of vessels scattered in the right hepatic lobe, which are consistent with telangiectases (*arrows*). Early opacification of the HVs (*arrowhead*) arise from the presence of extensive intraparenchymal arteriovenous shunts. (*C*) Coronal interstitial phase image shows large enhancing lesions corresponding to confluent vascular masses (*arrows*). (*D*) Transverse hepatic arterial phase image in another patient depicts enlargement of the hepatic artery (*arrow*) and numerous telangiectases (*arrowheads*).

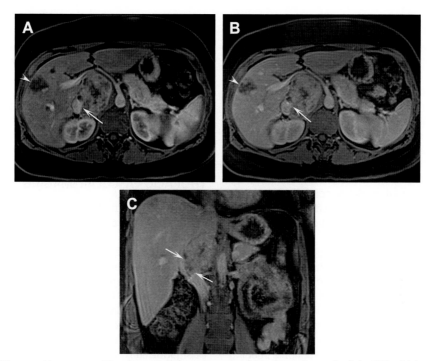

**Fig. 18.** A 36-year-old woman with primary leiomyosarcoma arising from the wall of the IVC with hepatic metastasis. (*A*) Transverse hepatic arterial phase and (*B*) venous phase postgadolinium 3D-GE images show a lobulated heterogeneous enhancing mass, embedded in the IVC (*arrow*), with large exophytic portion. A liver metastasis in segment 5 is also presented (*arrowhead*). (*C*) Coronal interstitial phase image shows the relationship of the mass and the extent of IVC involvement (*arrows*).

thrombus is crucial information for complete surgical resection.[7]

## PELVIC VASCULAR IMAGING

Respiratory artifacts are less of a problem in pelvic vascular imaging, and hence, standard 3D-GE sequences may result in acceptable image quality in patients who are unable to suspend respiration. In the setting of malignant diseases, this technique provides characterization of pelvic masses and vascular assessment that aids staging, surgical planning, and posttreatment surveillance.[40]

### Clinical Considerations

#### Pelvic veins
Dilation of pelvic vessels may occur as the result of various causes, such as venous obstruction (eg, IVC, iliac vein, and left renal vein), portal

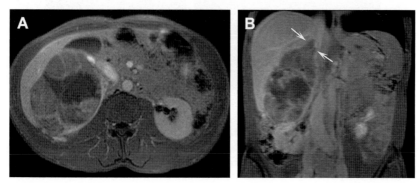

**Fig. 19.** A 43-year-old woman with adrenal cortical carcinoma with IVC invasion. (*A*) Transverse interstitial phase postgadolinium 3D-GE image shows a large right adrenal mass with peripheral nodular enhancement and central necrosis. (*B*) Coronal image shows tumor extension into the IVC (*arrows*).

hypertension, and increased blood flow in the presence of entities such as a pelvic neoplasm or Klippel-Trénaunay syndrome. Enlarged gonadal veins as well as retroperitoneal collaterals can be identified in case of venous obstruction. In the setting of portal hypertension, the portosystemic shunts can be observed in the pelvis, such as dilated rectal venous plexuses. Hypervascular pelvic tumors such as uterine leiomyomas, gestational trophoblastic neoplasms, and ovarian solid tumors may be associated with engorged draining or feeding pelvic vessels.[41] Klippel-Trénaunay syndrome is a rare complex congenital anomaly that is characterized by varicosities, venous malformations, soft tissue, and bone hypertrophy (**Fig. 20**).[41]

Pelvic congestion syndrome (PCS) is a controversial syndrome, defined as chronic pelvic pain that is associated with dilatation of ovarian veins as a result of retrograde venous flow through incompetent valves. It affects mainly premenopausal patients, suggesting a correlation between PCS and ovarian activity.[42] The criteria for diagnosing pelvic varices with cross-sectional imaging

are the presence of at least 4 ipsilateral tortuous parauterine veins of varying caliber, with at least 1 measuring more than 4 mm. in maximal diameter, or an ovarian vein diameter exceeding 8 mm.[42] MR imaging is an excellent modality to visualize engorgement of parauterine, paravaginal venous plexus, and dilated ovarian vessels. Early retrograde filling of a large tortuous gonadal vein may be shown on immediate postgadolinium 3D-GE (**Fig. 21**).

## THORACIC VASCULAR IMAGING

MR imaging of intrathoracic vessels is challenging because of cardiac and respiratory pulsation artifacts, magnetic susceptibility effects, and artifacts at air–soft tissue interfaces. Moreover, there is decreased acceptance by chest physicians, because of both greater artifacts and lower spatial resolution than CT. The development of faster sequences in conjunction with 3-T MR systems has significantly improved image quality. The intrathoracic vessels can be adequately shown using postgadolinium 3D-GE soft tissue sequences

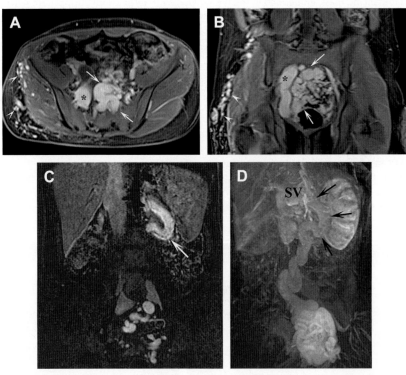

**Fig. 20.** A 21-year-old woman with Klippel-Trénaunay syndrome. (*A*) Transverse and (*B*) coronal interstitial phase postgadolinium 3D-GE image shows tortuous dilated pelvic venous plexus (*arrows*) and abnormally enlarged right internal iliac vein (*asterisk*). Dilated vessels are also apparent within subcutaneous tissue and extending into the right gluteus muscle (*arrowheads*). (*C*) Coronal venous phase contrast-enhanced MR angiography source image and (*D*) MIP reconstruction image, obtained in a coronal plane, show a large abdominopelvic varix connecting the pelvic varices with the splenic vein (SV) (*arrows*).

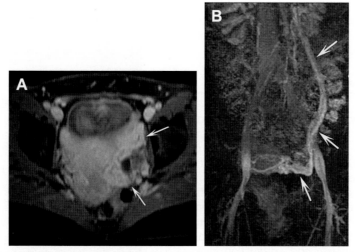

**Fig. 21.** A 51-year-old woman with a history of bilateral lower extremity varicosities. (*A*) Transverse interstitial phase postgadolinium 3D-GE image shows engorgement of parauterine venous plexus (*arrows*). (*B*) MIP reconstruction image obtained in the coronal plane shows filling of a large left ovarian vein (*arrows*).

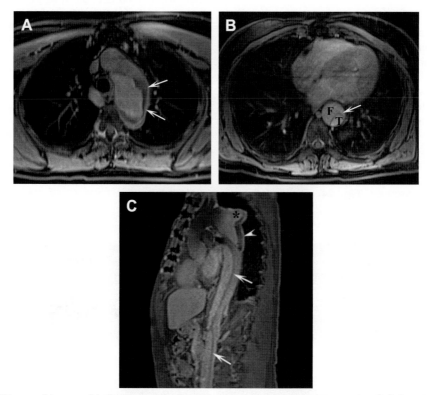

**Fig. 22.** A 55-year-old man with Stanford type B aortic dissection. (*A*) Transverse postgadolinium 3D-GE image obtained at the level of the aortic arch shows low signal intensity mural wall thrombus (*arrows*). (*B*) The lower tomographic image at the level of descending thoracic aorta shows a hypointense intimal flap (*arrow*), which separates the true (T) and false (F) lumens. (*C*) Oblique sagittal postgadolinium 3D-GE image shows the extent of intimal flap (*arrows*), mural thrombus (*arrowhead*), and focal eccentric aneurysm originating from posterior surface of the aortic arch (*asterisk*).

and contrast-enhanced MR angiography sequences. These sequences are beneficial in evaluating intrathoracic vessels and mediastinum as well as lung parenchyma.[23]

## Clinical Considerations

### Thoracic aorta

MR imaging has increasingly become the first-line imaging modality for the evaluation of thoracic aorta in medically stable patients.[43] The use of postgadolinium 3D-GE for assessment of aortic morphology and adjacent structures used in combination with contrast-enhanced MR angiography has achieved comprehensive evaluation of various diseases of the thoracic aorta. Indications for MR imaging of the thoracic aorta include evaluation of aortic aneurysm, aortic dissection, intramural hematoma, penetrating atherosclerotic ulceration, and congenital anomalies (**Figs. 22** and **23**). Postgadolinium 3D-GE implementation allows evaluation of the aortic wall, such as inflammatory aortitis.[1] Fat-saturated pregadolinium 3D-GE facilitates showing intramural hematoma, which appears as hyperintensity on T1-weighted images.[43]

### Pulmonary arteries and pulmonary thromboembolic disease

Contrast-enhanced 3D-GE images provided more sensitive detection of pulmonary embolism (73%) compared with conventional bolus-triggered 3D MR pulmonary angiography (55%).[44] The central, lobar, segmental, and subsegmental pulmonary arteries are well shown with sufficient image quality on postgadolinium 3D-GE sequences.[23] These sequences can detect pulmonary embolism in the main and segmental pulmonary arteries and show parenchyma diseases (**Fig. 24**). Postgadolinium

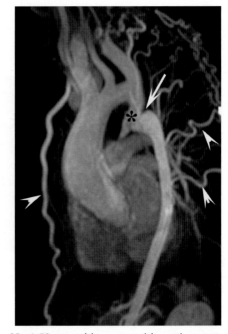

**Fig. 23.** A 53-year-old woman with aortic coarctation. Oblique sagittal MIP reconstruction image shows a short segment abrupt narrowing of the thoracic descending aorta (*arrow*) just distal to the left subclavian artery with a patent ductus arteriosus (*asterisk*). There are dilated intercostal and internal mammary arteries (*arrowheads*).

3D-GE sequences are a good alternative imaging modality to CT for the evaluation of pulmonary embolism in young patients. In patients with contraindication to GBCAs or who are pregnant, b-SSFP sequences, performed without intravenous contrast and with imaging in multiple planes, may be an adequate approach for pulmonary embolism.

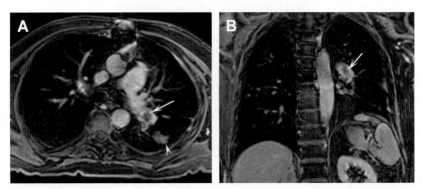

**Fig. 24.** A 76-year-old man with renal cell carcinoma with pulmonary embolism. (*A*) Transverse and (*B*) coronal postgadolinium 3D-GE images show the embolus as a filling defect located in the segmental artery of the left lower lobe (*arrow, A, B*). Pulmonary metastasis in the superior segment of the left lower lobe is noted (*arrowhead*).

## SUMMARY

Because of recent technological advances, vascular imaging with MR imaging has achieved high clinical usefulness. Robust thin-section 3D-GE tissue-imaging sequences have contributed greatly to improved diagnostic MR evaluation of patients with vascular abnormality. The use of high T1-relaxitivity GBCA with long vascular dwell times is suitable to improve the performance of body vascular imaging. Motion-resistant protocols enable adequate vascular imaging in patients who are unable to suspend respiration well. Non–contrast-enhanced MR angiography technique is preferable to gadolinium-enhanced 3D-GE in the setting of pregnancy and severely impaired renal function.

## REFERENCES

1. Sakamoto I, Sueyoshi E, Uetani M. MR imaging of the aorta. Radiol Clin North Am 2007;45(3):485–97.

2. Bradbury MS, Kavanagh PV, Bechtold RE. Mesenteric venous thrombosis: diagnosis and noninvasive imaging. Radiographics 2002;22:527–41.

3. Aslam R, Yeh BM, Yee J. MR imaging evaluation of the hepatic vasculature. Magn Reson Imaging Clin N Am 2010;18:515–23.

4. Sahani D, Mehta A, Blake M, et al. Preoperative hepatic vascular evaluation with CT and MR angiography: implications for surgery. Radiographics 2004;24:1367–80.

5. Shirkhoda A, Konez O, Shetty A, et al. Contrast-enhanced MR angiography of the mesenteric circulation: a pictorial essay. Radiographics 1998;18:851–61.

6. Park HS, Lee JM, Choi HK, et al. Preoperative evaluation of pancreatic cancer: comparison of gadolinium-enhanced dynamic MRI with MR cholangiopancreatography versus MDCT. J Magn Reson Imaging 2009;30:586–95.

7. Choyke PL, Walther MM, Wagner JR, et al. Renal cancer: preoperative evaluation with dual-phase three-dimensional MR angiography. Radiology 1997;205(3):767–71.

8. Vogt FM, Goyen M, Debatin JF. MR angiography of the chest. Radiol Clin North Am 2003;41:29–41.

9. Martin DR, Semelka RC, Chapman A, et al. Nephrogenic systemic fibrosis versus contrast-induced nephropathy: risks and benefits of contrast-enhanced MR and CT in renally impaired patients. J Magn Reson Imaging 2009;30:1350–6.

10. Ramalho M, Altun E, Heredia V, et al. Liver MR imaging: 1.5T versus 3T. Magn Reson Imaging Clin N Am 2007;15:321–47.

11. Erturk SM, Bayarri AA, Herrmann KA, et al. Use of 3.0-T MR imaging for evaluation of the abdomen. Radiographics 2009;29:1547–63.

12. Mihai G, Simonetti OP, Thavendiranathan P. Noncontrast MRA for the diagnosis of vascular disease. Cardiol Clin 2011;29:341–50.

13. Ivancevic MK, Geerts L, Weadock W, et al. Technical principles of MR angiography methods. Magn Reson Imaging Clin N Am 2009;17:1–11.

14. Miyazaki M, Isoda H. Non-contrast-enhanced MR angiography of the abdomen. Eur J Radiol 2011; 80:9–23.

15. Lanzman RS, Kropil P, Schmitt P, et al. Nonenhanced free-breathing ECG-gated steady-state free precession 3D MR angiography of the renal arteries: comparison between 1.5 T and 3T. AJR Am J Roentgenol 2010;194:794–8.

16. Ho VB, Corse WR. MR angiography of the abdominal aorta and peripheral vessels. Radiol Clin North Am 2003;41:115–44.

17. Glockner JF. Three-dimensional gadolinium-enhanced MR angiography: applications for abdominal imaging. Radiographics 2001;21:357–70.

18. Carroll TJ, Grist TM. Technical developments in MR angiography. Radiol Clin North Am 2002;40:921–51.

19. Kroencke TJ, Wasser MN, Pattynama PM, et al. Gadobenate dimeglumine-enhanced MR angiography of the abdominal aorta and renal arteries. AJR Am J Roentgenol 2002;179:1573–82.

20. Michaely HJ, Attenberger UI, Kramer H, et al. Abdominal and pelvic MR angiography. Magn Reson Imaging Clin N Am 2007;15:301–14.

21. Glockner JF, Hu HH, Stanley DW, et al. Parallel MR imaging: a user's guide. Radiographics 2005;25: 1279–97.

22. Hany TF, Schmidt M, Davis CP, et al. Diagnostic impact of four postprocessing techniques in evaluating contrast-enhanced three-dimensional MR angiography. AJR Am J Roentgenol 1998;170:907–12.

23. Altun E, Heredia V, Pamuklar E, et al. Feasibility of post-gadolinium three-dimensional gradient-echo sequence to evaluate the pulmonary arterial vasculature. Magn Reson Imaging 2009;27:1198–207.

24. Altun E, Semelka RC, Dale BM, et al. Water excitation MPRAGE: an alternative sequence for postcontrast imaging of the abdomen in noncooperative patients at 1.5 Tesla and 3.0 Tesla MRI. J Magn Reson Imaging 2008;27:1146–54.

25. Azevedo RM, de Campos R, Ramalho M, et al. Free-breathing 3D T1-weighted gradient-echo sequence with radial data sampling in abdominal MRI: preliminary observations. AJR Am J Roentgenol 2011;197: 650–7.

26. Kanematsu M, Semelka RC, Leonardou P, et al. Hepatocellular carcinoma of diffuse type: MR imaging findings and clinical manifestations. J Magn Reson Imaging 2003;18:189–95.

27. Liu Q, Lu JP, Wang F, et al. Three-dimensional contrast-enhanced MR angiography of aortic dissection: a pictorial essay. Radiographics 2007;27:1311–21.

28. Liu Q, Lu JP, Wang F, et al. Visceral artery aneurysms: evaluation using 3D contrast-enhanced MR angiography. AJR Am J Roentgenol 2008;191:826–33.

29. Sanyal R, Remer EM. Radiology of the retroperitoneum: case-based review. AJR Am J Roentgenol 2009;192:S112–7.

30. Hagspiel KD, Leung DA, Angle JF, et al. MR angiography of the mesenteric vasculature. Radiol Clin North Am 2002;40:867–86.

31. Shih MP, Hagspiel KD. CTA and MRA in mesenteric ischemia: part I, role in diagnosis and differential diagnosis. AJR Am J Roentgenol 2007;188:452–61.

32. Danet IM, Semelka RC, Braga L. MR imaging of diffuse liver disease. Radiol Clin North Am 2003; 41:67–87.

33. Bader TR, Braga L, Beavers KL, et al. MR imaging findings of infectious cholangitis. Magn Reson Imaging 2001;19:781–8.

34. Torabi M, Hosseinzadeh K, Federle MP. CT of nonneoplastic hepatic vascular and perfusion disorders. Radiographics 2008;28:1967–82.

35. Brancatelli G, Federle MP, Grazioli L, et al. Benign regenerative nodules in Budd-Chiari syndrome and other vascular disorders of the liver: radiologic-pathologic and clinical correlation. Radiographics 2002;22:847–62.

36. Carette MF, Nedelcu C, Tassart M, et al. Imaging of hereditary hemorrhagic telangiectasia. Cardiovasc Intervent Radiol 2009;32:745–57.

37. Scardapane A, Ianora S, Sabba C, et al. Dynamic 4D MR angiography versus multislice CT angiography in the evaluation of vascular hepatic involvement in hereditary hemorrhagic teleangiectasia. Radiol Med 2012;117:29–45.

38. Willinek WA, Hadizadeh D, von Falkenhausen M, et al. Magnetic resonance (MR) imaging and MR angiography for evaluation and follow-up of hepatic artery banding in patients with hepatic involvement of hereditary hemorrhagic telangiectasia. Abdom Imaging 2006;31:694–700.

39. Kaufman LB, Yeh BM, Breiman RS, et al. Inferior vena cava filling defects on CT and MRI. AJR Am J Roentgenol 2005;185:717–26.

40. Huertas CP, Brown MA, Semelka RC. MR imaging evaluation of the adnexa. Magn Reson Imaging Clin N Am 2007;14:471–87.

41. Umeoka S, Koyama T, Tagashi K, et al. Vascular dilatation in the pelvis: identification with CT and MR imaging. Radiographics 2004;24:193–208.

42. Ganeshan A, Upponi S, Hon LQ, et al. Chronic pelvic pain due to pelvic congestion syndrome: the role of diagnostic and interventional radiology. Cardiovasc Intervent Radiol 2007;30:1105–11.

43. Lohan DG, Krishnam M, Saleh R, et al. MR imaging of the thoracic aorta. Magn Reson Imaging Clin N Am 2008;16:213–34.

44. Kalb B, Sharma P, Tigges S, et al. MR imaging of pulmonary embolism: diagnostic accuracy of contrast-enhanced 3D MR pulmonary angiography, contrast-enhanced low-flip angle 3D GRE, and non-enhanced free-induction FISP sequences. Radiology 2012;263:271–8.

# Functional MR Imaging of the Abdomen

Kumar Sandrasegaran, MD

## KEYWORDS

- Functional magnetic resonance imaging • Diffusion-weighted imaging
- Intravoxel incoherent motion • Tumor response assessment • Magnetic resonance perfusion
- Dynamic contrast-enhanced magnetic resonance imaging • Magnetic resonance elastography

## KEY POINTS

- The potential benefits of diffusion-weighted magnetic resonance (MR) imaging and intravoxel incoherent motion are discussed.
- The challenges facing the clinical use of dynamic contrast-enhanced (DCE) MR imaging and its usefulness in assessing tumor therapy are discussed.
- The latest literature on MR elastography for abdominal disease is outlined.
- Functional MR imaging gives quantitative measurements and is increasingly being used in clinical practice.
- DCE MR imaging is still undergoing research as to how it may be incorporated in clinical practice. Studies have shown potential use of quantitative DCE MR imaging parameters, such as $K^{trans}$, in predicting outcome of cancer therapy.
- MR elastography is considered to be a useful tool in staging liver fibrosis.
- Other indications for these techniques are being investigated.
- A major issue with all functional MR imaging techniques is the lack of standardization of the protocol.

## INTRODUCTION

Traditionally, abdominal magnetic resonance (MR) imaging has been performed using T2-weighted sequences and pregadolinium-enhanced and postgadolinium-enhanced T1-weighted sequences. These sequences have been used to detect and characterize focal masses and assess treatment response of malignant lesions. Functional MR imaging techniques assess specific physiologic processes in normal and diseased organs. Unlike conventional MR imaging sequences, which are usually reported qualitatively based on the varying brightness of tissue, functional MR imaging techniques give quantitative data. Of the many functional MR imaging techniques,

diffusion-weighted imaging (DWI), intravoxel incoherent motion (IVIM), MR elastography, and T1-weighted dynamic contrast-enhanced (DCE) MR imaging are the most likely to find clinical use at present or in the near future in abdominal imaging. These techniques are discussed.

## DWI

Since its use for stroke detection in the early 1990s, DWI has evolved into a mature functional MR imaging technique with neuroradiology applications. With more recent advances in MR imaging hardware, DWI is becoming a tool for investigating abdominal disease, particularly in the liver. The attractions of DWI include the addition of qualitative

No relevant financial disclosures.
Department of Radiology, Indiana University School of Medicine, 550 N University Blvd, UH 0279, Indianapolis, IN 46202, USA
*E-mail address:* ksandras@iupui.edu

Radiol Clin N Am 52 (2014) 883–903
http://dx.doi.org/10.1016/j.rcl.2014.02.018

and quantitative functional information to conventional anatomic sequences, small scan times allowing the incorporation of DWI into routine clinical protocols, and the lack of need for gadolinium chelates. Nevertheless, abdominal DWI faces many challenges, and more research is needed to identify its clinical usefulness.

## Basic Concepts

DWI is an MR technique that investigates the random thermally induced Brownian movement of the water molecules. In the normal aqueous extracellular space, diffusion of water molecules is relatively unrestricted. On the other hand, diffusion of water molecules is restricted within cells because of the presence of macromolecules, organelles, and cell membrane. Diffusion may become restricted if there is a relative increase in intracellular volume, such as in highly cellular tumors, or if collagen molecules are deposited in the extracellular space, such as in liver fibrosis. Necrosis of cells with destruction of cell membrane is likely to lead to an increase in diffusion.

DWI is based on a T2-weighted sequence, with 1 major difference. A pair of additional (motion-sensitizing) gradients are applied on either side of the 180° refocusing radiofrequency pulse

(**Fig. 1**). For relatively static water molecules, the phase shift caused by the first gradient is reversed by the second gradient, leading to relatively no signal loss. However, for mobile water molecules, the effect of the first gradient is not completely reversed by the second gradient, resulting in reduced signal on DWI.[1] The degree of diffusion weighting is given by a factor known as the b value (see **Fig. 1**). The b value is mainly determined by the amplitude of the motion-sensitizing gradients, and to a lesser degree, by the duration of the gradients and the time interval between them. DWI performed with differing b values is used to construct quantitative maps, as described later.

## Optimizing Technique

Single-shot spin-echo echo-planar (SS-EPI) sequence is the most widely used DWI technique (see **Fig. 1**). Advantages include a short acquisition time and relatively high signal-to-noise ratio (SNR).[2] On the other hand, EPI sequence provides a limited spatial resolution, and it is highly sensitive to susceptibility variations. To improve image quality, technical innovations in hardware and in acquisition techniques may be used, including the use of fat suppression and parallel imaging techniques. Newer techniques of DWI include

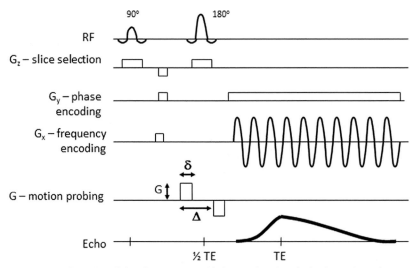

**Fig. 1.** DWI sequence. DWI is a T2-weighted sequence with long echo time (TE). The unique feature of DWI is the application of 2 motion-probing bipolar gradients on either side of the refocusing 180° pulse. The amplitude of the gradients (G), their duration ($\delta$), and interval between gradients ($\Delta$) determine the degree of diffusion weighting. This factor is quantitatively expressed by a parameter b, where $b = \gamma^2 G^2 \delta^2 (\Delta - \delta/3)$ and $\gamma$ is the gyromagnetic ratio (a constant). Protons in water molecules that have no net motion during the first gradient acquire phase shifts that are canceled out by the second gradient. Thus, the application of the diffusion gradients does not diminish the resultant echo. On the other hand, protons in water molecules that have moved during the application of the first gradient experience greater phase shifts, which are not canceled by the second gradient. This phenomenon results in a net loss of signal that is dependent on the degree on molecular motion. In single-shot echo-planar sequence, the frequency-encoding gradients are constantly changed to enable coverage of the entire volume after a single 90° pulse. RF, radiofrequency.

half-Fourier acquisition of single-shot turbo spin-echo (HASTE), and radial k-space acquisitions, such as periodically rotated overlapping parallel lines with enhanced reconstruction (PROPELLER) sequence.

SS-EPI may be performed as a breath-hold, respiratory-gated, or free breathing sequence. Breath-hold technique is the fastest, with the scan usually completed in less than 1 minute. Disadvantages of this acquisition include low SNR, poor spatial resolution, and limitation on the maximum possible b value (typically <500 s/mm$^2$).[1,3] Free breathing DWI take about 2 to 3 minutes to acquire, whereas respiratory-gated sequences take up to 7 minutes to complete.[2] These 2 techniques allow scanning with b values as high as 1000 s/mm$^2$ and acquire twice as many slices as the breath-hold sequence (typically 20 slices compared with 10 slices for breath-hold technique).[1] Cardiac gating helps identification of left hepatic lobe lesions, but substantially increases acquisition time and is not usually used.[4]

## Apparent Diffusion Coefficient

DWI is acquired with at least 2 different b values. With low b values, typically less than 200 s/mm$^2$, lesions with high T2 values appear hyperintense, regardless of their diffusion properties, because of the effect of T2 on the image contrast. This phenomenon is termed T2 shine through (**Fig. 2**) and is seem in the normal gall balder, benign cystic lesions, and hemangioma. On DWI with high b values, tissue with unrestricted diffusion, such as the normal extracellular space, shows signal loss. On the other hand, tissue with high cellularity, and therefore restricted diffusion, appears hyperintense (**Fig. 3**). Interpretation of DWI requires the generation of apparent diffusion coefficient (ADC) maps. These maps are automatically generated by commercial MR workstations, pixel by pixel, using the formula: ADC = $[\ln(SI_1/SI_2)]/(b_2 - b_1)$, where ln is the natural logarithm, $SI_1$ and $SI_2$ are the signal intensities of the pixel on DWI images with b values $b_1$ and $b_2$, respectively (see **Fig. 2**).

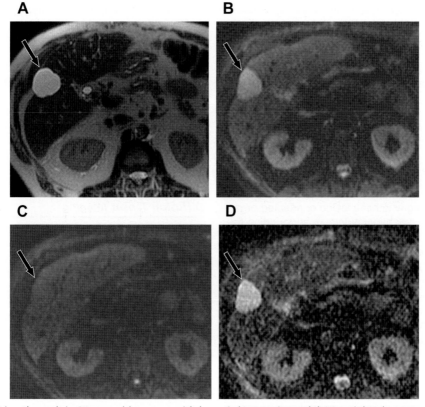

**Fig. 2.** T2 shine through in 35-year-old woman with hepatic hemangioma. (*A*) T2-weighted sequence shows the lesion (*arrow*) to be hyperintense. (*B*) DWI with b value of 50 s/mm$^2$ is T2 weighted, and the hemangioma (*arrow*) remains bright because of its high T2 value, a phenomenon known as T2 shine through. (*C*) On DWI with b value of 800 s/mm$^2$, the lesion (*arrow*) shows reduced intensity (compared with *B*). (*D*) On the apparent diffusion coefficient (ADC) map, the hemangioma (*arrow*) is hyperintense, indicating that it has relatively unrestricted diffusion. A region of interest placed over the lesion gives its mean ADC value.

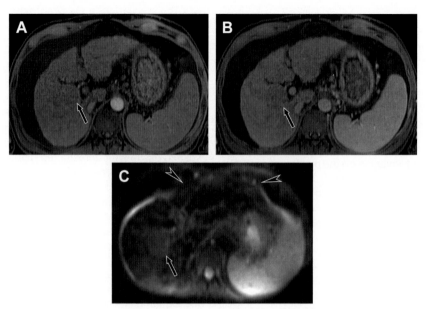

**Fig. 3.** 47-year-old man with cirrhosis. (*A*) On arterial phase image, a 3-cm isointense lesion (*arrow*) is seen. (*B*) On venous phase, the lesion (*arrow*) is mildly hypointense. The appearances are not typical of hepatocellular cancer (HCC) and may have led to a diagnosis of a benign hepatic nodule. (*C*) On DWI with b = 500 s/mm², the lesion (*arrow*) is hyperintense, suggesting that it has restricted diffusion. This finding is worrisome for highly cellular HCC. The lesion was biopsied and found to be a well-differentiated HCC. Note the distortion of anatomy in the anterior abdomen (*arrowheads*) in DWI image, because of sensitivity of SS-EPI to susceptibility effects from colonic gas.

The term apparent is used in ADC because the true coefficient cannot be measured using MR imaging. ADC is higher than true diffusion coefficient because of confounding effects of diffusion effect from molecules other than water, microscopic perfusion, eddy currents, and field inhomogeneity.[5]

### Qualitative and Quantitative Analysis of DWI

DWI is assessed qualitatively in clinical practice, by determining whether a lesion or affected organ is hypointense or hyperintense to surrounding tissue on both low and high b value sequences. ADC values may be estimated by drawing regions of interest (ROIs) in both abnormal and normal tissue. Quantitative measurements have not found routine clinical use, partly because of variability of results caused by differences in MR imaging hardware and the lack of standardized DWI protocol. In addition, there may be a substantial (about 10%) interobserver and baseline variability of ADC measurements.[6–13]

### IVIM

In conventional DWI, microscopic perfusion and diffusion are combined into a single measurement, the ADC. IVIM is a theoretical model that attempts to separate capillary microcirculation (perfusion) from molecular diffusion by using multiple b values. Multiple parameters for diffusion and perfusion may be obtained by IVIM (**Fig. 4**). The widespread use of IVIM is hampered by the time to obtain images sets with multiple b value sequences (typically ≥6) and the current lack of vendor software to analyze the data. Scan times are in the order of 10 to 20 minutes if respiratory compensation is used.

### Diffusion Tensor Imaging

In most abdominal organs, water molecules diffuse approximately equally in all directions. For instance, the ADC measurements from diffusion tensor imaging (DTI) techniques in most organs are similar to those obtained by conventional DWI methods. This situation is not true in the kidneys, in which the arrangement of tubules in a radial direction causes preferential diffusion in some planes (anisotropy). DTI has an established role in studying disease affecting white matter tracts in the brain. It has limited applications in the abdomen.

### Applications of DWI

In the next sections, the potential uses of DWI in diseases of the liver, pancreas, urinary tract, and bowel are discussed.

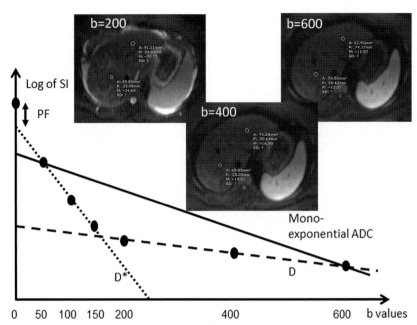

**Fig. 4.** IVIM is performed using multiple b values, typically more than 6. The graph shows the log of signal intensity (SI) (y-axis) of the same pixel in the right lobe of liver obtained at different b values (in s/mm$^2$: x-axis). A monoexponential gradient (ADC) may be obtained using signal intensities on high and low b values. Using only results from high b value (typically >200 s/mm$^2$) sequences, a true diffusion coefficient (D) may be estimated. This coefficient is likely to be a closer estimate of diffusion component to molecular motion. Using only results from low b value (typically <200 s/mm$^2$) sequences, the pseudodiffusion (or perfusion coefficient or D*) may be obtained. Low b values are sensitive to perfusion, which explains why signal intensity rapidly reduces when b value is increased from zero to about 200 s/mm$^2$. Note that the magnitude of D* is greater than D. The slope of D* is affected by small errors in measuring signal intensity and so shows greater interobserver variability. The perfusion fraction (PF) is another estimate of how much perfusion contributes to molecular motion.

### Diffuse liver disease

Deposition of collagen in extracellular space with increasing fibrosis reduces ADC. However, many studies have shown that, although it may be possible to separate normal liver from end-stage fibrosis (cirrhosis), intermediate grades of fibrosis cannot be discerned.[14–17] Therefore, this technique does not replace liver biopsy, which remains the gold standard for determining the stage of liver fibrosis. Studies on patients after orthotopic liver transplantation have shown that DWI or ADC measurements do not reliably differentiate parenchymal complications, such as rejection, recurrent viral hepatitis, or recurrent fibrosis.[18,19] One of the difficulties in parsing various studies on DWI is the different techniques used, leading to lack of standardization of ADC measurements.

ADC values have been shown to reduce with increasing hepatic steatosis. However, DWI is unlikely to become a tool for diagnosing hepatic steatosis, because other MR imaging techniques exist for this purpose. DWI does not reliably diagnose hepatic inflammation and is unlikely to be useful in the assessment of nonalcoholic fatty liver disease.

A few studies[20–23] have shown that perfusion or diffusion coefficients from IVIM are reduced in advanced fibrosis compared with normal liver. Nevertheless, it is not clear how useful these parameters are in individual patients to classify early and intermediate stages of fibrosis. Hepatic fat may not affect perfusion parameters (D* and perfusion fraction [PF]).[24] An animal study has shown reduction in perfusion parameters with the onset of steatohepatitis, distinguishing inflammation from steatosis.[25] This finding needs further verification.

### Focal liver masses

Early reports indicated that ADC values can differentiate benign cysts and hemangioma from malignant lesions.[26] However, this differentiation is easy with other standard sequences. ADC values of benign solid lesions, such as focal nodular hyperplasia or adenoma, and malignant lesions, such as metastases, show considerable overlap.[27–32] DWI is inferior to postgadolinium series on a head-to-head comparison for detecting liver lesions, particularly metastases.[33–36] Nevertheless, DWI plays a useful role in highlighting some small lesions that may be difficult to discern on contrast-enhanced sequences (**Fig. 5**). The combined use of DWI and contrast-enhanced sequences has a higher sensitivity for detecting liver metastases compared with either sequence on its own.[33–35,37] DWI may be particularly helpful in detecting small hypervascular neuroendocrine metastases that may not be well seen in postcontrast studies, especially if a high-quality arterial phase is not obtained.[38] Even in patients with hypovascular liver metastases, DWI may help increase confidence that a small indeterminate lesion is malignant if the lesion is hyperintense on high b value sequence and hypointense on ADC map. DWI is a useful sequence in patients who cannot receive gadolinium because of renal dysfunction or other reasons, because it is clearly superior to T2-weighted sequences in detecting liver metastases.[39–41]

In cirrhotic patients, DWI is inferior to contrast-enhanced MR imaging for hepatocellular cancer (HCC) detection.[42] Nevertheless, it helps to identify some lesions that do not have typical arterial enhancement or subsequent washout (see **Fig. 3**).[43–46] DWI helps to differentiate small well-differentiated HCC, which tend to be hyperintense on DWI, from dysplastic nodules [47–51] and vascular pseudolesions,[47,52–54] both of which are isointense on all DWI sequences. DWI is also helpful in identifying infiltrative poorly differentiated HCC, which are often difficult to diagnose on contrast-enhanced sequences.[55] However, DWI is not useful for differentiating the histologic grade of HCC[56–61] or differentiating malignant and benign portal vein thrombosis in patients with HCC and cirrhosis.[62]

## Liver tumor response assessment

Traditional anatomic methods, such as tumor size and even tumor enhancement patterns, do not show evidence of response or lack thereof, for several weeks or months after treatment. Because newer biological agents used for treating liver tumors are expensive, it would be useful to predict response at an earlier stage, for instance within 1 month of onset of treatment (**Fig. 6**). There has been much interest in whether DWI may provide earlier accurate assessment of tumor response. After therapy, tumors initially show increased cellular size over 48 to 72 hours because of cytotoxic edema.[5] This finding typically would be expected to reduce ADC, because the ratio of intracellular/extracellular volume in a voxel would increase. Subsequently, cellular necrosis and an increase in ADC are expected. Many studies do show a pattern of reduced ADC followed by an increase in ADC in tumors treated with biological therapy. Nevertheless, there are many challenges in the use of DWI in this clinical situation. ADC measurements of the same individual without treatment show baseline variability. Thus, any change that is ascribable to therapy must be

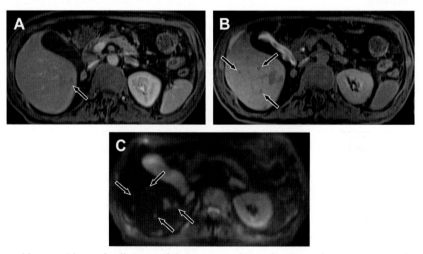

**Fig. 5.** 69-year-old man with renal cell cancer. (*A*) Contrast-enhanced venous phase sequence using gadoxetate disodium (Eovist, Bayer HealthCare, Whippany, NJ) shows possible metastases (*arrow*) in the posterior right lobe of liver. (*B*) Hepatobiliary phase at 20 minutes after contrast injection shows several small hypointense lesions (*arrows*) not previously seen. (*C*) DWI with b value of 800 s/mm² shows that the lesions (*arrows*) have restricted diffusion, consistent with metastases. Both DWI and the hepatobiliary phase of gadoxetate help to identify small metastases that may not be visible on other sequences. This technique is particularly useful if hepatic segmental resection is considered for metastatic disease.

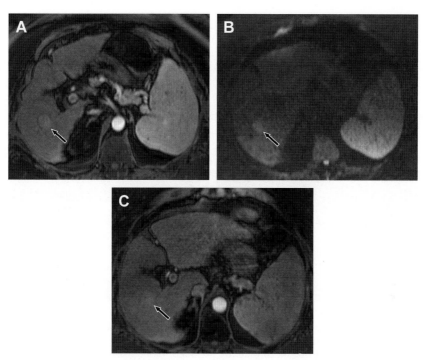

**Fig. 6.** 58-year-old woman with HCC treated with stereotactic body radiation therapy. (*A*) Pretreatment arterial phase image shows 2-cm hypervascular mass (*arrow*), which showed washout (venous phase image not shown), consistent with HCC. (*B*) On DWI with b value of 600 s/mm², the lesion (*arrow*) is hyperintense, indicating restricted diffusion. Lesion ADC was measured as $1.02 \times 10^{-3}$ mm²/s. (*C*) Imaging 1 month after treatment shows that the lesion (*arrow*) is still hypervascular and stable in size. Lesion ADC was measured as $1.47 \times 10^{-3}$ mm²/s. The substantial increase in ADC suggests tumor cellular necrosis. The lesion responded to therapy and was no longer seen at 6-month follow-up (not shown).

clearly above and beyond this variability. However, there is no consensus on what is the extent of baseline variability. Studies do not concur on the degree of ADC change that would predict response.[63–67] The discrepancies in study results may relate to scan protocol, tumor histology, and the treatment offered. In addition, the timing of the change in ADC is not clear. Some studies show normalization of ADC about a month after therapy.

It has been suggested that metastases that show high ADCs before treatment may be associated with more adverse response to chemotherapy.[66,68,69] The rationale may be that necrotic and hypoxic tumors may be less likely to respond to conventional and antiangiogenic therapy. However, other studies have not found this predictive value of pretreatment ADC.[63,67,70,71] No clear consensus may be drawn on the value of ADC measurements on tumor biology and assessing treatment response.

### Pancreatic disease

ADC values for the normal pancreas have been reported to range from 1.0 to $2.0 \times 10^{-3}$ mm²/s.[72]

The tail of pancreas shows slightly lower ADC values than the head and body.

DWI has not been shown to delineate the size or aggressiveness of pancreatic adenocarcinoma.[73,74] ADC values have not been shown to be useful in differentiating pancreatic cancer from mass-forming chronic pancreatitis.[75–79] Both entities show a reduction in ADC compared with the normal pancreas, but with substantial overlap in ADC values between each other (**Fig. 7**). Hyperintensity on DWI is a helpful sign in diagnosing a small hypervascular neuroendocrine tumors (NET) of the pancreas, although DWI is not particularly sensitive to small NET.[80] This sign also helps to differentiate NET from accessory splenic tissue in the pancreatic tail.[81] DWI is not useful in differentiating the histologic grade of mucinous cystic tumors of the pancreas (intraductal mucinous neoplasm and mucinous cystic neoplasm) and differentiating mucinous and serous cystic tumors.[82–84]

The use of DWI in diagnosing autoimmune pancreatitis (AIP) has been reported in a few studies. In focal or regional AIP, sites of inflammation have lower ADC than the unaffected gland.

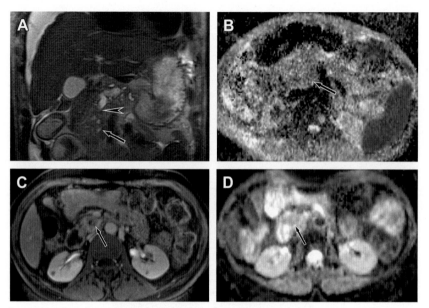

**Fig. 7.** DWI of mass-forming chronic pancreatitis (CP) and pancreatic cancer in 2 different patients. (*A, B*) 45-year-old man with abdominal pain. Coronal T2-weighted image (*A*) and axial ADC (*B*) show an enlarged head of pancreas (*arrow*) with an abrupt duct cutoff (*arrowhead, A*). ADC of pancreatic head was measured as $1.25 \times 10^{-3}$ mm$^2$/s. Because cancer could not be confidently excluded, patient underwent Whipple surgery and was found to have CP. (*C, D*) 70-year-old woman with pancreas cancer. Axial postgadolinium image (*C*) shows an ill-defined hypoenhancing mass (*arrow*). Axial ADC (*D*) shows hypointensity (*arrow*) at site of cancer. The tumor ADC was measured as $1.02 \times 10^{-3}$ mm$^2$/s. The uninvolved pancreas showed ADC of $1.76 \times 10^{-3}$ mm$^2$/s. In individual patients, it is not possible to reliably use ADC to distinguish between CP and pancreatic cancer.

ADC values also increase after response to steroids and may be a potential method of assessing treatment response.[79,85–87]

### Bowel disease

Peristaltic motion and the high susceptibility of echo-planar sequences to magnetic field heterogeneity and chemical shift limit are limiting factors for DWI assessment of bowel disease.[2] Early studies[88–92] have shown DWI to be an adjunct to conventional MR enterography sequences in detecting sites of inflammation in Crohn disease as hyperintense foci in DWI sequences with low ADC values. It is unclear if DWI helps to change management in the evaluation of inflammatory bowel disease.

Considerable attention has been paid to the usefulness of DWI in staging and assessing treatment response of locally advanced rectal cancer. DWI may help increase accuracy of T stage when combined with T2-weighted sequences and may add confidence in predicting tumor clearance of mesorectal fascia.[93,94] Studies[95–98] have shown that low ADC before treatment may suggest a higher likelihood of complete response to therapy. Early and substantial increase in ADC is likely to be a factor in suggesting good response.[95,97–101] Nevertheless, the cutoff ADC values reported vary between studies, reflecting the need to standardize DWI technique. Mucinous tumors tend to have high ADC values and may be mistaken for benign lesions.[100,102]

### Renal disease

The normal ADC values vary considerably across studies, depending on scanner hardware, imaging parameters, and patient's hydration status.[103,104] A wide variation of renal ADC values have been reported, ranging from 1.5 to $5.5 \times 10^{-3}$ mm$^2$/s.[105] Cortex has a higher mean ADC compared with the medulla. It is important to perform DWI before gadolinium administration for assessing renal disease, because contrast enhancement may affect renal ADC measurements, unlike with other abdominal organs.[106,107] Renal dysfunction, particularly chronic renal failure, causes reduced cortical ADC values. More importantly, foci of infarction and pyelonephritis show reduced ADC values and hyperintensity of DWI sequences.[105]

In general, more cellular renal neoplasm would be expected to have a lower ADC. However, there is substantial overlap of ADC values between benign and malignant solid renal tumors.[108,109] It is usually not possible to differentiate the grade of clear-cell renal cell cancer (RCC) or differentiate clear-cell histology from papillary-type RCC (**Fig. 8**).[109] Increasingly, treatment options, such as observation, ablation, and partial or radical nephrectomy, are being based on the histologic grade of the tumor. DWI is unlikely to replace biopsy for assessment of tumor histology. As with a solid renal mass, DWI has not been found to be useful in determining if an adrenal lesion is benign or malignant.[110–112]

### Prostate cancer

Prostate cancer is the most common neoplasm of men. Transrectal ultrasound-guided (TRUS) biopsy is used to biopsy the gland to diagnose cancer. Prostate MR imaging is usually performed to stage cancer. Traditionally, T2-weighted sequences are obtained, with or without an endorectal coil. Most (70%) tumors are in the peripheral zone and appear hypointense on T2-weighted MR imaging. DWI is able to show cancer in the peripheral zone, usually with a higher sensitivity and specificity than T2-weighted sequences (**Fig. 9**). However, studies vary significantly in the usefulness of DWI, with reported sensitivity as low as 40%. In the central gland, DWI is probably superior to T2-weighted sequence, but there is a large overlap in ADC values of benign hyperplasia, prostatitis, and cancer.[113–115] An important point to note is that ADC values of normal prostate vary from about 1.30 to 2.00 $\times$ 10$^{-3}$ mm$^2$/s in different studies and are dependent on the MR imaging platform used.[116] There is some evidence that very high b values in the range of 1200 to 2000 s/mm$^2$ may improve diagnostic sensitivity.[117,118] DWI may help guide biopsy, particularly by localizing potential tumor in the apical and anterior aspects of prostate.[119] In our practice, MR imaging and DWI images are fused with TRUS images to guide repeat biopsies, when the initial set of biopsies were negative, in cases with strong clinical suspicion of prostate cancer. ADC values have an inverse correlation with aggressiveness of cancer, as measured by the Gleason score. Nevertheless, there is substantial overlap of ADC values for different Gleason scores, making DWI and ADC measurements unhelpful in predicting tumor biology in individual patients.[120–122]

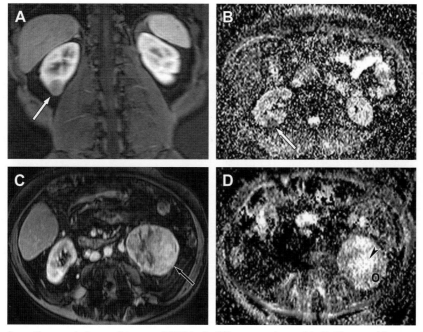

**Fig. 8.** DWI of papillary and clear-cell types of RCC in 2 different patients. (*A, B*) 43-year-old man with papillary RCC. Coronal postgadolinium image (*A*) shows a partially exophytic right renal mass (*arrow*) that enhances homogenously and hypointensely. These findings are typical of papillary RCC. Axial ADC map (*B*) shows the lesion (*arrow*). ADC was measured as 1.58 $\times$ 10$^{-3}$ mm$^2$/s. (*C, D*) 80-year-old woman with clear-cell RCC. Axial postgadolinium image (*C*) shows a heterogeneously enhancing large mass (*arrow*) in left kidney. (*D*) ADC of its central portion (*arrowhead*) was measured as 2.75 $\times$ 10$^{-3}$ mm$^2$/s. The more solid region (*O*) showed an ADC of 1.56 $\times$ 10$^{-3}$ mm$^2$/s. In most tumors, the most reproducible DWI measurement is the minimum ADC, which corresponds to the most cellular tissue. The overlap in ADC values of different solid renal tumors does not permit reliable differentiation.

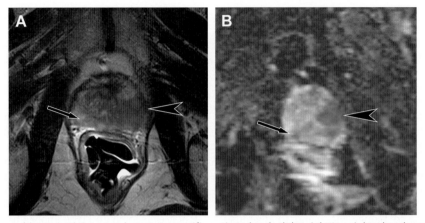

**Fig. 9.** 55-year-old man with increased prostate-specific antigen levels. (*A*) Axial T2-weighted endorectal prostate MR imaging image shows a 1.6-cm hypointensity (*arrowhead*) in the left peripheral zone, worrisome for cancer. No convincing lesion was seen in the right peripheral zone. There was only vague hypointensity (*arrow*). (*B*) Axial ADC map at same level shows hypointense foci in the left (*arrowhead*) and right (*arrow*) zones. Surgical pathology showed bilateral tumors.

Once a tumor is diagnosed, ADC values may help in determining seminal vesicle invasion in some cases.[123] Generally, they do not add substantial information to T2-weighted images in assessing extracapsular invasion.[116,124,125]

DTI has been studied for differentiating benign and malignant prostatic lesions and in determining extent of neurovascular invasion.[126] Early results are conflicting. Studies show a higher,[127–129] lower,[130] or similar[131] fractional anisotropy (FA) in cancer compared with background tissue. It is also unclear if the FA of peripheral zone is the same or different compared with transitional zone. IVIM has also been used to show diffusion and perfusion aspects of prostate cancer. Again, there are conflicting data as to whether PF and perfusion-related diffusion coefficient (D*) of tumors is higher or lower than normal tissue.[132–134] Further investigation of DTI and IVIM in prostate cancer is required to clarify these discrepancies.

DWI is helpful in assessing tumor recurrence after ablation, radiation, or high-intensity focused ultrasonographic therapy.[135,136] After therapy, the gland shows reduced intensity on T2-weighted images obscuring recurrent tumor.[137,138] The zonal anatomy may become indistinct. Hyperintense foci on high b value DWI images, at site of original tumor, are likely to indicate tumor recurrence.

DWI is sometimes helpful in detecting malignant involvement despite normal size of node. Even although ADC values of malignant nodes are on average lower than those of benign nodes, there is overlap of ADC values of reactive and malignant adenopathy. In our practice, we report on nodes that are hyperintense on high b value sequences and show an ADC value less than

$1.00 \times 10^{-3}$ mm$^2$/s as being concerning for metastatic disease.

### Summary of DWI

One of the main difficulties in widespread clinical use of DWI is the reliance of quantitative measurements on the scan protocol. Standardization of DWI protocols is necessary. Nevertheless, it has become clear that qualitative assessment of signal intensities on high and low b value sequence helps to improve lesion detection. Lesions that remain hyperintense on high b value images and that show low signal on ADC maps are worrisome for malignant lesions. Prospective multicenter research is required to determine if ADC values may be used to predict and assess response to therapy for malignant lesions.

### MR PERFUSION

Assessment of tumor perfusion has become an important technique, particularly with the advent of antiangiogenic therapy. Computed tomography (CT) perfusion has many advantages over MR perfusion. These advantages include rapid scan time of CT (with the entire abdomen and pelvis covered easily within a few seconds) and the almost direct correlation between Hounsfield measurements and tissue iodine concentration. However, CT perfusion is radiation intensive. MR perfusion, on the other hand, is a more difficult technique to undertake, as discussed later. MR perfusion techniques include DCE MR imaging, dynamic susceptibility contrast (DSC) imaging, and arterial spin labeling (ASL). DSC investigates changes in T2* as a result of first pass of gadolinium through tissue and gives information regarding vessel density, mean transit time, and relative blood volume. ASL uses magnetically labeled blood as an endogenous tracer.[139] ASL and DSC techniques are well established in neuroradiology. However, they are in the early stages of development for abdominal applications and are not further discussed. On the other hand, there is a substantial amount of literature on abdominopelvic applications of DCE MR imaging, which is discussed later.

## DCE MR Imaging Technique

The basis of DCE MR imaging is the acquisition of multiple image sets, every few seconds, through the tumor or as much of the organ as possible, after gadolinium injection. The first 90 seconds of postcontrast acquisition is important, because this corresponds to the rapid increase in gadolinium concentration in the extracellular space. Scanning is typically carried on until 5 minutes after contrast injection, although there is less need for high temporal resolution after the first 90 to 120 seconds of data acquisition.

Semiquantitative perfusion parameters are obtained from signal intensity versus time curve. Such measurements, which include onset time (time to arrival of gadolinium after start of injection), maximal initial slope, maximal signal intensity, and washout gradient (**Fig. 10**), are dependent on the scanner hardware, sequence used, and patient's cardiovascular status. Although easy to obtain, these measurements are difficult to compare between different studies.

Quantitative methods try to overcome patient and scanner variability. These methods are more difficult to perform and require additional steps (**Table 1**). The most important quantitative parameter yielded by DCE MR imaging is $K^{trans}$, which is the volume transfer constant between plasma and the extravascular extracellular space and is usually expressed as per minute (see **Fig. 10**). Another parameter that may be derived from quantitative DCE MR imaging is the volume of extravascular extracellular space per unit tissue volume, expressed as a unit-less ratio between 0 and 1. Further details of quantitative DCE MR imaging are discussed elsewhere.[140–142]

## Challenges in DCE MR Imaging

The selection of imaging parameters is important to optimize the opposing demands of spatial resolution, anatomic coverage, and temporal resolution. There are different techniques used for image acquisition, from two-dimensional to three-dimensional T1-weighted gradient-echo sequences and newer cyclic k-space techniques. There is debate as to whether a generic arterial input function is equivalent to one derived from imaging the patient. In addition, pharmacokinetic models used for fitting image data have built-in assumptions that may not be accurate for the clinical situation. For instance, the commonly used Toft model assumes that the vascular supply to liver metastases is arterial, which may not be entirely correct.[141] As with DWI, there needs to be further standardization of quantitative DCE MR imaging technique. This strategy is necessary to reduce the interobserver and baseline variability in quantitative parameters.[143–145]

We are attempting to incorporate abdominal DCE MR imaging in clinical studies. With newer three-dimensional T1-weighted sequences, the entire liver may be imaged in 5 to 8 seconds. Three such image sets may be obtained per breath-hold. The scan is paused during the 5-second to 7-second period of free breathing in between the breath-holds. At about 35 seconds after contrast injection, it is necessary to acquire a clinically diagnostic high-quality arterial phase sequence, which typically lasts 15 seconds. This procedure entails the loss of 2 or 3 DCE MR imaging data points. The multiple breath-holds in the first 90 seconds do require motivated patients and MR technologists. Despite the many difficulties in performing DCE MR imaging, we believe that it may become a clinical MR imaging sequence in the near future.

## Uses of DCE MR Imaging

In the abdomen, DCE MR imaging has been used in the study of cancers of the liver, pancreas, kidneys, prostate, cervix, and rectum. An increase in $K^{trans}$ after therapy has been suggested to indicate response to therapy for rectal[146] and pancreatic[147] cancers (see **Fig. 10**). Studies also suggest that high pretreatment $K^{trans}$ or substantial (>40%) reduction in $K^{trans}$ after therapy correlates with longer progression-free survival in cancers of the cervix,[148] and kidneys.[149,150] Several studies have looked at the value of DCE MR imaging in predicting aggressiveness of prostate cancer. The results are discordant[151,152] and may be related to the difference in scan protocol and postprocessing techniques. Further research is required before DCE MR imaging may be considered to be a clinical tool.

## MR ELASTOGRAPHY

MR elastography is based on the principle that disease processes, such as fibrosis or the presence

**A**

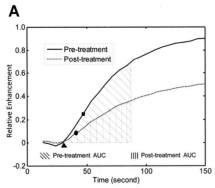

▲ Indicate contrast agent arrival time (at 28.2 s)
■ Indicate the maximal slope for pre-treatment (0.098 mmol/L/s)
● Indicate the maximal slope for post-treatment (0.045 mmol/L/s)

**B**

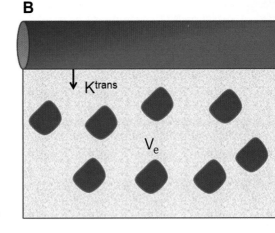

**C**

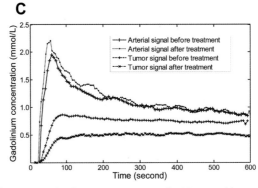

**Fig. 10.** DCE MR imaging. (*A*) Semiquantitative DCE parameters in 67-year-old man with pancreatic cancer before and after sorafenib and gemcitabine therapy. The area under the curve (AUC) at 90 seconds after contrast was 21.1 mmol/L/s pretreatment and 11.1 mmol/L/s after treatment. The reduction in semiquantitative parameters after treatment suggests that antiangiogenic therapy has reduced the leakiness of tumor vessels. However, these measurements cannot be used to compare different patients because they are dependent on the scan protocol and the cardiovascular status of patients. (*B*) Diagram of 2-compartment (Toft) model used in quantitative DCE MR imaging. This model assumes that gadolinium diffuses from the vascular space (*red tube*) to the extracellular extravascular space (EES) (*blue textured region*). The proportion of EES in a unit volume of tissue is denoted as $v_e$. The rate of transfer of contrast from plasma to EES is the volume transfer contrast or $K^{trans}$. This model assumes that gadolinium distributes evenly in the EES, the flux between plasma and EES is proportional to concentration differences, the EES volume does not change during acquisition, and the T1 relaxivity is proportional to gadolinium concentration. (*C*) Quantitative parameters in the same patient as in (*A*). To model quantitative DCE MR imaging parameters, it may be necessary to obtain the gadolinium concentration in the major supplying vessel. The gadolinium concentrations of tumor and artery were fed into the pharmacokinetic model and pretreatment and posttreatment $K^{trans}$ of 1.27/min and 0.37/min were obtained.

of certain tumors, may change tissue stiffness. The basic steps in MR elastography are:

1. Application of a sheer wave that deforms the organ of interest. The sheer wave is created by a pneumatically powered acoustic driver, which is appropriately placed on the patient's skin. The typical frequency range of the acoustic sheer wave is 40 to 120 kHz.
2. Acquisition of gradient-echo sequence that use motion-sensitizing gradients to detect the tissue response (displacement or velocity) to the sheer waves. The wavelength and velocity of the sheer wave increase with tissue stiffness.
3. Elastograms or quantitative stiffness maps are generated by postprocessing of the raw data. These maps give the tissue stiffness in kilopascals or the velocity of sheer wave in meters per second on a pixel-by-pixel basis. Organ/tumor stiffness is measured by placing appropriate ROIs on the elastogram maps.

## Applications of MR Elastography

Initial studies on the diagnostic value of MR elastography in predicting liver fibrosis have been promising. Liver stiffness measured by MR

**Table 1**
**Steps in quantitative DCE MR imaging**

| DCE MR Imaging Step | Explanation | Additional Comments |
|---|---|---|
| Convert MR signal intensity to tissue gadolinium concentration | Requires T1 mapping or the use of phantoms with different gadolinium concentration | Many methods of T1 mapping. Typically multiple gradient-echo sequence obtained with different flip angles |
| High temporal resolution image sets through the lesion or organ of interest | Highest temporal resolution (typically <8 s per acquisition) is optimal. After 90 s, temporal resolution need not be high and data points may be further apart. Scanning typically carried out to 5 min after contrast injection | If arterial input function is required, scan needs to include aorta and main portal vein (for liver studies). Low molecular weight gadolinium (0.1 mmol/kg) injected at 2 mL/s followed by saline flush |
| Motion correction | May be applied to free breathing technique or to breath-holds to ensure level of diaphragm in each image set is identical | In our experience, proprietary motion correction software work best with breath-hold techniques |
| Measuring arterial input function (AIF) | AIF needed to model image data and reduce interpatient variability of perfusion parameters. May be a generic AIF (provided by third-party vendor software) or be individually derived from scan. Latter requires obtaining ROIs on each image set from the aorta ± portal vein | It is unclear if generic AIFs (which are the average of AIFs from studies performed in similar patients) are equivalent to those individually calculated for the patient |
| Obtaining signal intensities of lesion/ organ from each image acquisition | May be semiautomatic or manual (but time-consuming) | At present, manual techniques probably have more accurate result than semiautomatic techniques |
| Pharmacokinetic modeling | Required to obtain robust quantitative DCE MR imaging parameters, such as $K^{trans}$ | Two-compartment models typically used. Modeling is performed by third-party software |

elastography correlates well with histologic staging of fibrosis (from F0 or normal liver to F1 and F2 or mild fibrosis, F3 or severe fibrosis, and F4 or cirrhosis).[153,154] The overlap of MR elastography data between different fibrosis stages is minimal (unlike the situation with DWI), indicating the potential clinical value.[155] MR elastography has been validated for assessing fibrosis with different causes of chronic liver disease.[156–159] However, the cutoff values for different fibrosis stages may be dependent on the cause. For instance, in primary sclerosing cholangitis, higher liver stiffness values are seen on (transient) elastography[160] than in viral hepatitis or alcoholic liver disease.[156,157,159] It is likely that MR elastography may eliminate the need for serial liver biopsies in some patients (eg, patients with coagulopathy). Even if liver biopsy is undertaken, MR elastography may help guide the site of biopsy

(**Fig. 11**).[161] MR elastography has advantages over ultrasonographic elastography; MR elastography has a higher technical success rate in obese patients and those with ascites.[162]

MR elastography has also been investigated in differentiating benign and malignant liver lesions. One study[163] has shown a substantially higher stiffness for malignant lesions compared with benign lesions, with a cutoff value of 5 kPa, indicating malignant nature of the mass. This finding needs further verification. Initial studies showed that MR elastography is sensitive to onset of parenchymal disease in liver transplant[164] but may not differentiate between rejection and onset of recurrent viral hepatitis.[165] The use of MR elastography in renal transplants is being assessed.[166] In addition, MR elastography has been attempted in the assessment of breast lesions, myocardial contractility, and prostate cancer.[167–169]

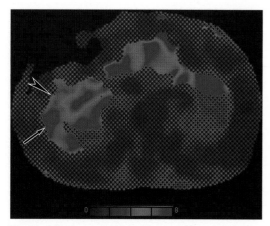

**Fig. 11.** MR elastography in 44-year-old man with hepatitis C. MR elastography was performed because it was part of routine liver MR imaging protocol. Elastogram shows variable stiffness of the liver with regions in the posterior right lobe (*arrow*) showing stiffness measurements of 8 kPa. This finding corresponds to cirrhosis (fibrosis grade 4). The site of anterior right lobe (*arrowhead*), which is the traditional biopsy site, does not show F4 fibrosis. Appropriately targeted ultrasound-guided biopsy showed F4 fibrosis.

## SUMMARY

Despite enormous quantity of research being undertaken in determining the use of functional MR imaging techniques in the abdomen, the clinical usefulness of these techniques is still limited to a few indications. Many challenges need to be overcome:

1. Vendors need to standardize their sequences, so that quantitative measurements are not dependent on the hardware used.
2. Multicenter prospective studies on interobserver and intraobserver variability as well as baseline variation of quantitative parameters need to be undertaken to determine what change in the parameters values may be considered abnormal.
3. Scan times for some of these newer techniques need to be substantially reduced if they are to become feasible in a busy clinical practice.

As radiology evolves over the next decade, it is probable that quantitative measurements from DWI, MR perfusion, and MR elastography will become part of routine clinical practice.

## REFERENCES

1. Taouli B, Koh DM. Diffusion-weighted MR imaging of the liver. Radiology 2010;254(1):47–66.
2. Schmid-Tannwald C, Oto A, Reiser MF, et al. Diffusion-weighted MRI of the abdomen: current value in clinical routine. J Magn Reson Imaging 2013; 37(1):35–47.
3. de Souza DA, Parente DB, de Araujo AL, et al. Modern imaging evaluation of the liver: emerging MR imaging techniques and indications. Magn Reson Imaging Clin N Am 2013;21(2):337–63.
4. Koh DM, Takahara T, Imai Y, et al. Practical aspects of assessing tumors using clinical diffusion-weighted imaging in the body. Magn Reson Med Sci 2007;6(4):211–24.
5. Culverwell AD, Sheridan MB, Guthrie JA, et al. Diffusion-weighted MRI of the liver–interpretative pearls and pitfalls. Clin Radiol 2013;68(4):406–14.
6. Barral M, Soyer P, Ben Hassen W, et al. Diffusion-weighted MR imaging of the normal pancreas: reproducibility and variations of apparent diffusion coefficient measurement at 1.5- and 3.0-Tesla. Diagn Interv Imaging 2013;94(4):418–27.
7. Bilgili MY. Reproductibility of apparent diffusion coefficients measurements in diffusion-weighted MRI of the abdomen with different B values. Eur J Radiol 2012;81(9):2066–8.
8. Colagrande S, Pasquinelli F, Mazzoni LN, et al. MR-diffusion weighted imaging of healthy liver parenchyma: repeatability and reproducibility of apparent diffusion coefficient measurement. J Magn Reson Imaging 2010;31(4):912–20.
9. Corona-Villalobos CP, Pan L, Halappa VG, et al. Agreement and reproducibility of apparent diffusion coefficient measurements of dual-B-value and multi-B-value diffusion-weighted magnetic resonance imaging at 1.5 Tesla in phantom and in soft tissues of the abdomen. J Comput Assist Tomogr 2013;37(1):46–51.
10. Heijmen L, Ter Voert EE, Nagtegaal ID, et al. Diffusion-weighted MR imaging in liver metastases of colorectal cancer: reproducibility and biological validation. Eur Radiol 2013;23(3):748–56.
11. Kim SY, Lee SS, Byun JH, et al. Malignant hepatic tumors: short-term reproducibility of apparent diffusion coefficients with breath-hold and respiratory-triggered diffusion-weighted MR imaging. Radiology 2010;255(3):815–23.
12. Lu TL, Meuli RA, Marques-Vidal PM, et al. Interobserver and intraobserver variability of the apparent diffusion coefficient in treated malignant hepatic lesions on a 3.0T machine: measurements in the whole lesion versus in the area with the most restricted diffusion. J Magn Reson Imaging 2010; 32(3):647–53.
13. Rosenkrantz AB, Oei M, Babb JS, et al. Diffusion-weighted imaging of the abdomen at 3.0 Tesla: image quality and apparent diffusion coefficient reproducibility compared with 1.5 Tesla. J Magn Reson Imaging 2011;33(1):128–35.
14. Bulow R, Mensel B, Meffert P, et al. Diffusion-weighted magnetic resonance imaging for staging

liver fibrosis is less reliable in the presence of fat and iron. Eur Radiol 2012;23(5):1281–7.

15. Sandrasegaran K, Akisik FM, Lin C, et al. Value of diffusion-weighted MRI for assessing liver fibrosis and cirrhosis. AJR Am J Roentgenol 2009;193(6):1556–60.

16. Watanabe H, Kanematsu M, Goshima S, et al. Staging hepatic fibrosis: comparison of gadoxetate disodium-enhanced and diffusion-weighted MR imaging–preliminary observations. Radiology 2011;259(1):142–50.

17. Tonan T, Fujimoto K, Qayyum A. Chronic hepatitis and cirrhosis on MR imaging. Magn Reson Imaging Clin N Am 2010;18(3):383–402, ix.

18. Regev A, Molina E, Moura R, et al. Reliability of histopathologic assessment for the differentiation of recurrent hepatitis C from acute rejection after liver transplantation. Liver Transpl 2004;10(10):1233–9.

19. Sandrasegaran K, Ramaswamy R, Ghosh S, et al. Diffusion-weighted MRI of the transplanted liver. Clin Radiol 2011;66(9):820–5.

20. Chow AM, Gao DS, Fan SJ, et al. Liver fibrosis: an intravoxel incoherent motion (IVIM) study. J Magn Reson Imaging 2012;36(1):159–67.

21. Hayashi T, Miyati T, Takahashi J, et al. Diffusion analysis with triexponential function in liver cirrhosis. J Magn Reson Imaging 2013;38(1):148–53.

22. Luciani A, Vignaud A, Cavet M, et al. Liver cirrhosis: intravoxel incoherent motion MR imaging–pilot study. Radiology 2008;249(3):891–9.

23. Patel J, Sigmund EE, Rusinek H, et al. Diagnosis of cirrhosis with intravoxel incoherent motion diffusion MRI and dynamic contrast-enhanced MRI alone and in combination: preliminary experience. J Magn Reson Imaging 2010;31(3):589–600.

24. Lee JT, Liau J, Murphy P, et al. Cross-sectional investigation of correlation between hepatic steatosis and IVIM perfusion on MR imaging. Magn Reson Imaging 2012;30(4):572–8.

25. Joo I, Lee JM, Yoon JH, et al. Nonalcoholic fatty liver disease: intravoxel incoherent motion diffusion-weighted MR imaging–an experimental study in a rabbit model. Radiology 2014;270(1):131–40.

26. Bruegel M, Holzapfel K, Gaa J, et al. Characterization of focal liver lesions by ADC measurements using a respiratory triggered diffusion-weighted single-shot echo-planar MR imaging technique. Eur Radiol 2008;18(3):477–85.

27. Cieszanowski A, Anysz-Grodzicka A, Szeszkowski W, et al. Characterization of focal liver lesions using quantitative techniques: comparison of apparent diffusion coefficient values and T2 relaxation times. Eur Radiol 2012;22(11):2514–24.

28. Li Y, Chen Z, Wang J. Differential diagnosis between malignant and benign hepatic tumors using apparent diffusion coefficient on 1.5-T MR imaging: a meta analysis. Eur J Radiol 2012;81(3):484–90.

29. Miller FH, Hammond N, Siddiqi AJ, et al. Utility of diffusion-weighted MRI in distinguishing benign and malignant hepatic lesions. J Magn Reson Imaging 2010;32(1):138–47.

30. Onur MR, Cicekci M, Kayali A, et al. The role of ADC measurement in differential diagnosis of focal hepatic lesions. Eur J Radiol 2012;81(3):e171–6.

31. Parikh T, Drew SJ, Lee VS, et al. Focal liver lesion detection and characterization with diffusion-weighted MR imaging: comparison with standard breath-hold T2-weighted imaging. Radiology 2008;246(3):812–22.

32. Sandrasegaran K, Akisik FM, Lin C, et al. The value of diffusion-weighted imaging in characterizing focal liver masses. Acad Radiol 2009;16(10):1208–14.

33. Chung WS, Kim MJ, Chung YE, et al. Comparison of gadoxetic acid-enhanced dynamic imaging and diffusion-weighted imaging for the preoperative evaluation of colorectal liver metastases. J Magn Reson Imaging 2011;34(2):345–53.

34. Hardie AD, Naik M, Hecht EM, et al. Diagnosis of liver metastases: value of diffusion-weighted MRI compared with gadolinium-enhanced MRI. Eur Radiol 2010;20(6):1431–41.

35. Lowenthal D, Zeile M, Lim WY, et al. Detection and characterisation of focal liver lesions in colorectal carcinoma patients: comparison of diffusion-weighted and Gd-EOB-DTPA enhanced MR imaging. Eur Radiol 2011;21(4):832–40.

36. Shimada K, Isoda H, Hirokawa Y, et al. Comparison of gadolinium-EOB-DTPA-enhanced and diffusion-weighted liver MRI for detection of small hepatic metastases. Eur Radiol 2010;20(11):2690–8.

37. Kenis C, Deckers F, De Foer B, et al. Diagnosis of liver metastases: can diffusion-weighted imaging (DWI) be used as a stand alone sequence? Eur J Radiol 2012;81(5):1016–23.

38. d'Assignies G, Fina P, Bruno O, et al. High sensitivity of diffusion-weighted MR imaging for the detection of liver metastases from neuroendocrine tumors: comparison with T2-weighted and dynamic gadolinium-enhanced MR imaging. Radiology 2013;268(2):390–9.

39. Chandarana H, Taouli B. Diffusion-weighted MRI and liver metastases. Magn Reson Imaging Clin N Am 2010;18(3):451–64, x.

40. Schmid-Tannwald C, Thomas S, Ivancevic MK, et al. Diffusion-weighted MRI of metastatic liver lesions: is there a difference between hypervascular and hypovascular metastases? Acta Radiol 2013. [Epub ahead of print].

41. Soyer P, Boudiaf M, Place V, et al. Preoperative detection of hepatic metastases: comparison of diffusion-weighted, T2-weighted fast spin echo and gadolinium-enhanced MR imaging using surgical and histopathologic findings as standard of reference. Eur J Radiol 2011;80(2):245–52.

42. Park MS, Kim S, Patel J, et al. Hepatocellular carcinoma: detection with diffusion-weighted versus contrast-enhanced magnetic resonance imaging in pretransplant patients. Hepatology 2012;56(1):140–8.

43. Park MJ, Kim YK, Lee MW, et al. Small hepatocellular carcinomas: improved sensitivity by combining gadoxetic acid-enhanced and diffusion-weighted MR imaging patterns. Radiology 2012;264(3):761–70.

44. Piana G, Trinquart L, Meskine N, et al. New MR imaging criteria with a diffusion-weighted sequence for the diagnosis of hepatocellular carcinoma in chronic liver diseases. J Hepatol 2011;55(1):126–32.

45. Qu JR, Li HL, Shao NN, et al. Additional diffusion-weighted imaging in the detection of new, very small hepatocellular carcinoma lesions after interventional therapy compared with conventional 3 T MRI alone. Clin Radiol 2012;67(7):669–74.

46. Xu PJ, Yan FH, Wang JH, et al. Added value of breathhold diffusion-weighted MRI in detection of small hepatocellular carcinoma lesions compared with dynamic contrast-enhanced MRI alone using receiver operating characteristic curve analysis. J Magn Reson Imaging 2009;29(2):341–9.

47. Kim DJ, Yu JS, Kim JH, et al. Small hypervascular hepatocellular carcinomas: value of diffusion-weighted imaging compared with "washout" appearance on dynamic MRI. Br J Radiol 2012;85(1018):e879–86.

48. Kim JE, Kim SH, Lee SJ, et al. Hypervascular hepatocellular carcinoma 1 cm or smaller in patients with chronic liver disease: characterization with gadoxetic acid-enhanced MRI that includes diffusion-weighted imaging. AJR Am J Roentgenol 2011;196(6):W758–65.

49. Kim YK, Lee WJ, Park MJ, et al. Hypovascular hypointense nodules on hepatobiliary phase gadoxetic acid-enhanced MR images in patients with cirrhosis: potential of DW imaging in predicting progression to hypervascular HCC. Radiology 2012;265(1):104–14.

50. Lee MH, Kim SH, Park MJ, et al. Gadoxetic acid-enhanced hepatobiliary phase MRI and high-B-value diffusion-weighted imaging to distinguish well-differentiated hepatocellular carcinomas from benign nodules in patients with chronic liver disease. AJR Am J Roentgenol 2011;197(5):W868–75.

51. Xu PJ, Yan FH, Wang JH, et al. Contribution of diffusion-weighted magnetic resonance imaging in the characterization of hepatocellular carcinomas and dysplastic nodules in cirrhotic liver. J Comput Assist Tomogr 2010;34(4):506–12.

52. Fruehwald-Pallamar J, Bastati-Huber N, Fakhrai N, et al. Confident non-invasive diagnosis of pseudolesions of the liver using diffusion-weighted imaging at 3T MRI. Eur J Radiol 2012;81(6):1353–9.

53. Motosugi U, Ichikawa T, Sou H, et al. Distinguishing hypervascular pseudolesions of the liver from hypervascular hepatocellular carcinomas with gadoxetic acid-enhanced MR imaging. Radiology 2010;256(1):151–8.

54. Vandecaveye V, De KF, Verslype C, et al. Diffusion-weighted MRI provides additional value to conventional dynamic contrast-enhanced MRI for detection of hepatocellular carcinoma. Eur Radiol 2009;19(10):2456–66.

55. Rosenkrantz AB, Lee L, Matza BW, et al. Infiltrative hepatocellular carcinoma: comparison of MRI sequences for lesion conspicuity. Clin Radiol 2012;67(12):e105–11.

56. An C, Park MS, Jeon HM, et al. Prediction of the histopathological grade of hepatocellular carcinoma using qualitative diffusion-weighted, dynamic, and hepatobiliary phase MRI. Eur Radiol 2012;22(8):1701–8.

57. Heo SH, Jeong YY, Shin SS, et al. Apparent diffusion coefficient value of diffusion-weighted imaging for hepatocellular carcinoma: correlation with the histologic differentiation and the expression of vascular endothelial growth factor. Korean J Radiol 2010;11(3):295–303.

58. Muhi A, Ichikawa T, Motosugi U, et al. High-B-value diffusion-weighted MR imaging of hepatocellular lesions: estimation of grade of malignancy of hepatocellular carcinoma. J Magn Reson Imaging 2009;30(5):1005–11.

59. Nakanishi M, Chuma M, Hige S, et al. Relationship between diffusion-weighted magnetic resonance imaging and histological tumor grading of hepatocellular carcinoma. Ann Surg Oncol 2012;19(4):1302–9.

60. Nishie A, Tajima T, Asayama Y, et al. Diagnostic performance of apparent diffusion coefficient for predicting histological grade of hepatocellular carcinoma. Eur J Radiol 2011;80(2):e29–33.

61. Sandrasegaran K, Tahir B, Patel A, et al. The usefulness of diffusion-weighted imaging in the characterization of liver lesions in patients with cirrhosis. Clin Radiol 2013;68(7):708–15.

62. Sandrasegaran K, Tahir B, Nutakki K, et al. Usefulness of conventional MRI sequences and diffusion-weighted imaging in differentiating malignant from benign portal vein thrombus in cirrhotic patients. AJR Am J Roentgenol 2013;201(6):1211–9.

63. Sun YS, Cui Y, Tang L, et al. Early evaluation of cancer response by a new functional biomarker: apparent diffusion coefficient. AJR Am J Roentgenol 2011;197(1):W23–9.

64. Chung JC, Naik NK, Lewandowski RJ, et al. Diffusion-weighted magnetic resonance imaging to predict response of hepatocellular carcinoma to chemoembolization. World J Gastroenterol 2010;16(25):3161–7.

65. Mannelli L, Kim S, Hajdu CH, et al. Serial diffusion-weighted MRI in patients with hepatocellular carcinoma: prediction and assessment of response to transarterial chemoembolization. Preliminary experience. Eur J Radiol 2012;82(4):577–82.

66. Cui Y, Zhang XP, Sun YS, et al. Apparent diffusion coefficient: potential imaging biomarker for prediction and early detection of response to chemotherapy in hepatic metastases. Radiology 2008; 248(3):894–900.

67. Dudeck O, Zeile M, Wybranski C, et al. Early prediction of anticancer effects with diffusion-weighted MR imaging in patients with colorectal liver metastases following selective internal radiotherapy. Eur Radiol 2010;20(11):2699–706.

68. Koh DM, Scurr E, Collins D, et al. Predicting response of colorectal hepatic metastasis: value of pretreatment apparent diffusion coefficients. AJR Am J Roentgenol 2007;188(4):1001–8.

69. Yuan Z, Ye XD, Dong S, et al. Role of magnetic resonance diffusion-weighted imaging in evaluating response after chemoembolization of hepatocellular carcinoma. Eur J Radiol 2010;75(1):e9–14.

70. Kubota K, Yamanishi T, Itoh S, et al. Role of diffusion-weighted imaging in evaluating therapeutic efficacy after transcatheter arterial chemoembolization for hepatocellular carcinoma. Oncol Rep 2010;24(3):727–32.

71. Sahin H, Harman M, Cinar C, et al. Evaluation of treatment response of chemoembolization in hepatocellular carcinoma with diffusion-weighted imaging on 3.0-T MR imaging. J Vasc Interv Radiol 2012;23(2):241–7.

72. Herrmann J, Schoennagel BP, Roesch M, et al. Diffusion-weighted imaging of the healthy pancreas: ADC values are age and gender dependent. J Magn Reson Imaging 2013;37(4):886–91.

73. Fukukura Y, Takumi K, Kamimura K, et al. Pancreatic adenocarcinoma: variability of diffusion-weighted MR imaging findings. Radiology 2012; 263(3):732–40.

74. Rosenkrantz AB, Matza BW, Sabach A, et al. Pancreatic cancer: lack of association between apparent diffusion coefficient values and adverse pathological features. Clin Radiol 2013;68(4): e191–7.

75. Muhi A, Ichikawa T, Motosugi U, et al. Mass-forming autoimmune pancreatitis and pancreatic carcinoma: differential diagnosis on the basis of computed tomography and magnetic resonance cholangiopancreatography, and diffusion-weighted imaging findings. J Magn Reson Imaging 2012;35(4):827–36.

76. Sandrasegaran K, Nutakki K, Tahir B, et al. Use of diffusion-weighted MRI to differentiate chronic pancreatitis from pancreatic cancer. AJR Am J Roentgenol 2013;201(5):1002–8.

77. Huang WC, Sheng J, Chen SY, et al. Differentiation between pancreatic carcinoma and mass-forming chronic pancreatitis: usefulness of high B value diffusion-weighted imaging. J Dig Dis 2011;12(5): 401–8.

78. Wiggermann P, Grutzmann R, Weissenbock A, et al. Apparent diffusion coefficient measurements of the pancreas, pancreas carcinoma, and mass-forming focal pancreatitis. Acta Radiol 2012; 53(2):135–9.

79. Hur BY, Lee JM, Lee JE, et al. Magnetic resonance imaging findings of the mass-forming type of autoimmune pancreatitis: comparison with pancreatic adenocarcinoma. J Magn Reson Imaging 2012; 36(1):188–97.

80. Bakir B, Salmaslioglu A, Poyanli A, et al. Diffusion weighted MR imaging of pancreatic islet cell tumors. Eur J Radiol 2010;74(1):214–20.

81. Jang KM, Kim SH, Lee SJ, et al. Differentiation of an intrapancreatic accessory spleen from a small (<3-cm) solid pancreatic tumor: value of diffusion-weighted MR imaging. Radiology 2013;266(1): 159–67.

82. Wang Y, Miller FH, Chen ZE, et al. Diffusion-weighted MR imaging of solid and cystic lesions of the pancreas. Radiographics 2011;31(3):E47–64.

83. Mottola JC, Sahni VA, Erturk SM, et al. Diffusion-weighted MRI of focal cystic pancreatic lesions at 3.0-Tesla: preliminary results. Abdom Imaging 2012;37(1):110–7.

84. Sandrasegaran K, Akisik FM, Patel AA, et al. Diffusion-weighted imaging in characterization of cystic pancreatic lesions. Clin Radiol 2011;66(9):808–14.

85. Kamisawa T, Takuma K, Anjiki H, et al. Differentiation of autoimmune pancreatitis from pancreatic cancer by diffusion-weighted MRI. Am J Gastroenterol 2010;105(8):1870–5.

86. Taniguchi T, Kobayashi H, Nishikawa K, et al. Diffusion-weighted magnetic resonance imaging in autoimmune pancreatitis. Jpn J Radiol 2009; 27(3):138–42.

87. Oki H, Hayashida Y, Oki H, et al. DWI findings of autoimmune pancreatitis: comparison between symptomatic and asymptomatic patients. J Magn Reson Imaging 2013. http://dx.doi.org/10.1002/jmri.24508.

88. Buisson A, Joubert A, Montoriol PF, et al. Diffusion-weighted magnetic resonance imaging for detecting and assessing ileal inflammation in Crohn's disease. Aliment Pharmacol Ther 2013;37(5):537–45.

89. Kinner S, Blex S, Maderwald S, et al. Addition of diffusion-weighted imaging can improve diagnostic confidence in bowel MRI. Clin Radiol 2014; 69(4):372–7.

90. Neubauer H, Pabst T, Dick A, et al. Small-bowel MRI in children and young adults with Crohn disease: retrospective head-to-head comparison of

contrast-enhanced and diffusion-weighted MRI. Pediatr Radiol 2013;43(1):103–14.

91. Oto A, Kayhan A, Williams JT, et al. Active Crohn's disease in the small bowel: evaluation by diffusion weighted imaging and quantitative dynamic contrast enhanced MR imaging. J Magn Reson Imaging 2011;33(3):615–24.

92. Ream JM, Dillman JR, Adler J, et al. MRI diffusion-weighted imaging (DWI) in pediatric small bowel Crohn disease: correlation with MRI findings of active bowel wall inflammation. Pediatr Radiol 2013;43(9):1077–85.

93. Feng Q, Yan YQ, Zhu J, et al. T-Staging of Rectal Cancer: Accuracy of Diffusion-Weighted Imaging Compared with T2-Weighted Imaging on 3.0 Tesla MRI. J Dig Dis 2014;15(4):188–94.

94. Park MJ, Kim SH, Lee SJ, et al. Locally advanced rectal cancer: added value of diffusion-weighted MR imaging for predicting tumor clearance of the mesorectal fascia after neoadjuvant chemotherapy and radiation therapy. Radiology 2011;260(3):771–80.

95. Cai G, Xu Y, Zhu J, et al. Diffusion-weighted magnetic resonance imaging for predicting the response of rectal cancer to neoadjuvant concurrent chemoradiation. World J Gastroenterol 2013;19(33):5520–7.

96. Jung SH, Heo SH, Kim JW, et al. Predicting response to neoadjuvant chemoradiation therapy in locally advanced rectal cancer: diffusion-weighted 3 Tesla MR imaging. J Magn Reson Imaging 2012;35(1):110–6.

97. Lambrecht M, Vandecaveye V, De Keyzer F, et al. Value of diffusion-weighted magnetic resonance imaging for prediction and early assessment of response to neoadjuvant radiochemotherapy in rectal cancer: preliminary results. Int J Radiat Oncol Biol Phys 2012;82(2):863–70.

98. Sun YS, Zhang XP, Tang L, et al. Locally advanced rectal carcinoma treated with preoperative chemotherapy and radiation therapy: preliminary analysis of diffusion-weighted MR imaging for early detection of tumor histopathologic downstaging. Radiology 2010;254(1):170–8.

99. Ippolito D, Monguzzi L, Guerra L, et al. Response to neoadjuvant therapy in locally advanced rectal cancer: assessment with diffusion-weighted MR imaging and 18FDG PET/CT. Abdom Imaging 2012;37(6):1032–40.

100. Kim SH, Lee JM, Hong SH, et al. Locally advanced rectal cancer: added value of diffusion-weighted MR imaging in the evaluation of tumor response to neoadjuvant chemo- and radiation therapy. Radiology 2009;253(1):116–25.

101. Song I, Kim SH, Lee SJ, et al. Value of diffusion-weighted imaging in the detection of viable tumour after neoadjuvant chemoradiation therapy in patients with locally advanced rectal cancer: comparison with T2 weighted and PET/CT imaging. Br J Radiol 2012;85(1013):577–86.

102. Nural MS, Danaci M, Soyucok A, et al. Efficiency of apparent diffusion coefficients in differentiation of colorectal tumor recurrences and posttherapeutical soft-tissue changes. Eur J Radiol 2013;82(10):1702–9.

103. Muller MF, Prasad PV, Bimmler D, et al. Functional imaging of the kidney by means of measurement of the apparent diffusion coefficient. Radiology 1994;193(3):711–5.

104. Thoeny HC, De Keyzer F, Oyen RH, et al. Diffusion-weighted MR imaging of kidneys in healthy volunteers and patients with parenchymal diseases: initial experience. Radiology 2005;235(3):911–7.

105. Bittencourt LK, Matos C, Coutinho AC Jr. Diffusion-weighted magnetic resonance imaging in the upper abdomen: technical issues and clinical applications. Magn Reson Imaging Clin N Am 2011;19(1):111–31.

106. Saito K, Araki Y, Park J, et al. Effect of Gd-EOB-DTPA on T2-weighted and diffusion-weighted images for the diagnosis of hepatocellular carcinoma. J Magn Reson Imaging 2010;32(1):229–34.

107. Wang CL, Chea YW, Boll DT, et al. Effect of gadolinium chelate contrast agents on diffusion weighted MR imaging of the liver, spleen, pancreas and kidney at 3 T. Eur J Radiol 2011;80(2):e1–7.

108. Erbay G, Koc Z, Karadeli E, et al. Evaluation of malignant and benign renal lesions using diffusion-weighted MRI with multiple B values. Acta Radiol 2012;53(3):359–65.

109. Sandrasegaran K, Sundaram CP, Ramaswamy R, et al. Usefulness of diffusion-weighted imaging in the evaluation of renal masses. AJR Am J Roentgenol 2010;194(2):438–45.

110. Kilickesmez O, Inci E, Atilla S, et al. Diffusion-weighted imaging of the renal and adrenal lesions. J Comput Assist Tomogr 2009;33(6):828–33.

111. Miller FH, Wang Y, McCarthy RJ, et al. Utility of diffusion-weighted MRI in characterization of adrenal lesions. AJR Am J Roentgenol 2010;194(2):W179–85.

112. Sandrasegaran K, Patel AA, Ramaswamy R, et al. Characterization of adrenal masses with diffusion-weighted imaging. AJR Am J Roentgenol 2011;197(1):132–8.

113. Hoeks CM, Hambrock T, Yakar D, et al. Transition zone prostate cancer: detection and localization with 3-T multiparametric MR imaging. Radiology 2013;266(1):207–17.

114. Jung SI, Donati OF, Vargas HA, et al. Transition zone prostate cancer: incremental value of diffusion-weighted endorectal MR imaging in tumor detection and assessment of aggressiveness. Radiology 2013;269(2):493–503.

115. Hoeks CM, Vos EK, Bomers JG, et al. Diffusion-weighted magnetic resonance imaging in the prostate transition zone: histopathological validation using magnetic resonance-guided biopsy specimens. Invest Radiol 2013;48(10):693–701.

116. Koh DM, Sohaib A. Diffusion-weighted imaging of the male pelvis. Radiol Clin North Am 2012;50(6):1127–44.

117. Ueno Y, Kitajima K, Sugimura K, et al. Ultra-high B-value diffusion-weighted MRI for the detection of prostate cancer with 3-T MRI. J Magn Reson Imaging 2013;38(1):154–60.

118. Metens T, Miranda D, Absil J, et al. What is the optimal B value in diffusion-weighted MR imaging to depict prostate cancer at 3T? Eur Radiol 2012;22(3):703–9.

119. Komai Y, Numao N, Yoshida S, et al. High diagnostic ability of multiparametric magnetic resonance imaging to detect anterior prostate cancer missed by transrectal 12-core biopsy. J Urol 2013;190(3):867–73.

120. Chang JH, Lim Joon D, Lee ST, et al. Diffusion-weighted MRI, C-choline PET and F-fluorodeoxyglucose pet for predicting the Gleason score in prostate carcinoma. Eur Radiol 2014;24(3):715–22.

121. Peng Y, Jiang Y, Yang C, et al. Quantitative analysis of multiparametric prostate MR images: differentiation between prostate cancer and normal tissue and correlation with Gleason score–a computer-aided diagnosis development study. Radiology 2013;267(3):787–96.

122. Bittencourt LK, Barentsz JO, de Miranda LC, et al. Prostate MRI: diffusion-weighted imaging at 1.5T correlates better with prostatectomy Gleason grades than TRUS-guided biopsies in peripheral zone tumours. Eur Radiol 2012;22(2):468–75.

123. Soylu FN, Peng Y, Jiang Y, et al. Seminal vesicle invasion in prostate cancer: evaluation by using multiparametric endorectal MR imaging. Radiology 2013;267(3):797–806.

124. Rosenkrantz AB, Chandarana H, Gilet A, et al. Prostate cancer: utility of diffusion-weighted imaging as a marker of side-specific risk of extracapsular extension. J Magn Reson Imaging 2013;38(2):312–9.

125. Somford DM, Hamoen EH, Futterer JJ, et al. The predictive value of endorectal 3 Tesla multiparametric magnetic resonance imaging for extraprostatic extension in patients with low, intermediate and high risk prostate cancer. J Urol 2013;190(5):1728–34.

126. Panebianco V, Barchetti F, Sciarra A, et al. In vivo 3D neuroanatomical evaluation of periprostatic nerve plexus with 3T-MR diffusion tensor imaging. Eur J Radiol 2013;82(10):1677–82.

127. Gibbs P, Pickles MD, Turnbull LW. Diffusion imaging of the prostate at 3.0 Tesla. Invest Radiol 2006;41(2):185–8.

128. Gurses B, Kabakci N, Kovanlikaya A, et al. Diffusion tensor imaging of the normal prostate at 3 Tesla. Eur Radiol 2008;18(4):716–21.

129. Li C, Chen M, Li S, et al. Diffusion tensor imaging of prostate at 3.0 Tesla. Acta Radiol 2011;52(7):813–7.

130. Manenti G, Carlani M, Mancino S, et al. Diffusion tensor magnetic resonance imaging of prostate cancer. Invest Radiol 2007;42(6):412–9.

131. Kozlowski P, Chang SD, Meng R, et al. Combined prostate diffusion tensor imaging and dynamic contrast enhanced MRI at 3T–quantitative correlation with biopsy. Magn Reson Imaging 2010;28(5):621–8.

132. Dopfert J, Lemke A, Weidner A, et al. Investigation of prostate cancer using diffusion-weighted intravoxel incoherent motion imaging. Magn Reson Imaging 2011;29(8):1053–8.

133. Pang Y, Turkbey B, Bernardo M, et al. Intravoxel incoherent motion MR imaging for prostate cancer: an evaluation of perfusion fraction and diffusion coefficient derived from different B-value combinations. Magn Reson Med 2013;69(2):553–62.

134. Shinmoto H, Tamura C, Soga S, et al. An intravoxel incoherent motion diffusion-weighted imaging study of prostate cancer. AJR Am J Roentgenol 2012;199(4):W496–500.

135. Panebianco V, Barchetti F, Sciarra A, et al. Prostate cancer recurrence after radical prostatectomy: the role of 3-T diffusion imaging in multi-parametric magnetic resonance imaging. Eur Radiol 2013;23(6):1745–52.

136. Roy C, Foudi F, Charton J, et al. Comparative sensitivities of functional MRI sequences in detection of local recurrence of prostate carcinoma after radical prostatectomy or external-beam radiotherapy. AJR Am J Roentgenol 2013;200(4):W361–8.

137. Donati OF, Jung SI, Vargas HA, et al. Multiparametric prostate MR imaging with T2-weighted, diffusion-weighted, and dynamic contrast-enhanced sequences: are all pulse sequences necessary to detect locally recurrent prostate cancer after radiation therapy? Radiology 2013;268(2):440–50.

138. Futterer JJ. Imaging of recurrent prostate cancer. Radiol Clin North Am 2012;50(6):1075–83.

139. Essig M, Shiroishi MS, Nguyen TB, et al. Perfusion MRI: the five most frequently asked technical questions. AJR Am J Roentgenol 2013;200(1):24–34.

140. Do RK, Rusinek H, Taouli B. Dynamic contrast-enhanced MR imaging of the liver: current status and future directions. Magn Reson Imaging Clin N Am 2009;17(2):339–49.

141. Haider MA, Farhadi FA, Milot L. Hepatic perfusion imaging: concepts and application. Magn Reson Imaging Clin N Am 2010;18(3):465–75, x.

142. Paldino MJ, Barboriak DP. Fundamentals of quantitative dynamic contrast-enhanced MR imaging. Magn Reson Imaging Clin N Am 2009;17(2):277–89.

143. Garpebring A, Brynolfsson P, Yu J, et al. Uncertainty estimation in dynamic contrast-enhanced MRI. Magn Reson Med 2013;69(4):992–1002.

144. Heye T, Merkle EM, Reiner CS, et al. Reproducibility of dynamic contrast-enhanced MR imaging. Part II. Comparison of intra- and interobserver variability with manual region of interest placement versus semiautomatic lesion segmentation and histogram analysis. Radiology 2013;266(3):812–21.

145. Ng CS, Raunig DL, Jackson EF, et al. Reproducibility of perfusion parameters in dynamic contrast-enhanced MRI of lung and liver tumors: effect on estimates of patient sample size in clinical trials and on individual patient responses. AJR Am J Roentgenol 2010;194(2):W134–40.

146. Gollub MJ, Gultekin DH, Akin O, et al. Dynamic contrast enhanced-MRI for the detection of pathological complete response to neoadjuvant chemotherapy for locally advanced rectal cancer. Eur Radiol 2012;22(4):821–31.

147. Akisik MF, Sandrasegaran K, Bu G, et al. Pancreatic cancer: utility of dynamic contrast-enhanced MR imaging in assessment of antiangiogenic therapy. Radiology 2010;256(2):441–9.

148. Andersen EK, Hole KH, Lund KV, et al. Pharmacokinetic parameters derived from dynamic contrast enhanced MRI of cervical cancers predict chemoradiotherapy outcome. Radiother Oncol 2013;107(1):117–22.

149. De Bruyne S, Van Damme N, Smeets P, et al. Value of DCE-MRI and FDG-PET/CT in the prediction of response to preoperative chemotherapy with bevacizumab for colorectal liver metastases. Br J Cancer 2012;106(12):1926–33.

150. Hahn OM, Yang C, Medved M, et al. Dynamic contrast-enhanced magnetic resonance imaging pharmacodynamic biomarker study of sorafenib in metastatic renal carcinoma. J Clin Oncol 2008;26(28):4572–8.

151. Oto A, Yang C, Kayhan A, et al. Diffusion-weighted and dynamic contrast-enhanced MRI of prostate cancer: correlation of quantitative MR parameters with Gleason score and tumor angiogenesis. AJR Am J Roentgenol 2011;197(6):1382–90.

152. Vos EK, Litjens GJ, Kobus T, et al. Assessment of prostate cancer aggressiveness using dynamic contrast-enhanced magnetic resonance imaging at 3 T. Eur Urol 2013;64(3):448–55.

153. Venkatesh SK, Yin M, Ehman RL. Magnetic resonance elastography of liver: technique, analysis, and clinical applications. J Magn Reson Imaging 2013;37(3):544–55.

154. Godfrey EM, Mannelli L, Griffin N, et al. Magnetic resonance elastography in the diagnosis of hepatic fibrosis. Semin Ultrasound CT MR 2013;34(1):81–8.

155. Wang QB, Zhu H, Liu HL, et al. Performance of magnetic resonance elastography and diffusion-weighted imaging for the staging of hepatic fibrosis: a meta-analysis. Hepatology 2012;56(1):239–47.

156. Ichikawa S, Motosugi U, Ichikawa T, et al. Magnetic resonance elastography for staging liver fibrosis in chronic hepatitis C. Magn Reson Med Sci 2012;11(4):291–7.

157. Venkatesh SK, Wang G, Lim SG, et al. Magnetic resonance elastography for the detection and staging of liver fibrosis in chronic hepatitis B. Eur Radiol 2014;24(1):70–8.

158. Kovac JD, Dakovic M, Stanisavljevic D, et al. Diffusion-weighted MRI versus transient elastography in quantification of liver fibrosis in patients with chronic cholestatic liver diseases. Eur J Radiol 2012;81(10):2500–6.

159. Bensamoun SF, Leclerc GE, Debernard L, et al. Cutoff values for alcoholic liver fibrosis using magnetic resonance elastography technique. Alcohol Clin Exp Res 2013;37(5):811–7.

160. Corpechot C, Gaouar F, El Naggar A, et al. Baseline values and changes in liver stiffness, measured by transient elastography, are associated with fibrosis severity and outcomes of patients with primary sclerosing cholangitis. Gastroenterology 2013. http://dx.doi.org/10.1053/j.gastro.2013.12.030.

161. Perumpail RB, Levitsky J, Wang Y, et al. MRI-guided biopsy to correlate tissue specimens with MR elastography stiffness readings in liver transplants. Acad Radiol 2012;19(9):1121–6.

162. Huwart L, Sempoux C, Vicaut E, et al. Magnetic resonance elastography for the noninvasive staging of liver fibrosis. Gastroenterology 2008;135(1):32–40.

163. Garteiser P, Doblas S, Daire JL, et al. MR elastography of liver tumours: value of viscoelastic properties for tumour characterisation. Eur Radiol 2012;22(10):2169–77.

164. Lee VS, Miller FH, Omary RA, et al. Magnetic resonance elastography and biomarkers to assess fibrosis from recurrent hepatitis C in liver transplant recipients. Transplantation 2011;92(5):581–6.

165. Crespo S, Bridges M, Nakhleh R, et al. Non-invasive assessment of liver fibrosis using magnetic resonance elastography in liver transplant recipients with hepatitis C. Clin Transplant 2013;27(5):652–8.

166. Lee CU, Glockner JF, Glaser KJ, et al. MR elastography in renal transplant patients and correlation with renal allograft biopsy: a feasibility study. Acad Radiol 2012;19(7):834–41.

167. Kolipaka A, Aggarwal SR, McGee KP, et al. Magnetic resonance elastography as a method to estimate myocardial contractility. J Magn Reson Imaging 2012;36(1):120–7.

168. Sahebjavaher RS, Baghani A, Honarvar M, et al. Transperineal prostate MR elastography: initial

in vivo results. Magn Reson Med 2013;69(2): 411–20.

169. Siegmann KC, Xydeas T, Sinkus R, et al. Diagnostic value of MR elastography in addition to contrast-enhanced MR imaging of the breast-initial clinical results. Eur Radiol 2010;20(2):318–25.

# Index

*Note:* Page numbers or article titles are in **boldface** type.

Radiol Clin N Am 52 (2014) 905–911
http://dx.doi.org/10.1016/S0033-8389(14)00074-8
0033-8389/14/$ – see front matter © 2014 Elsevier Inc. All rights reserved.

radiologic.theclinics.com

# Moving?

## Make sure your subscription moves with you!

To notify us of your new address, find your **Clinics Account Number** (located on your mailing label above your name), and contact customer service at:

Email: journalscustomerservice-usa@elsevier.com

800-654-2452 (subscribers in the U.S. & Canada)
314-447-8871 (subscribers outside of the U.S. & Canada)

Fax number: 314-447-8029

**Elsevier Health Sciences Division**
**Subscription Customer Service**
**3251 Riverport Lane**
**Maryland Heights, MO 63043**

*To ensure uninterrupted delivery of your subscription, please notify us at least 4 weeks in advance of move.

ELSEVIER